The Placenta

The Placenta

and its Maternal Supply Line

Effects of Insufficiency on the Fetus

Edited by Dr. P. Gruenwald

University Park Press
Baltimore

Published in the USA and Canada by
UNIVERSITY PARK PRESS
Chamber of Commerce Building
Baltimore, Maryland, 21202

Library of Congress Cataloging in Publication Data

Gruenwald, Peter, 1912–
  The placenta and its maternal supply line.

  1. Placenta.   2. Placenta—Diseases.   3. Maternal–
fetal exchange.   I. Title.   [DNLM: 1. Maternal–
fetal exchange.   2. Placenta.   WQ212 G886p]
  RG591.G78   1975   618.3   74–30155
  ISBN 0–8391–0806–0

Copyright © 1975 Dr. P. Gruenwald

First published 1975

MTP MEDICAL AND TECHNICAL PUBLISHING CO. LTD.
St Leonard's House
St Leonardgate, Lancaster, Lancs.

Printed and bound in Great Britain

Foreword

The most important single ingredient for fetal welfare is clearly oxygen. And the most important place for that oxygen to be delivered is the fetal brain. In the complex pathway from maternal nostril to fetal brain the placenta, its membranes and cord occupy a prominent position. This prominence, plus the ready availability to the tissues, has led to a great deal of investigation and study. It has also led to some oversimplification and an occasional false analogy. The writer himself recalls using the illustration of an hermetically sealed room with a single occupant and a slowly closing porthole to illustrate 'placental insufficiency'.

Dr Peter Gruenwald, a pioneer in studies of oxygenation in the fetus and newborn, is presenting this volume in an effort to counteract some of these oversimplifications. His title, 'The Placenta', carries the important subtitle 'And Its Maternal Supply Line' and reminds us that respiratory gas exchange in the placenta itself is not the entire key to fetal oxygenation. Indeed, speaking of fetal deprivation, he points out: 'If fetal size were regulated within such narrow limits by placental size (and function), this would presuppose a placenta at the border of its functional capacity. . . . There is no reason to believe that this is the case.'

Eighteen distinguished placentologists have contributed to this volume and all are to be commended on the clarity of their presentations. They do not, in all instances, agree, but this is as it should be. Complete agreement is usually only reached at the lowest common denominator and the easygoing platitude.

It has been an active research field in the past decade and this volume serves admirably to bring the reader up to date. The expanding armamentarium of the laboratory—ranging from the electron microscope to radio immune assays, from ultrasonics to binding site analysis—has been brought to bear on the study of the maternal–fetal relationship. Many of the authors, however, point to the fact that our areas of ignorance are still extensive. This book is not the finish line for research in the fetal supply line, in other words, but rather represents a milestone along a continuing path. As such it is exceedingly valuable.

ALLAN C. BARNES, M.D.
Vice President
The Rockefeller Foundation

Contents

List of Contributors

Karlis Adamsons, M.D., Ph.D.
Professor of Obstetrics and Gynecology and Professor of Pharmacology, Mount Sinai School of Medicine of The City University of New York, New York, NY 10029, U.S.A.

W. Aherne
Senior Lecturer in Pathology, Royal Victoria Infirmary, Newcastle upon Tyne, NE1 4LP, U.K.

Silvio Aladjem, M.D., F.A.C.O.G.
Associate Professor of Obstetrics and Gynecology, Abraham Lincoln Medical School, University of Illinois at the Medical Center, Chicago, IL 60612, U.S.A.

Professor Dr. Volker Becker
Direktor des Pathologischen Instituts der Universität Erlangen-Nürnberg, 8520 Erlangen, Germany

Yves W. Brans, M.D.
Instructor in Pediatrics, The University of Alabama in Birmingham, Birmingham, AL 35294, U.S.A.

Stuart Campbell, M.R.C.O.G.
Senior Lecturer, Institute of Obstetrics and Gynaecology, University of London, Queen Charlotte's Hospital for Women, London, U.K.

George Cassady, M.D.
Professor of Pediatrics and Associate Professor of Obstetrics; Director, Division of Perinatal Medicine, The University of Alabama in Birmingham, Birmingham, AL 35294, U.S.A.

Joseph Dancis, M.D.
Professor of Pediatrics, New York University Medical Center School of Medicine, New York, NY 10016, U.S.A.

Stephen J. DeVoe, M.D.
Instructor in Obstetrics and Gynecology, University of Pennsylvania School of Medicine, Philadelphia, PA 19104, U.S.A. (Presently at the Naval Regional Medical Center, Charleston, SC)

Shirley G. Driscoll, M.D.
Pathologist (Lying-in Division), Boston Hospital for Women; Associate Professor of Pathology, Harvard Medical School, Boston, MA 02115, U.S.A.

H. Fox, M.D., M.R.C.Path.
Senior Lecturer in Pathology, University of Manchester; Honorary Consultant Pathologist, United Manchester Hospitals, Manchester M13 9PT, U.K.

Peter Gruenwald, M.D.
Associate Professor of Pathology and Clinical Associate Professor of Pediatrics, Hahnemann Medical College and Hospital, Philadelphia, PA 19102, U.S.A.

Jonathan T. Lanman, M.D.
Associate Director, The Population Council, The Rockefeller University, New York, NY 10021; Professor of Pediatrics, New York University Medical Center School of Medicine, New York, NY 10016, U.S.A.

Ronald E. Myers, M.D., Ph.D.
Director, Laboratory of Perinatal Physiology, National Institute of Neurological Diseases and Stroke, National Institutes of Health, Bethesda, MD 20014, U.S.A.

Henning Schneider, M.D.
Clinical Instructor of Obstetrics and Gynecology, New York University Medical Center School of Medicine, New York, NY 10016, U.S.A.

Richard H. Schwarz, M.D.
Professor of Obstetrics and Gynecology and Director of the Jerrold R. Golding Division of Fetal Medicine, University of Pennsylvania School of Medicine, Philadelphia, PA 19104, U.S.A.

Rosemarie B. Thau, Ph.D.
Staff Scientist, Biomedical Division, The Population Council, New York, NY 10021, U.S.A.

Ralph M. Wynn, M.D.
Professor and Head, Department of Obstetrics and Gynecology, Abraham Lincoln Medical School, University of Illinois at the Medical Center, Chicago, IL 60612, U.S.A.

CHAPTER 1

Introduction— The Supply Line of the Fetus; Definitions Relating to Fetal Growth

Peter Gruenwald

Research and clinical experience relating to the normal and the deficient supply line of the fetus have only recently led to the accumulation of a substantial body of information. This is mostly in the stage of original communications. There are as yet no generally accepted teachings on the normal and pathological placenta, and the supply line coming to it from the mother. The point has been reached at which a volume can be compiled that may serve as a textbook on the subject. Leading research workers have been invited to present their own views, along with those of others which they consider significant. This necessarily involves disagreements and contradictions which have been partly eliminated by mutual consent, and partly left standing, indicating that we are far from concensus on some aspects. It is hoped that sufficient evidence and references are provided to enable the reader to reach his own conclusions.

Since the placenta is but one of two major links in the supply line of mammalian fetuses, it is necessary to discuss the other, maternal component as an equal partner. (The term supply line will be used here whenever no distinction between maternal and placental component is intended or known. It will also be assumed without being mentioned specifically that the same route serves the movement of wastes and other substances in the other direction.)

The effects of a deranged supply line on the fetus, and eventually the child, need to be considered because they are the principal reason for our interest in the supply line. Also, these effects are, particularly in man, often the only yard stick by which to measure adequacy of the fetal environment. The more adequately we can apprehend and interpret the reactions of the fetus to variations in the supply line, the more we will learn about our principal subject. For this reason, a seemingly excessive part of the book will deal with the aspects of fetal growth which relate directly or by inference to fetal 'nutrition'.

Comparative aspects will be discussed very briefly in Chapters 2 and 3, largely in order to acquaint the reader with the staggering variety of placental form and function in mammals, including those groups which are of direct interest to us as laboratory models, pets and farm animals.

The Thorny Road to Knowledge of the Fetal Supply Line

In addition to wide interspecies differences which limit our ability to transfer experimental results to man, the protected environment of the fetus renders study difficult. Merely exposing the conceptus to view or to testing devices may lead to severely abnormal conditions. The delivered human placenta has been treated with disrespect, perhaps because it is too readily available. It is the only human tissue that may be discarded with impunity even in the highly regulated setting of American hospitals where a splinter removed from a patient's arm must be sent to the pathologist for examination. Any hope of obtaining clinically or scientifically useful information by examining the placenta hinges on the correlation with adequate clinical data. These data are often not available, but even when they are, the circumstances leading to fetal difficulties or neonatal disease are apparent in the placenta to a limited extent. This will become apparent as we consider non-placental causes of fetal distress, and will be summarised in the last chapter.

Interest in the fetal supply line increased in recent years when it became common knowledge that intra-uterine growth retardation, presumably caused by deprivation, is a fairly common occurrence and has far-reaching consequences for the fetus and infant. Appreciation of the basic principles of fetal needs and growth might have occurred long ago, had it not been for a series of three misconceptions that prevented our colleagues from asking, and consequently answering, the proper questions. These misconceptions will be pointed out in order that we may learn a lesson, and be careful to say just what we mean, and mean just what we say.

First came the idea that the fetus is an *immensely successful parasite* that obtains from the maternal organism whatever it needs for normal growth and development, even at the risk of causing maternal deprivation. If this were true the status of the mother would, short of catastrophic illness, have no effect on the fetus. That it is not so will become apparent as the maternal part of the supply line is discussed in Chapters 9 and 11.

The second misleading concept was that of *prematurity based on birth weight*. The practice of setting apart infants weighing at birth 2500 g or less, was accepted in 1950 by the World Health Organization[1] for the legitimate purpose of identifying them for special care on the basis of a readily obtainable criterion. The unfortunate use of the term *prematurity* for this group led the great majority of workers to believe that these were really premature infants, and conversely that true prematurity is the only significant cause of low birth weight. This prevented for many years the recognition of fetal growth retardation. True there were cries in the wilderness, such as the statement of McKeown and Gibson[2] in 1951: '. . . as a means of identifying an entity suitable for inquiry, [the use of weight as an index of maturity] could hardly be less satisfactory . . .'; yet immense efforts were expended in studies of properties, handicaps, or sequelae of 'prematurity' determined solely by weight. It was not until the early 60s that studies of birth weight in relation to gestational age came into their own right, thus paving the way for recognising and studying abnormal fetal growth. It has been suggested that the further use of the term prematurity be avoided since it has been so extensively misused. We will therefore speak of pre-term *v.* small-for-dates infants. More on definitions of groups of newborn infants will be found later in this chapter.

As soon as fetal growth retardation was recognised as a frequent sequel of deprivation another slogan was thoughtlessly used, namely *placental insufficiency*, and I must confess to being one of those who did. No elaborate and sophisticated studies are needed to find that the role of the placenta proper in causing deprivation of the fetus is small compared with that of the maternal supply line to the placenta. Here again a poor term threatened to retard progress: If true placental insufficiency were the cause of fetal deprivation, little or nothing could be done about it, and the condition would be of no practical medical interest. If however this slogan is avoided and the prominent role of the maternal organism is recognised, then a wide field opens up for investigation, treatment and perhaps prevention. This we hope will be substantiated in some of the chapters to follow.

It is essential to define the border of the placental and maternal components of the fetal supply line[3]. Since the conceptus is enclosed in the maternal organism, anything reaching or leaving it must somehow traverse maternal fixed tissues or blood. We are not certain that all this exchange takes place at the placenta proper; some may occur across fetal membranes and reference to this will be made from time to time. Conditions prior to the establishment of the definitive placenta will also be mentioned briefly, but will not concern us a great deal.

Composition and flow of maternal blood in the intervillous space determine what is offered the placenta for transfer. They are under maternal control and, therefore, properly constitute maternal factors (Figure 1.1). Placental components of the supply line reside within the villi which are part of the conceptus. True placental insufficiency would limit transfer

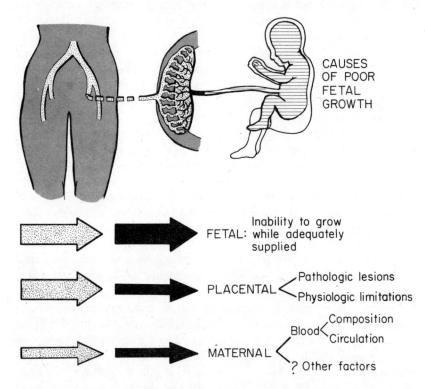

Figure 1.1 Fetal, placental, and maternal factors which may cause poor fetal growth. (From Gruenwald, P. (1971). *Obstet. Gynecol.*, **37**, 906, by permission of Harper & Row)

across the villous trophoblast, which is the interface between maternal and fetal compartments, in the presence of adequate flow and composition of maternal blood. Some changes in the placenta which reduce the area of exchange, e.g. infarcts, are secondary to maternal circulatory disturbances in the intervillous space (Chapter 12).

One of the arguments in favour of limitation of fetal growth by the placenta has been the close correlation of fetal and placental size, yet when one examines this carefully it indicates nothing of this sort. If fetal size were regulated within such narrow limits by placental size (and function) this would presuppose a placenta at the border of its functional capacity or else it could not have that influence. There is no reason to believe that this is the case. On the other hand, the placenta as part of the conceptus may well be regulated in its growth along with, or by, the fetus. This is a more plausible explanation of the size relationship.

The Placental Component of the Fetal Supply Line

As has just been suggested, and will be explained in more detail in Chapter 6, it would be quite difficult to obtain compelling evidence that any aspect of placental transfer function is normally near the limits of its functional capacity and can, under abnormal circumstances short of drastic experiments, be the limiting factor in the supply line. The fact that the placenta transmits only as much of a given substance as is utilised by the fetus is readily explained by an equilibrium between maternal and fetal blood streams (Chapter 6) maintained by replacement of what the fetus withdraws. Yet, lack of knowledge of specific instances of limitation or insufficiency is surely due, at least in part, to our failure to know where to look for them or how to recognise them. Such knowledge may come forth in the future. Suggestions of structural changes that might produce placental insufficiency are found in Chapters 12 and 14. The most likely circumstance in which to find true placental insufficiency would be prolonged pregnancy when both aging changes and failure to keep up with fetal growth could have this effect. Even this has not been demonstrated to reduce placental function below the needed limit, and it may well be the maternal supply line that the fetus outgrows. All in all, it is unlikely that placental insufficiency in the strict sense as defined here will ever emerge as a major factor in limitation of the fetal supply line.

The Maternal Component of the Fetal Supply Line

It has been well established by experiments that foreign substances introduced into the maternal circulation appear in the fetal blood, or have demonstrable effects on the fetus. Similarly, the concentration of normal constituents in the mother has been raised or lowered, with corresponding changes in the fetal blood or other effects on the fetus. Yet we have little knowledge of specific substances, apart from oxygen, which might under circumstances of human reproduction become deficient in the mother's circulation to the point of limiting fetal well-being. In malnutrition, for instance, effects on the fetus are known, but the nature of the specific substances which are the limiting factors in fetal nutrition has not been established. These problems will be dealt with in Chapters 10 and 11.

In contrast, circulatory abnormalities have been extensively implicated, with more or less compelling evidence, in insufficiency of the supply line in human pregnancy and in animal experiments. In fact, much of what we know about fetal deprivation can be traced to the mechanical aspects of maternal circulation in the intervillous space, as will be shown in Chapter 9. In addition, certain maternal characteristics, many of them not usually considered as diseases, are known to produce or predispose to fetal deprivation, as discussed in Chapter 11.

It is thus clear that the search for causes of fetal deprivation, usually apparent as growth retardation, must be made primarily in the maternal organism. Placenta and fetus account for but a small proportion of instances of deprivation *in utero*. In the present volume an effort will be made to separate placental and maternal causes of fetal deprivation, but this cannot always be carried through. In some instances the mechanism of action is not known, and in some others primary abnormalities of maternal circulation are complicated by secondary pathological changes in the placenta. Yet, conceptually as well as for practical medical reasons it is important to maintain this distinction whenever possible.

Fetal Growth Retardation

While this volume is not primarily concerned with the fetus itself, it is necessary to consider in some detail the conditions under which growth retardation occurs, since this is the best and often the only indicator of an inadequate supply line. If one arbitrarily contrasts growth on the one hand, and maturation on the other, it is obvious that the latter is of far greater biological significance: it determines the physiological capabilities of the organism such as the ability to adapt at birth to extrauterine life. Maturation is much less inhibited by deprivation than is growth. Thus, the small-for-dates infant lacks the handicaps of pre-term birth (but has some of its own). If, in spite of this, we pay so much attention to growth, it is because it is readily assessed in the form of weight in relation to age, but more importantly because it is the more sensitive indicator of deprivation.

Fetal growth may be retarded either when the fetus is unable to grow normally in the presence of a normal supply line, or when the supply line is less than adequate (Figure 1.1). Since the greater part of fetal weight accrues during the second half of gestation and since an inadequate supply line is unlikely to exist in earlier stages, factors which inhibit the fetal growth potential independent of the supply line will be defined arbitrarily as being inherent in the fetus at mid-gestation. It matters little whether this line is drawn somewhat more to one side or the other. These fetal factors include genetic as well as environmental conditions, even though they have reached the conceptus via the mother at an earlier stage. The largest group is that of malformed fetuses. While not all malformed fetuses have a reduced growth potential, they do as a group. Subnormal growth may be the only discernible manifestation of maldevelopment, as is suggested by growth-retarded and otherwise well-formed littermates of malformed fetuses in animal experiments with teratogens. This leads imperceptibly into the field of dwarfism without associated structural defects. How many of these undergrown fetuses are included among the deprived ones because they are not visibly malformed or otherwise diseased, is not known. It is generally believed that their number is not sufficiently great to lead to statistical errors. At postmortem examination fetal deprivation can be differentiated from other states by organ weights and histological criteria (Chapter 19). The second group of fetuses with a reduced growth potential includes those with chronic disease. The cause is usually infection such as by rubella or cytomegalovirus. The borderline against malformation is partially obliterated by the fact that some infections produce malformations. Finally, there is runt disease as a result of graft-versus-host reaction due to maternal lymphocytes reaching the fetus in certain experimental circumstances[4]. No comparable condition has been identified in man.

It is very likely that genetic traits affect body growth independent of the supply line. The difficulties of pin-pointing genetic factors in man and even in experimental animals have been discussed by Brent and Jensch[5]. As has been mentioned, it is unlikely that genetic factors as the only variable are responsible for many infants satisfying the criteria of small-for-dates birth. In a multiple regression analysis of the data of the Collaborative Perinatal Study of the National Institute of Neurological Diseases and Blindness, Naylor and Myrianthopoulos[6] determined that a sizable proportion of the difference in birth weights between Whites and Negroes in the United States, namely about 130 g, is determined by genetic rather than environmental factors. A genetic difference of this magnitude is not in agreement with data from Negro middle class populations, and could conceivably be the result of different effects of various environmental factors on the two populations, for reasons other than genetic. Yet the possibility of significant genetic differences does exist, as is also suggested by wide variations of mean birth weights among populations such as those tabulated from the literature by McClung[7]. The sex difference of fetal growth may or may not be genetically mediated. The category of fetuses with an intrinsically reduced growth potential, indicated on the right side of Figure 1.1, is mentioned here only because it must be excluded from all considerations of growth retardation due to deprivation.

Fetal growth is inhibited in a number of clinical and experimental situations in which it is likely or certain that deprivation rather than reduction of the growth potential is involved. In some instances we have vague knowledge of the cause, but not the details or mechanism: in maternal malnutrition, for instance, it is not known which specific substances are deficient to the point of limiting fetal growth. In another example, multiple pregnancy, we surmise a maternal cause of growth retardation, but the limiting factors are also unknown (Chapter 11).

Definition of Abnormal Fetal Growth

Since growth is much more sensitive to deprivation than is maturation, it will be the basis of our considerations. For this reason, criteria of abnormal growth must first be established. Normal standards can be obtained in two ways: empirically from the population to which the individual probands belong or another population that one has reason to believe is similar in fetal growth; or else by extrapolation of the unconstrained portions of empirical data to arrive at a universally valid optimal standard (see below). The latter has not been used extensively, and differs from the former only in that period late in pregnancy in which deceleration of growth occurs, that is, near and past term[8]. No matter which standard is used, an infant is recognised as small-for-dates if the birth weight is below mean -2 standard deviations or below the tenth centile for the respective week of gestation. The latter criterion selects 3–4 times as many infants as small-for-dates as does the former. Usher and McLean[9] found that infants below mean -2 standard deviations (or the third centile) are at much greater risk than those between the third and tenth centile, and therefore suggest the use of the more stringent standard. On the other hand, it should not be thought that those above the third centile are all normally grown.

Empirical standards have been determined for many populations; examples are given in Table 1.1 and Figure 1.2. All are very similar early in the third trimester. Differences in the latter part of the third trimester depend largely on the time of onset of growth deceleration. These differences are presumed to relate to the time when the fetal supply line becomes insufficient to support the full growth potential. If this is true, extrapolation of the straight and universally valid part of the curve through the last weeks of pregnancy should indicate how the fetus would grow if its growth potential could be realised without inhibition (Table 1.1, Figure 1.2). This concept is supported by the observation of McKeown and Record[10] that the infant returns to a curve with the same slope after birth when it has adjusted to extra-uterine life and is well supplied.

Table 1.1. Birth weights during the third trimester from six sources with standard deviations (where available), **and extrapolated weights**

Nearest week of gestation	Denver	Baltimore	Montreal	Portland	Britain	Amsterdam	Extrapolated
28	1150	1050±310	1113±150	1172±344		1249	
29	1268	1200±350	1228±165	1322±339	1165±540	1336	
30	1392	1380±370	1373±175	1529±474	1250±450	1419	
31	1537	1560±400	1540±200	1757±495	1575±445	1604	
32	1661	1750±410	1727±225	1881±437	1870±550	1808	
33	1844	1950±420	1900±250	2158±511	2015±640	1989	
34	2117	2170±430	2113±280	2340±552	2200±670	2203	
35	2385	2390±440	2347±315	2518±468	2410±675	2389	
36	2618	2610±440	2589±350	2749±490	2680±640	2642	
37	2809	2830±440	2868±385	2989±466	2895±560	2909	
38	2946	3050±450	3133±400	3185±450	3070±500	3163	
39	3076	3210±450	3360±430	3333±444	3225±465	3298	3250±450
40	3178	3280±450	3480±460	3462±456	3360±455	3444	3460±490
41	3266	3350±450	3567±475	3569±468	3450±460	3539	3670±520
42	3307	3400±460	3513±480	3637±482	3510±480	3619	3880±540
43		3410±490	3416±465	3660±502	3500±510	3642	4090±570
44		3420±500	3384±485	3619±515	3495±510	3694	4300±600

Denver (Lubchenco et al.[23]): original data corrected for erroneous dates interpolated here from completed weeks.

Baltimore (Gruenwald[11]): original data corrected for erroneous dates and smoothed.

Montreal (Usher and McLean[9]): original data smoothed; except for 40 weeks, no group has more than 27 cases.

Portland, Oregon (Babson et al.[19]).

Britain (Butler and Alberman[25]): interpolated here from completed weeks.

Amsterdam (Kloosterman[26]).

Extrapolated: Derived from a straight line (Figure 1.2, E) characterised by the averages of the regression coefficients and intercepts of the portions between 30 and 36 weeks of the six sets of data in this table. The slopes are nearly identical and the intercepts at 39 weeks are all within 190 g. The help of Dr O. DeLisser with these calculations is gratefully acknowledged. An equivalent of standard deviation was set arbitrarily at 14% of weight, as it is in the Baltimore data from 39 to 42 weeks.

Several considerations must be kept in mind when using 'fetal growth curves'. They are birth-weight curves and not true growth curves since they are derived from different neonates born after various gestation times. It is abnormal to be born early in the third trimester, and the possibility exists that the products of such births are abnormal. Since, however, the functional reserve of the supply line is greater early in pregnancy than later, such abnormality probably does not affect fetal growth in a significant number of instances. Late in the third trimester the number of those normally born

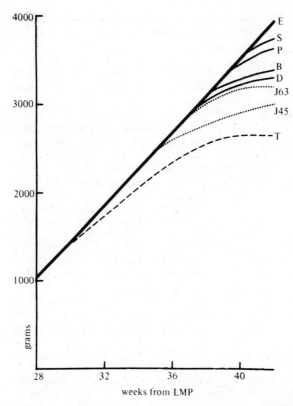

Figure 1.2 Highly smoothed birth-weight curves of several populations, shown to demonstrate departure from a common, straight line at various gestational ages with resulting differences in weight at term. E, extrapolated curve; S, Sweden (Lindell, A. (1956). *Acta Obstet. Gynaec. Scand.*, **35**, 136; P, Portland, Oregon[19]; B, Baltimore[11]; D, Denver[23]; J63 and J45, Japan 1963–64 and 1945–46, respectively (Gruenwald, P., Funakawa, H., Mitani, S., Nishimura, T., and Takeuchi, S. (1967). *Lancet*, **i**, 1026); T, Twins representing a group with a high proportion of small-for-dates infants

greatly exceeds abnormal ones. It is therefore surmised that birth-weight curves are representative of fetal growth. The only true longitudinal growth curves are those of the biparietal diameter of the skull obtained by ultrasound. It is gratifying to see to what extent these resemble our birth-weight curves as is apparent, for instance, by comparing Figures 1.2 and 17.6a, or the dotted line in Figure 1.5 with Figure 17.9.

Some of the sets of birth-weight data show peculiar high values for the early part of the third trimester. When weights are plotted for a given week, the distribution has either a very broad peak, or is bimodal with a lower peak at a weight expected 4 weeks later. All evidence suggests that this is an artefact due to the last menstrual period recorded as 4 weeks too late, and correction has been made for this[11, 12]. The extent of this error varies inversely with the quality of prenatal interviewing, and the error is nearly absent from certain sets of data[13].

Several organisations have published deliberations on terminology related to fetal growth. One set of definitions deals with the lower limit of perinatal death *v.* abortion; this concerns us here only marginally, to the extent that it affects mortality statistics. Two major stumbling blocks in this area have been (1) the primary use of gestational age which is so often unknown in early termination of pregnancy, and (2) the undue status of neonatal death accorded some very small, previable fetuses because they gasped or moved a limb. A recent report of the World Health Organization[14] (quoted with permission) made realistic suggestions which are given here even though they have not yet achieved official status: it was recommended that body weight rather than gestational age be the primary criterion, and that:—

(i) all fetuses and infants delivered weighing 500 g or more be registered, irrespective of whether they are alive or dead;
(ii) deliveries of fetuses weighing less than 500 g be considered abortions, whether there are signs of life or not; and
(iii) for the purpose of standard perinatal mortality statistics for international reporting, only those births weighing 1000 g or more be included.

I believe that this recommendation deserves universal support.

With regard to later stages, the World Health Organization who had previously endorsed the term *premature* for all infants born with a weight of 2500 g or less, stated in 1961[15] that this was inappropriate because not all of these infants are premature, and suggested the term *infant of low birth weight* for the same group to be identified for special care. This term was found cumbersome by some, and was misused as synonymous with small-for-dates by others. Subsequently, the American Academy of Pediatrics[24] suggested that newborn infants be characterised as pre-term (up to 38 weeks), term (38–42 weeks) or post-term (beyond 42 weeks) births. This was indicated in a diagram, but not strictly defined. Furthermore, infants are to be designated as small, appropriate, or large for gestational age with respect to borderlines set at the 10th and 90th centiles of weight for the respective week of gestation. No specific values were prescribed, and the use of 2 standard deviations or the third centile was not ruled out. Weight groups are to be characterised by their limits in grams rather than by terms which are so readily misused.

Later, the Second European Congress of Perinatal Medicine[16] published similar guidelines, except that the borderline between pre-term and term birth was defined clearly at less than 37 weeks, and that of post-term birth at 42 weeks or more. Standards of adequacy for gestational age should be quoted specifically, such as 'below 5th centile for boys, Aberdeen 1968'. This is significant particularly when the position of a given infant is examined relative to growth standards that are broad, or derived from a different

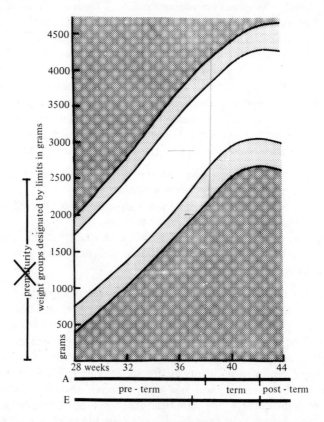

Figure 1.3 Diagram illustrating recently suggested methods of characterising newborn infants by birth weight and gestational age. The heavily stippled areas include weights above or below 2 standard deviations from the mean, the lightly stippled areas the additional ranges if the 10th and 90th centiles are used as criteria of small and large-for-gestational-age, using data from Portland, Oregon[19]. At the bottom, the ranges of pre-term, term, and post-term birth are given as suggested (A) by the American Academy of Pediatrics[24], and (E) by the Second European Congress of Perinatal Medicine[16]. Use of the term *prematurity* to indicate a birth weight below 2501 g, or in any other sense, should be avoided because of past misuse

population. Tanner and Thomson[17] devised standards based on Aberdeen data, taking into account sex, parity, and the mother's height and weight. Thomson[18] showed an example in which an infant on the borderline of abnormal weight for gestational age by indiscriminate standards, turned out to be of average weight when these factors were considered.

The standards just described and their differences are shown in Figure 1.3, using as an example the data of Babson et al.[19]. Also, a scoring system based on standard deviations has been suggested; this simplifies terminology in certain contexts[20]. These scores, and their comparison with centiles[21], are seen in Figure 1.4. Similar scores can be used for placenta or organ weights, by either gestational age or body weight.

Most data relating birth weight to gestational age have been presented

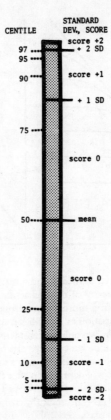

Figure 1.4 Comparison of centiles and scores based on standard deviation. (Slightly modified from Gruenwald, P. (1970). *Adv. Reprod. Physiol.*, **2**, by permission of Academic Press)

in the form of graphs and tables. While graphs are more impressive when trends are considered, tables allow the placing of individual cases more accurately and quickly. It is important to distinguish birth weight curves from curves indicating centiles or other fractions that might serve to identify abnormal growth. The former presumably represent stages of growth of individual fetuses, normal or abnormal, whereas the latter (such as the borders of the shaded areas in Figure 1.3) do not. This difference was confused by Dunn and Butler[22] in their *gestogram* in which each line connects the same centiles at various gestational ages, and is yet presented as a 'fetal growth line' indicating 'growth velocity'. Graphs depicting normal or abnormal growth should actually appear more like Figure 1.5, based on evidence in this chapter and on actual longitudinal growth data in Chapter

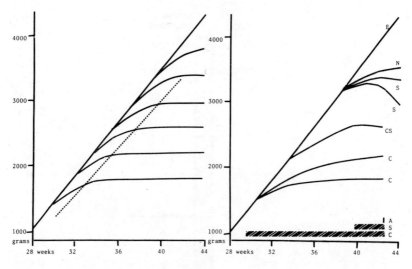

Figure 1.5 Diagrams of the effects of timing and severity of deprivation on fetal grow Timing depends in part on severity of the deficiency as the fetus outgrows a severely deficient supply line earlier than a more adequate one. The effect of time of onset of deprivation causing eventual cessation of growth, on weight at or past term is shown on the left. The upper two curved lines would be considered as normal in Western countries; the next two represent the usual in some other parts of the world. The remaining two probably represent few if any populations, but rather cases of severe deprivation. On the right, the effect of varying degrees of deprivation after the same time of onset of deceleration is shown, at the top for infants who had developed sufficient subcutaneous fat to lose weight when severely deprived: (N) normal; (S) two degrees of subacute fetal distress. Near the bottom, the two lines marked (C) show chronic fetal distress of two degrees, arising when the fetus cannot yet lose weight by wasting. (CS) is an intermediate form, with late onset of chronic distress when wasting has become possible, producing a 'combination form' of chronic and subacute distress

17. The only circumstance in which the gestogram may apply, is that of normally supplied fetuses with different growth potentials, as indicated by the dotted line in Figure 1.5. Consideration must also be given to the downward trend of some lines late in gestation, indicating the possibility of wasting when limitation by the supply line is severe.

The straight course of the usual growth curve in the third trimester prior to deceleration should not be construed as indicating proportional growth of the fetus in all of its parts. Firstly, an equal weekly increment indicates a decreasing growth rate. Secondly, body proportions change, as indicated by the weight/length index as an example (Figure 1.6). Thus, these equal increments of body weight are almost fortuitous, but they are useful for practical purposes.

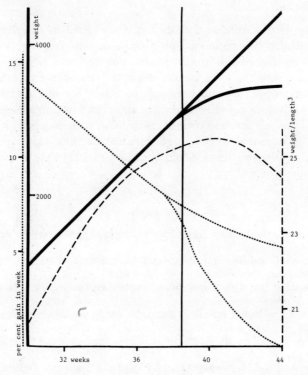

Figure 1.6 Birth-weight curves (heavy lines — Baltimore empiric data below, and extrapolated curve above), growth rates from these curves (dotted lines), and body weight/length³ from data of the National Birthday Trust Fund[25]. All curves are heavily smoothed and only indicate trends. (From Gruenwald, P. (1970). In: *Physiology of the Perinatal Period*, Vol. 1. (U. Stave, editor). Courtesy of Appleton-Century-Crofts, Publishing Division of Prentiss–Hall, Inc., Englewood Cliffs, New Jersey)

When the gestational age is not known or is questioned in a given case, tests during pregnancy (Chapters 16, 17) or on the neonate (Chapter 19) are used to ascertain the state of maturity. Estimates based on routine prenatal examination are less reliable.

Several studies have shown that differences between populations in mean birth weight are usually due to variations of fetal growth rather than gestational age. In the absence of information on gestational age in a population (not in individuals) one may therefore assume *tentatively* that fetal growth is the cause of differences which in turn may involve genetic factors and/or the supply line. Confirmation by gestational age studies is, of course, desirable.

Fetal Wasting

In subacute fetal distress as described in more detail in Chapter 19, and found particularly in prolonged pregnancy, the late onset of deprivation results in wasting of full-length infants, but not in a weight deficit of sufficient magnitude to place these infants in the small-for-dates category. In severe instances the long, thin, wasted appearance is quite spectacular, but there are to date no objective criteria to apprehend such infants as a group including lesser degrees, and correlate their status with maternal or placental factors. The abnormal weight/length index as discussed in Chapter 19, as well as measurements of skin-fold thickness should make it possible to delineate this group.

References

1. World Health Organization (1950). Final report, expert group on prematurity. *Wld. Hlth. Org. Tech. Rep. Series* 27
2. McKeown, T. and Gibson, J. R. (1951). Observations on all birth (23,970) in Birmingham, 1947. IV: 'Premature birth'. *Brit. Med. J.*, **2**, 513
3. Gruenwald, P. (1971). Fetal deprivation and placental insufficiency. *Obst. Gynec.*, **37**, 906
4. Beer, A. E. and Billingham, R. E. (1973). Maternally acquired runt disease. *Science*, **179**, 240
5. Brent, R. L. and Jensch, R. P. (1967). Intra-uterine growth retardation. *Advan. Teratol.*, **2**, 140
6. Naylor, A. F. and Myrianthopoulos, N. C. (1967). The relation of ethnic and socio-economic factors to human birth-weight. *Ann. Hum. Genet.*, **31**, 71
7. McClung, J. (1969). *Effects of High Altitude on Human Birth: Observations on Mothers, Placentas, and the Newborn in two Peruvian Populations.* (Cambridge: Harvard University Press)
8. Gruenwald, P. (1964). The fetus in prolonged pregnancy. *Amer. J. Obst. Gynec.*, **89**, 503

9. Usher, R. and McLean, F. (1969). Intrauterine growth of liveborn Caucasian infants at sea level: standards obtained from measurements in 7 dimensions of infants born between 25 and 44 weeks of gestation. *J. Ped.*, **74**, 901

10. McKeown, T. and Record, R. G. (1953). The influence of placental size on foetal growth in man, with special reference to multiple pregnancy. *J. Endocrinol.*, **9**, 418

11. Gruenwald, P. (1966). Growth of the human fetus. I. Normal growth and its variation. *Amer. J. Obst. Gynec.*, **94**, 1112

12. Neligan, G. (1965). A community study of the relationship between birth weight and gestational age. *Clinics Develop. Med.*, **19**, 28

13. Gruenwald, P. (1970). Intra-uterine growth. *Pediatrics*, **46**, 815

14. World Health Organization (1972). Report of the Consultation on Methodology of Reporting and Analysis of Perinatal and Maternal Morbidity and Mortality (Document: ICD/72.3)

15. World Health Organization (1961). Expert Committee on Maternal and Child Health: Public health aspects of low birth weight. *Wld. Hlth. Org. Tech. Rep. Series*, 217

16. Second European Congress of Perinatal Medicine (1970). Working party to discuss nomenclature based on gestational age and birthweight. *Arch. Dis. Childh.*, **45**, 730

17. Tanner, J. M. and Thomson, A. M. (1970). Standards for birthweight at gestation periods from 32 to 42 weeks, allowing for maternal height and weight. *Arch. Dis. Childh.*, **45**, 566

18. Thomson, A. M. (1970). The evaluation of human growth patterns. *Amer. J. Dis. Child.*, **120**, 398

19. Babson, S. G., Behrman, R. E. and Lessel, R. (1970). Fetal growth: liveborn birth weights for gestational age of white middle class infants. *Pediatrics*, **45**, 937

20. Gruenwald, P. (1963). Chronic fetal distress and placental insufficiency. *Biol. Neonat.*, **5**, 215

21. Gruenwald, P. (1967). Growth of the human foetus. *Advan. Reprod. Physiol.*, **2**, 279

22. Dunn, P. M. and Butler, N. R. (1971). Intrauterine growth. A discussion of some of the problems besetting its measurement. In: *Biological Aspects of Demography*. Symposia of the Society for the Study of Human Biology, Vol. 10, p. 147. (W. Brass, editor) (London: Taylor and Francis)

23. Lubchenco, L. O., Hansman, C., Dressler, M. and Boyd, E. (1963). Intrauterine growth as estimated from liveborn birthweight data at 24 to 42 weeks of gestation. *Pediatrics*, **32**, 793

24. American Academy of Pediatrics (1967). Nomenclature for duration of gestation, birth weight and intra-uterine growth. *Pediatrics*, **39**, 935

25. Butler, N. R. and Alberman, E. D. (1969). *Perinatal Problems. The Second Report of the British Perinatal Mortality Survey.* (Edinburgh: Livingstone)

26. Kloosterman, J. G. (1966). Prevention of prematurity. *Nederl. Tijdschr. Verlosk. Gynaec.*, **66**, 361

CHAPTER 2

Principles of Placentation and Early Human Placental Development

Ralph M. Wynn

Defined broadly as a union of fetal and parental tissues for the purposes of physiological exchange, the placenta encompasses a great diversity of morphological types, of which the human haemochorial disc is but one specific variant. The unique morphological features of the placenta include its dual (fetal and parental) composition and its extracorporeal location; its unique functional characteristics include full growth and development within a limited life span and anatomical adaptations to diverse tasks that encompass transport of gases and metabolites to and from the fetus, elimination of waste products, and elaboration of steroid and protein hormones.

Types of Placentation

Details of comparative anatomy of the placenta and the evolution of viviparity are discussed in recent reviews by the author[1, 2]. This chapter deals only in broad outline with the variety of placental types, placing particular emphasis on the human condition.

Unilaminar placentation, the simplest form, consists of trophoblast (blastocystic ectoderm) in contact with maternal tissue, usually endometrium. Addition of endoderm forms a bilaminar blastocyst, the fetal component of simple bilaminar placentation. Development of mesoderm results in a trilaminar blastocyst; the vascularised trilaminar blastocyst is the essential fetal component common to all mammalian placentas[3-5]. The omphalopleure is the wall of the yolk sac. When the exocelom extends into the area of the yolk sac it separates the vascular splanchnopleure from the non-vascular

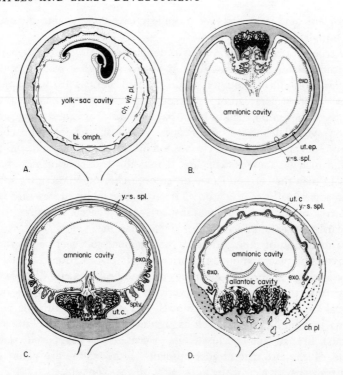

Figure 2.1 A. Schematic cross section of an early gestational sac of the black bear, illustrating central implantation, bilaminar omphalopleure (bi. omph.), and the early extensive vascular choriovitelline placenta (ch. vit. pl.)

B. Definitive arrangement of the placenta and fetal membranes in *Solenodon*, showing the discoidal chorioallantoic placenta antimesometrially, and the extensive completely inverted yolk sac placenta over the remaining area of contact between fetal and maternal tissues. Exocelom (exo.), uterine epithelium (ut. ep.), and yolk sac splanchnopleure (y.-s. spl.) are shown. (Redrawn from Wislocki)

C. Definitive arrangement of placenta and membranes in the guinea pig. The discoidal chorioallantoic placenta lies mesometrially. The bilaminar omphalopleure has degenerated over the entire antimesometrial area and the everted yolk sac splanchnopleure (y.-s. spl.) is in contact with the endometrium, forming a completely inverted yolk sac placenta over the antimesometrial hemisphere. Exocelom (exo.) is clearly illustrated. In the paraplacental area the splanchnopleure has numerous villi (spl. v.) that project into the uterine cavity (ut. c.)

D. Fetal membranes and placenta in the rabbit, showing the surviving chorionic placenta (ch. pl.) at the margin of the placental disc and the extensive inverted yolk sac placenta. Uterine cavity (ut. c.), exocelom (exo.), and yolk sac splanchnopleure (y.-s. spl.) are shown. The discoidal chorioallantoic placenta is situated mesometrially. The black dots in the decidua within the paraplacental zone represent free trophoblastic giant cells. (From *Amer. J. Obstet. Gynec.* **84**, 1570 (1962). Courtesy of Dr W. A. Wimsatt and the C. V. Mosby Company, St. Louis) somatopleure and transforms the more primitive yolk sac into the definitive splanchnopleuric stage (Figure 2.1).

The true chorion, which consists of trophoblast and mesenchymal tissue, is basically avascular. Although it is absent in higher rodents and man, avascular chorionic placentation occurs in many animals. It entails apposition of true chorion (extraembryonic somatopleure other than that of the amnion) to the endometrium. Its trophoblast may form multinucleate giant cells or syncytial masses. Secondarily avascular chorionic or chorioallantoamnionic placentation occurs in middle and late gestation in anthropoid apes and man. In some rodents and rabbits this true chorion may be functional. In man the chorion laeve, or 'smooth chorion', although apparently similar superficially to the true chorion of the rabbit, arises through devascularisation of the decidua capsularis and adjacent chorion to form secondarily avascular chorioamnionic placentation.

Vascularisation of the chorion by the vitelline (yolk sac) vessels results in choriovitelline placentation; in chorioallantoic placentation the fetal blood supply is received through allantoic, or umbilical, vessels. Choriovitelline placentation, the more primitive variety, is the principal means of fetomaternal exchange in most marsupials, and it coexists with the allantoic placenta in many Eutheria, such as lagomorphs (e.g. rabbits) and rodents (e.g. rats). In man true choriovitelline placentation is never well established because of the precocious development of the extra-embryonic celom, which prevents contact of the yolk sac with the trophoblast.

An entirely different form of yolk sac placentation occurs in mammals in which there is inversion of the germ layers. Such inverted yolk sac placentation occurs among the rodents, rabbits and hares, many bats and insectivores, and armadillos. No mesoderm develops in the abembryonic hemisphere of the blastocystic wall, the bilaminar omphalopleure therefore remaining a very thin membrane in contact with the uterus. The bilaminar omphalopleure may disappear entirely, or it may never develop, as in the guinea pig. In either case, the highly vascular embryonic hemisphere of the yolk sac is inserted into the abembryonic area, thus bringing its lining endoderm into very close relation with the uterine mucosa over a wide area. The inverted yolk sac placenta is undoubtedly of great physiological significance in many animals and must therefore be considered in extrapolation of all data concerning placental function that are derived from those species.

In the typical eutherian blastocyst the early segregation of ectodermal tissue destined to form the trophoblast limits the formation of the endoderm and the intra-embryonic mesoderm to a restricted group of cells. According to Mossman[3], formation of endoderm in all mammals is basically similar to that in the avian egg in that the cells are delaminated from the deep surface of the inner cell mass. These endodermal cells may, in part, become intimately related to the trophoblast in formation of the bilaminar yolk sac. The origin of the extra-embryonic mesoderm has generated considerable controversy. In the human placenta it may arise, at least in part, by delamination from the cytotrophoblast but comparative studies suggest that part of this layer may be derived from the same source as the intra-embryonic mesoderm.

Structural differences in placental form far outnumber the interspecific similarities, which, according to Mossman[4], comprise a somatopleuric amnion and chorion, a splanchnopleuric yolk sac and allantois, and, in all Eutheria (true placental mammals), a chorioallantoic placenta with vascular mesodermal villi and separation of the two blood streams by layers that probably include at least fetal endothelium and trophoblast. Mossman has provided a current account of the morphological adaptations of the fetal membranes to viviparity throughout the animal kingdom[6].

Chorioallantoic placentation

Because the chorioallantoic placenta is the principal organ of feto-maternal exchange in most higher mammals, including man, its classification, on the basis of gross shape, histological 'barrier', presence or absence of decidua, and other anatomical criteria, has been attempted frequently. However, frequent exceptions to all these criteria have been made. The definitive shape of the placenta is usually determined by the initial distribution of the villi over the chorionic surface, although, according to Wimsatt[5], the shape is occasionally secondarily derived. In the sow and mare the distribution of villi over almost the entire chorionic surface produces a diffuse placenta. In the cow and sheep, villi are restricted to separate tufts that are widely scattered over the chorion to form a cotyledonary, or multiplex, placenta. In most carnivores the grouping of villi in bands around the equator of the chorioallantoic sac results in a zonary placenta. In man, apes, rodents, bats, and most insectivores, the placenta forms a single disc; double discs may be commonly found in certain monkeys, such as the macaque. The definitive shape of the human placenta is a result of the disappearance of villi from all but a circumscribed locus on the chorion. Villi may arise primarily as outgrowths from the chorionic plate or secondarily from the basal plate as protrusions of cytotrophoblast that grow into a preformed syncytial mantle. The initially solid villous protrusions are subsequently vascularised by ingrowth of allantoic mesenchyme and vessels. Although deferred formation of villi usually results in a labyrinthine condition, the human placenta, according to Hamilton and Boyd[7], is derived from an earlier labyrinthine stage. Conversely, the lamelliform placenta of the carnivores represents a secondary modification of the original villous condition brought about by fusion of the small villous branches of the chorion[8].

Placentas may be classified also according to the presence or absence of a maternal (decidual) component. Examples of deciduate placentas are those of man and the guinea pig. Adeciduate placentas are common to such animals as the ungulates (e.g. cow) and carnivores (e.g. dog).

Strictly defined, the decidua is the gestational endometrium that is shed at parturition. It is thus imprecise to designate the transformed endometrium of the dog or sheep, e.g. as decidua. A decidual cell refers specifically to the transformed stromal cell of the pregnant endometrium. A decidual reaction usually refers to the typical endometrial stromal changes of the guinea pig or man but may include the epithelial plaque that is formed in the endometrium of the pregnant rhesus monkey.

The Grosser classification[9] retains its limited value in histological categorisation of placentas. It has, however, proved an increasingly inadequate means of predicting placental function. The shortcomings of the Grosser classification include its failure to account for anatomical variation within the placenta, changes accompanying placental ageing, and accessory placental organs. Its basic deficiency, however, is the implication that a reduction in the number of layers in the placental membrane is necessarily equivalent to increased placental efficiency. Although the transfer of substances that cross the placenta by simple diffusion is likely to be influenced by the thickness of the barrier, the Grosser scheme fails to take account of the physiological activity of the placental membranes, particularly with regard to enzymatic facilitation of transport, pinocytosis, and cytopempsis.

The minimal histological barrier in Grosser's original scheme comprised 3 fetal components: trophoblast, connective tissue, and endothelium. In the haemochorial placenta the trophoblast is exposed directly to the maternal blood. The persistence of maternal endothelium adds a fourth layer to form the endotheliochorial placenta. If, in addition, endometrial connective tissue remains, the postulated syndesmochorial placenta would result. When the endometrial epithelium enters into formation of a 6–layered membrane, the epitheliochorial condition prevails. On the basis of knowledge gained through electron microscopy this classification has been refined (see Chapter 4). The endotheliochorial placenta is much more likely to be 'vasochorial', since the maternal capillaries must be supported by some form of connective tissue. It is most unlikely, however, that this supporting tissue is a remnant of the original endometrium. It is more likely a product of the trophoblast or perhaps a manifestation of the reaction of trophoblast to endometrium. The classic syndesmochorial condition, as originally described in the sheep, goat, and cow, according to electron microscopic observations, represents

more nearly an epitheliochorial condition, since persistent remnants of
maternal uterine epithelia have been found. The classic syndesmochorial
condition, moreover, is unlikely to occur in the definitive placenta except
in limited areas, for there are no known species in which the main chorioallantoic mass is of this histological type.

The typical epitheliochorial placenta (Figure 2.2) is found among
Perissodactyla, Artiodactyla, Pholidota, Cetacea, Talpidae, and among the
primates, Lemuridae and Lorisidae. The vasochorial placenta with varying
contributions of endometrial stromal cells is found typically among the

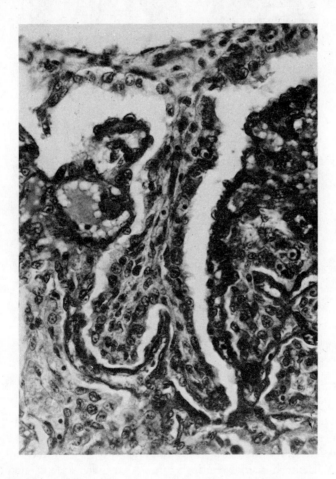

Figure 2.2 Epitheliochorial villous placenta of the mole *Parascalops*. × 280. (Courtesy of
Dr H. W. Mossman)

Carnivora (Figure 2.3). Recent re-examination of the hyena's placenta in this laboratory suggests that it too may be endotheliochorial rather than haemochorial, as previously reported[1]. The endotheliochorial or vasochorial

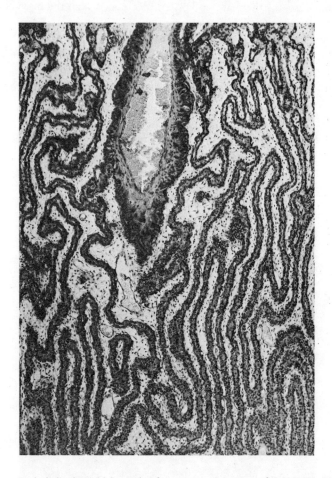

Figure 2.3 Endotheliochorial labyrinth of cat. × 45. (Courtesy of Dr H. W. Mossman)

condition is found also among members of the Bradypodidae, Soricidae, Chiroptera, Tubulidentata, and Proboscidea.

The haemochorial condition is subdivided into labyrinthine and villous types. A haemochorial labyrinth (Figure 2.4) is found among members of the Insectivora, Chiroptera, Hyracoidea, Tarsiidae, Rodentia, and Lagomorpha. The haemochorial villous condition is found among the higher

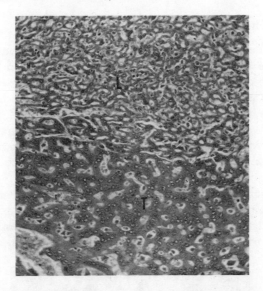

Figure 2.4 Haemochorial placenta of guinea pig, showing syncytiotrophoblastic labyrinth (L) and trophospongium (T). × 145

primates, Edentata, Insectivora, and certain isolated members of other groups.

The number of layers in the placenta fails, however, to provide an accurate index even of the ease of diffusion. For example, capillaries may indent both trophoblast and endometrium in an almost intra-epithelial location. Thus without changing the number of cellular layers the thickness of the membrane is significantly reduced.

Rigid histological classifications neglect transitions within the same placenta and fundamental differences in origin and function of numerous placental specialisations that appear superficially homologous or analogous. The human chorion laeve is perhaps analogous, but certainly not homologous, with the true chorion of the rabbit. Another example is the carnivore's placental haematoma, which may superficially resemble the true haemochorial condition. In the placental haematoma, however, stagnant blood extravasates between the chorion and the endometrial surface. This structure is histotrophic, i.e. it provides nutrition for the trophoblast from sources other than circulating blood. In contrast, the haemochorial placenta of man represents a true haemotrophic relation, since the nutrition is derived from circulating blood. A histotrophic phase precedes definitive formation of the haemotrophic condition during placental development.

The Haemochorial Condition

In a haemochorial labyrinth the trophoblast forms lamellae between the blood-filled spaces. In the villous placenta, such as that of man, there is an initial rupture of the maternal vessels by the trophoblast with escape of blood to form large sinusoids with trabeculae across the blood-filled spaces[5,7]. Wynn[1] illustrated the villous condition in a variety of taxonomically unrelated animals and confirmed the presence of numerous transitions from villous to labyrinthine forms, as seen particularly in the placentas of some New World monkeys (Figure 2.5). In the human placenta the villi are essentially free; the apparent intervillous connections are formed not by syncytiotrophoblast but by fibrinous adhesions resulting from organisation of minute haematomas. The labyrinthine condition is not different fundamentally; in the squirrel monkey, for example, the breakdown of syncytium converts the trabeculae in the affected areas to villi. In man there is no

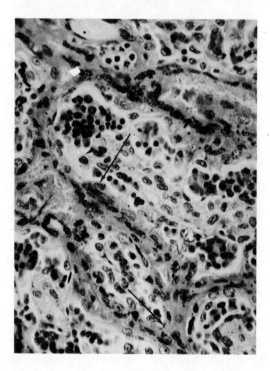

Figure 2.5 Haemochorial placenta of the squirrel monkey (*Saimiri sciureus*), showing individual villi connected by abundant intervillous syncytium (arrows), which creates a pseudolabyrinth. × 74

evidence of ontogenetic recapitulation of postulated phylogenetic development. Because the human placenta achieves a haemochorial status long before fetal vessels and mesenchyme appear, that is, before the formation of the definitive placenta, there are no recognised intermediate stages of development. The varieties of placentation among the anthropoids may be related to the differential activity of the ectoplacental trophoblast. In the platyrrhine (New World) monkeys, such as *Saimiri* and *Sanguinus*, there is less freedom of individual villi as a result of the initially broad attachment to the endometrium, but early and massive proliferation of trophoblast occurs. In the catarrhine (Old World) monkeys, such as the macaque[10] (Figure 2.6) and baboon[11], trophoblastic penetration is earlier and more extensive. Among anthropoids the most highly invasive trophoblast occurs in the early human blastocyst[12, 13] with the result that the chorionic villi lie free in the intervillous space in contact with maternal blood almost as soon as they are formed. The haemochorial condition appears to result from

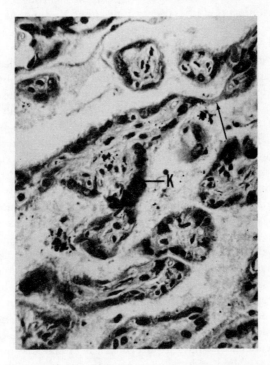

Figure 2.6 Haemochorial villous placenta of the bonnet monkey (*Macaca radiata*), showing syncytial knot (K) and intervillous junction (arrow). The freedom of individual villi approaches that in the human placenta. × 150

extensive erosion of maternal vessels associated with suppression of growth of maternal capillaries.

Development of the Human Placenta

The human placenta is basically a chorioallantoic structure, for although a vesicular allantois is absent, its precociously developed mesenchyme, which later forms the umbilical cord, gives rise *in situ* to the allantoic vessels that vascularise the chorion.

Decidua

Implantation and subsequent development of the human placenta depend on certain changes in the endometrium that culminate in the formation of the decidua. In the human being, complete conversion of the endometrium to decidua does not occur until several days after nidation, first appearing locally around blood vessels, and later spreading throughout the uterus. During development of the decidual reaction, the endometrial stromal elements enlarge to form polygonal or roundish decidual cells. The nuclei become round and vesicular, while the cytoplasm becomes clear, slightly basophilic, and surrounded by a translucent membrane. The decidua directly beneath the site of implantation forms the decidua basalis. Surrounding the ovum and separating it from the rest of the uterine cavity in the early months of gestation is the decidua capsularis, which forms as a result of deep implantation of the human ovum. The remainder of the pregnant uterus is lined by decidua parietalis. Since the ovum does not occupy the entire uterine cavity in the early months of pregnancy, there is a space between the capsular and parietal portions of the decidua. By the fourth month the growing ovum fills the uterine cavity; the capsularis and parietalis then fuse, obliterating the endometrial cavity. Capsular decidua is most prominent around the second month of pregnancy, consisting of stromal cells covered by a single layer of flattened epithelium without traces of glands; internally it contacts the chorion laeve. The decidua parietalis and the decidua basalis comprise 3 layers each; a surface, or a zona compacta; a middle portion, or zona spongiosa, with glands and numerous small blood vessels; and a zona basalis. The compacta and the spongiosa together form the zona functionalis. The basal zone remains after parturition and, except at the placental site, gives rise to new endometrium. As pregnancy advances, the epithelium of the decidua parietalis changes from cylindrical to cuboidal or flattened, at times even resembling endothelium. After the fourth month the parietalis gradually thins from its maximal height of 1 cm in the first trimester to 1–2 mm at term.

In the early months of pregnancy, ducts of uterine glands are found in the zona compacta, but they disappear toward term. The spongy layer consists of large, distended glands, which are often hyperplastic and separated by minimal stroma. The glands contribute to nourishment of the ovum during its histotrophic phase of development (before development of a placental circulation).

The decidua basalis enters into formation of the placenta itself. It differs from the rest of the decidua in two respects. First, the spongy zone consists mainly of arteries and widely dilated veins; by term, glands have virtually disappeared. Second, the basal decidua is invaded extensively by tropho-blastic giant cells[14]. Ageing of the decidua is accompanied by changes similar to those found during maturation of the placenta. Fibrinoid generally forms where trophoblast meets decidua. In the basal plate, the more or less continuous deposit of fibrinoid is known as Nitabuch's layer, and the inconstant deposition of a similar substance at the bottom of the intervillous space and surrounding the anchoring villi is known as Rohr's stria.

Yolk sac

The yolk sac, or umbilical vesicle, into which it develops, is quite prominent at the beginning of pregnancy. The embryo is at first a flattened disc, placed between amnion and yolk sac. As the embryo grows, it bulges into the amnionic sac, and the dorsal part of the yolk sac is incorporated into the body of the embryo to form the gut. The yolk sac may occasionally be recognised even in the mature placenta as a crumpled vascular sac, 3–5 mm in diameter, on the surface of the placental disc between amnion and chorion, or in the membranes just beyond the placental margin.

Allantois

The allantois may project into the base of the body stalk. Its precociously differentiated mesoderm forms the umbilical cord, which normally contains two arteries and one vein. The right umbilical vein disappears early, leaving only the original left vein. Sections of the cord frequently reveal, near its centre, a small duct of the umbilical vesicle. Sections just beyond the umbilical end of the cord, but never at the maternal end, occasionally reveal another duct, the remnant of the allantois.

Amnion

The amnion forms between the seventh and eighth days of development of the normal ovum. In the human being the amnion develops by cavitation. It is initially a small vesicle, which develops into a sac that covers the dorsal surface of the embryo. As the amnion enlarges, it gradually surrounds the embryo, which prolapses into its cavity. Distension of the sac brings it into contact with the internal surface of the chorion. Apposition of the mesoblasts of chorion and amnion occurs between the fourth and fifth months of gestation with the result that the extraembryonic celom is obliterated. The amnion and chorion, though normally slightly adherent, may always be separated easily, even at term.

The placenta proper

As early as 72 hours after fertilisation the 58-celled human blastocyst was observed to differentiate into 5 embryo-producing cells and 53 destined to form the trophoblast. On the 4th or 5th day after ovulation, when the morula, which is not more than 0·1–0·2 mm in diameter, enters the uterine cavity, the human endometrium is about 5 mm in thickness. The morula then lies free within the uterine cavity for about 2 or 3 days. Because of the earlier attachment of the ovum and perhaps because of the rapid penetration by the trophoblast (Figures 2.7 and 2.8), the human blastocyst is completely embedded in the endometrium by the 11th or 12th day[12] (Figure 2.9). This deep, or interstitial, implantation is associated with the development of a capsular decidua. The defect in the epithelium caused by blastocystic

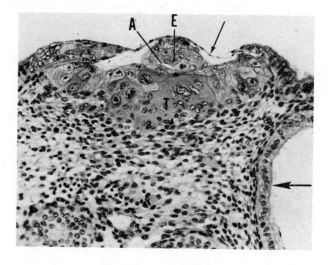

Figure 2.7 Human blastocyst at 78 days' gestation. Heavy arrow indicates a uterine gland. Light arrow points to outer wall of blastocyst. Trophoblast (T), embryonic disc (E), and amnionic cavity (A) are shown. The wall of the blastocyst facing the uterine cavity is thin. The portion of the blastocystic wall that faces the decidua is thickened, forming cytotrophoblast and syncytium. ×210. (Courtesy of Dr A. T. Hertig and the Carnegie Institution of Washington)

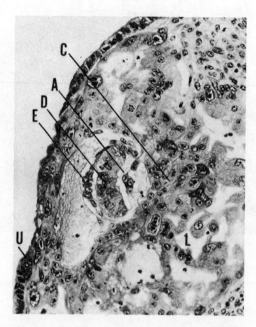

Figure 2.8 Section of 9-day human embryo, showing an early stage in formation of the trophoblastic lacunae (L). Uterine epithelium (U), endoderm (E), embryonic disc (D), amnionic cavity (A), and cytotrophoblast (C) are shown. × 210. (Courtesy of Dr A. T. Hertig and the Carnegie Institution of Washington)

penetration is gradually covered, at first by a coagulum of fibrin and later by the regrowth of adjacent endometrial epithelium.

During and after implantation there appear within the syncytiotrophoblast numerous vacuoles, the coalescence of which forms lacunae, which merge to form the primitive intervillous space[10]. Maternal venous sinuses are tapped early, but until the 14th or 15th day no maternal arterial blood enters the intervillous space. By about the 17th day (Figure 2.10), both maternal and placental blood vessels are functioning. The feto-placental circulation is not completed, however, until the intraembryonic blood vessels are connected with those of the chorion.

Villi may first be easily distinguished in the human placenta on or about the 12th day. The period between the 9th and the 20th days is characterised by intense growth and differentiation of the chorion. As a result, the tropho-blastic trabeculae, instead of remaining irregular, become orientated radially around the chorion as villi. The trabeculae then develop a cellular core as a result of multiplication of cytotrophoblastic elements on the deep, or

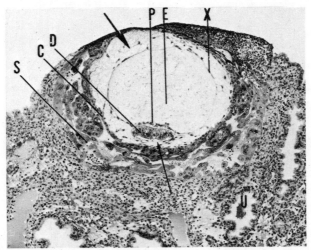

Figure 2.9 Human embryo of about 12 days' gestational age. Heavy arrow indicates extraembryonic mesoblast, and light arrow points to amnion. Primitive endoderm (P), embryonic disc (D), cytotrophoblast (C), syncytiotrophoblast (S), exocelomic cavity (E), and uterine gland (U) are seen. The inner surface of the cytotrophoblast is lined by mesoderm, which is condensed to form the exocelomic (Heuser's) membrane (X). × 70. (Courtesy of Dr A. T. Hertig and the Carnegie Institution of Washington)

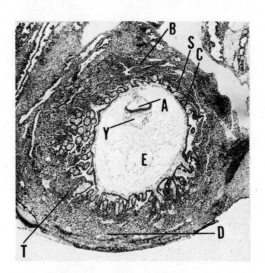

Figure 2.10 Human embryo at early villous stage (16 days' gestational age), showing amnion (A), yolk sac (Y), and large exocelomic cavity (E). Decidua basalis (B) and capsularis (D) are prominent. Secondary villus (S), chorion (C), and cytotrophoblast (T) of peripheral shell are seen. × 21 (Courtesy of Dr A. T. Hertig and the Carnegie Institution of Washington)

chorionic, surface. The highly modified trabeculae may then be designated primary villi. The villous stems later develop mesodermal cores, which convert primary into secondary villi. Vascularisation of the secondary villi transforms them into tertiary, or definitive villi, the principal organs of exchange in the human placenta.

Proliferation of cellular trophoblast at the tips of the villi forms the cytotrophoblastic cell columns, which are not invaded by mesenchyme but are anchored to decidua at the basal plate. The floor of the intervillous space consists of this cytotrophoblast from the cell columns in addition to peripheral syncytium and decidua of the basal plate. The chorionic plate, or roof of the intervillous space, comprises trophoblast externally and mesoderm internally. From the time that the cytotrophoblastic shell is completed, its periphery gives rise to masses of syncytium-like giant cells that extend through the decidua basalis into the myometrium[15].

Between the 18th and 19th days of development the blastocyst measures $6 \times 2 \cdot 5$ mm in diameter. The embryo is then at the primitive streak stage, having attained a maximal length of $0 \cdot 6$–$0 \cdot 7$ mm. The endoderm of this trilaminar embryo is continuous with the lining of the yolk sac. An intermediate layer of intra-embryonic mesoderm may be traced in continuity with the extra-embryonic mesoderm, which later forms part of the walls of the amnion and yolk sac and connects the embryonic structures to the chorionic mesoderm by the body stalk, or abdominal pedicle, the forerunner of the umbilical cord. At this stage the secondary or definitive yolk sac is completely lined by endoderm. External to the yolk sac is the fluid-filled exocelomic cavity, the early formation of which prevents approximation of the yolk sac and trophoblast in man and, hence, precludes formation of a choriovitelline placenta.

The greater part of the chorion, in contact with the decidua capsularis, loses its villi between the 3rd and 4th months of gestation and forms the smooth chorion, or chorion laeve. The villi on the side of the chorion toward the decidua basalis enlarge and become elaborately branched to form the chorion frondosum. By the 3rd month the decidua capsularis, which early in gestation covers the chorion laeve and projects into the uterine cavity, degenerates, along with its associated villi. With disappearance of the decidua capsularis the chorion laeve comes into contact with the parietal decidua of the opposite wall of the uterus. Within the smooth chorion, ghost villi may be found and, clinging to its surface, shreds of decidua.

Since the decidua basalis is only about 6 mm in depth at the time of implantation, once the cytotrophoblast has penetrated the deepest layer of the decidua, the continued growth of the normal placenta beyond the first trimester cannot be accomplished by further trophoblastic invasion. Increased thickness of the placenta is, therefore, the result of growth in length and size of the villi of the chorion frondosum with accompanying expansion of the intervillous space. Until the end of the 4th month, the placenta grows in thickness and circumference; thereafter, there is no appreciable increase in thickness, but growth in circumference continues almost throughout pregnancy.

Lobular architecture, fine structure (histological and electron microscopic), and morphometry of the placenta are described in the following three chapters.

References

1. Wynn, R. M. (1968). Morphology of the placenta. In: *Biology of Gestation*, Vol. I, p. 93 (N. S. Assali, editor) (New York: Academic Press)
2. Wynn, R. M. (1973). Fine structure of the placenta. In: *Handbook of Physiology*, Section 7: Endocrinology, Vol. II: Female Reproductive System, Part 2. p. 261. (R. O. Greep, editor) (Washington D.C.: American Physiological Society)
3. Mossman, H. W. (1937). Comparative morphogenesis of the fetal membranes and accessory uterine structures. *Contrib. Embryol.*, **26**, 129
4. Mossman, H. W. (1967). Comparative biology of the placenta and fetal membranes. In: *Fetal Homeostasis*, Vol. II, p. 13 (R. M. Wynn, editor) (New York: New York Academy of Science)
5. Wimsatt, W. A. (1962). Some aspects of the comparative anatomy of the mammalian placenta. *Amer. J. Obstet. Gynec.*, **84**, 1568
6. Mossman, H. W. (1974). Structural changes in vertebrate fetal membranes associated with the adoption of viviparity. In: *Obstetrics and Gynecology Annual*, Vol. 3, p. 7. (R. M. Wynn, editor) (New York: Appleton–Century–Crofts)
7. Hamilton, W. J. and Boyd, J. D. (1960). Development of the human placenta in the first three months of gestation. *J. Anat.*, **94**, 297
8. Amoroso, E. C. (1952). In: *Marshall's Physiology of Reproduction*, Vol. II, p. 127. (A. S. Parkes, editor) (London: Longmans)
9. Grosser, O. (1927). *Frühentwicklung, Eihautbildung und Placentation des Menschen und der Säugetiere* (Berlin: Springer)
10. Wislocki, G. B. and Streeter, G. L. (1938). On the placentation of the macaque (*Macaca mulatta*), from the time of implantation until the formation of the definitive placenta. *Contrib. Embryol.*, **27**, 1
11. Wynn, R. M., Panigel, M., and MacLennan, A. H. (1971). Fine structure of the placenta and fetal membranes of the baboon. *Amer. J. Obstet. Gynec.*, **109**, 638
12. Hertig, A. T. and Rock, J. (1941). Two human ova of the pre-villous stage, having an ovulation age of about eleven and twelve days respectively. *Contrib. Embryol.*, **29**, 127
13. Hertig, A. T. and Rock, J. (1945). Two human ova of the previllous stage having a developmental age of about seven and nine days respectively. *Contrib. Embryol.*, **31**, 65
14. Wynn, R. M. (1967). Fetomaternal cellular relations in the human basal plate: an ultrastructural study of the placenta. *Amer. J. Obstet. Gynec.*, **97**, 832
15. Boyd, J. D. and Hamilton, W. J. (1970). *The Human Placenta*. (Cambridge: Heffer)

CHAPTER 3

Lobular Architecture of Primate Placentas

Peter Gruenwald

In this chapter the following subjects will be considered: (1) placental size in absolute terms and relative to the uterus, including expansion of the placental site; (2) the structural and functional unit, the lobule, and its relation to maternal vessels opening into the intervillous space; (3) hypotheses regarding blood flow in the intervillous space and its role in the development of the lobule; and (4) the relationship of the lobule to pathological changes. These subjects are controversial, and it is only fair to warn the reader that the following presentation is based in large measure on my own observations and ideas. However, efforts will be made to document my views, and discuss opposing ones and their merits. Placentas of non-human primates will be mentioned because these animals are used in experimental work to an increasing extent, and their similarities and differences with regard to placentation should be appreciated.

In all haemochorial placentas of primates except Tarsiidae (other Prosimiae have epitheliochorial placentas), namely, those of Ceboidea (New World monkeys), Cercopithecoidea (Old World monkeys) and Hominoidea (apes and man) the placental site expands relative to the endometrial surface area[1] from the minute spot occupied at implantation to a size which has been estimated, e.g. to be $\frac{1}{4}$ of the surface of the conceptus in man[2] where, in contrast to other forms, this area does not represent the emdometrial cavity which is compressed and obliterated early on (Chapter 2).

Tarsiidae have the most primitive haemochorial placenta among primates. It consists of one lobule supplied by one maternal artery. The placenta site proper does not expand. The placenta grows beyond its attachment, thus assuming the shape of a button sewn to a garment[1]. The maternal artery continues into the placenta as a fibrin-lined channel similar to those to be described in Ceboidea.

In Simiae proper the establishment and expansion of the placental site depends to a considerable degree on the invasive properties of the tropho-blast, which increase from lower to higher forms. In Ceboidea (the prototype studied most extensively is the squirrel monkey, Saimiri) the trophoblast invading the endometrium spares at first the maternal vessels and their walls (Figure 3.1 (a)). The vessel walls disappear later while a layer of fibrin (? or fibrinoid) replaces them, so that in the mature state maternal blood is dis-tributed to the central portions of the lobules by perforated, fibrin-lined channels (Figure 3.1 (b))[1]. As in all Simiae, venous drainage is principally from the interlobular areas. Expansion of the placental site is at first by in-vasion of additional areas of endometrium by new trophoblastic outgrowth, and then by spread of the placenta to a moderate extent so as to stretch the underlying endometrium in a radial direction[1].

In Cercopithecoidea (the best studied forms are the rhesus monkey, *Macaca mulatta*, and the baboon, *Papio* sp.) implantation is also superficial, but the trophoblast immediately destroys maternal vessel walls, so that these vessels open where they reach the intervillous space. The placental site also increases by stretching, carrying along the nearby endometrium as in Ceboidea, but here some maternal vessels in that endometrium surrounding the original implantation site, are eventually opened up and thus supply the intervillous space[1]. In both Ceboidea and Cercopithecoidea the final number of arteries supplying a placental disc is about 10–15.

Among Hominoidea early stages of placentation are well known only in man. When the placental disc has been defined by degeneration of the villi over the rest of the chorion, this disc enlarges like in the forms just described, probably by a combination of stretching the decidua basalis, and attachment of this portion to the underlying decidua parietalis. In these peripheral areas the zona compacta covers an intact zona spongiosa, whereas no such regular arrangement is seen in the centre, the original implantation site (Figure 3.2 (a)). In later stages the decidua under the peripheral areas is extensively eroded (Figure 3.2 (b)) and large numbers of maternal vessels are tapped over the entire base of the placenta. These are not vessels carried along from the vicinity of the implantation site; they take a very short course from the myometrium across the thin remnants of decidua to the intervillous space. Thus, the human placenta receives maternal blood from several hundred arterioles supplied by both uterine arteries. Phylogenetically, it would seem at first glance that irrigation by maternal blood from perforated channels as it develops in Tarsiidae and Ceboidea, is the ideal system; yet it is too rigid to make possible the expansion needed in the course of evolution; thus, the

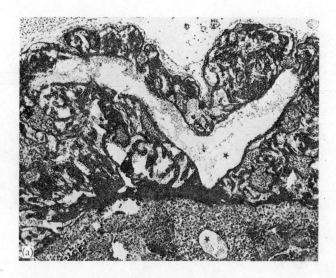

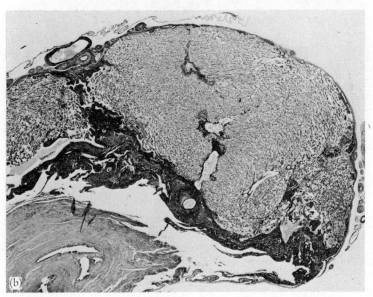

Figure 3.1 Sections of placentas of the squirrel monkey (*Saimiri*). In early stages (a) (from an 8·6 mm embryo) maternal arteries are at first spared (★) by the invading trophoblast. Later on (b) (from a term pregnancy) the maternal vessel wall has disappeared and only a deeply stained layer of fibrin remains. (From Gruenwald[1, 11], by permission of the Wistar Press)

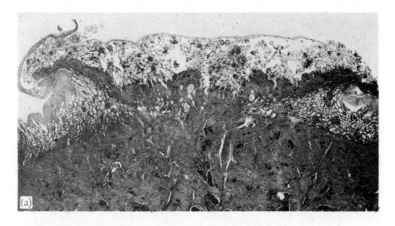

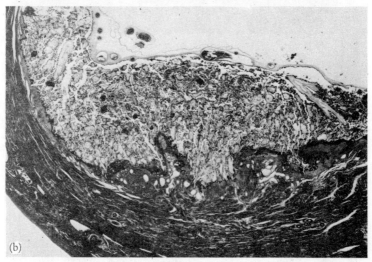

Figure 3.2 Early human placental disc, showing spread beyond the implantation site
(a) (from a 52-day pregnancy) and subsequent permeation and elimination of much of the
decidua, paving the way for tapping large numbers of additional uterine vessels (b) (from
an 87-day pregnancy, after Gruenwald[1], by permission of the Wistar Press). (Photo-
graphs courtesy Department of Embryology, Carnegie Institution of Washington)

irrigation system ceded to the more versatile one which culminated in man
(and probably all Hominoidea) in the availability of several hundred arterial
openings to supply the intervillous space.

Throughout development of mammalian embryos and fetuses the placenta
starts out larger than the embryo, but is outstripped by the fetus. This trend

continues so that during the third trimester the ratio of fetus to placenta in man changes from 5:1 to 7:1. This is not a measure of functional size since during that period the efficiency per unit weight increases as a result of maturation. The average weight relationship of fetus and placenta is seen in Figure 3.3. Growth of the diameter of the placenta during the second half of gestation was measured and illustrated by Boyd and Hamilton[3]. Morphometric data are given in Chapter 5.

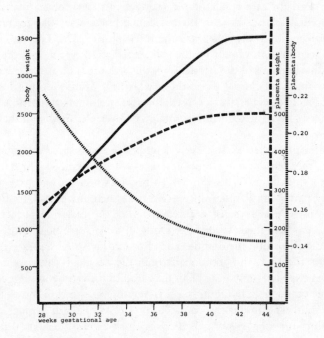

Figure 3.3 Weight of fetus and placenta, and ratio of the two during the third trimester. (From Gruenwald, P. (1963). Chronic fetal distress and placental insufficiency. *Biol. Neonat.*, **5**, 215, by permission of Karger, Basel)

As a result of continued invasion of the decidua at the base of the human placenta (which probably includes a larger area than the original decidua basalis, see Figure 3.2) there is usually only a thin layer left, and the course of the maternal arteries is accordingly short. Several changes normally occur in these arteries; these were ably summarized by Harris and Ramsey[4]. Cytotrophoblast invades the arteries, in man probably predominantly through the wall from the surrounding stroma, and in the rhesus monkey through the lumen. In man in particular, there is a spectacular fibrinoid degeneration of the wall. This may well be connected with the presence of cytotrophoblast as it is elsewhere in the placenta. Acute atherosis with fat-laden cells, fibrosis and fibrinoid necrosis in spiral arteries of the human placental bed have been described by Robertson *et al.*[23], and ultrastructural changes including the presence of trophoblast, fibrin and thrombi by Sheppard and Bonnar[24]. Many of these changes occur in normal pregnancy; the existence or distribution of lesions characteristic of pregnancy with hypertension is controversial[25]. Perhaps as a result of the changes just mentioned, many of the uteroplacental arteries have in their decidual portion sac-like terminations, often with multiple openings into the intervillous space. The degenerative changes seen in man cannot be the sole explanation of the low pressure in the decidual portions of the arteries since the pressure is similarly low in other species with haemochorial placentas in which the arteries do not have such lesions[26, 27]. It is generally accepted that the myometrial portions of the spiral arteries have the regulatory function of arterioles in spite of their much larger size.

In contrast to what has just been described as the normal thinning of the decidua, there occurs in some instances of spontaneous first-trimester abortion a thick layer of decidua which becomes necrotic and may result in confusing pathological appearances. One finds then, in addition to the ovum with the usual thin layer of decidua covering the maternal surface of the placenta, another, thick layer of necrotic decidua forming a more or less complete shell around the ovum[5]. The two may be passed separately (Figure 3.4 (a)) or together, and occasionally only the decidual 'cast' is seen if the ovum was expelled previously. This may lead to the erroneous suggestion of an ectopic pregnancy. In Figure 3.4 (b) a microscopic section shows the two structures almost completely separated by a cleft, but still in their original relationship. It is not known whether the thick layer of decidua is the basic abnormality causing abortion in these cases, or a secondary change in the decidua as abortion proceeds. No similar layer has been identified in normal early pregnancies examined *in situ*[5].

The structural and functional unit of the placenta, vaguely comparable to the liver lobule, is defined easily in some mammalian placentas, and with difficulty in others. In such placentas as that of the sheep, separate portions of placenta are scattered over the chorion, and have been called cotyledons. In primates this term is used, perhaps improperly, to designate portions of placental discs separated from one another on the maternal surface by clefts. Medical dictionaries and text books of embryology differ in the use of this word. In Hominoidea, the term cotyledon is most commonly used to indicate areas separated by clefts on the maternal surface; some human placentas have none of these. When well demarcated, these areas of the human

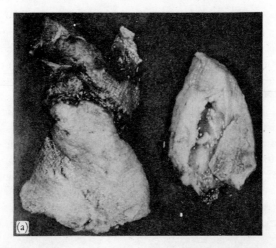

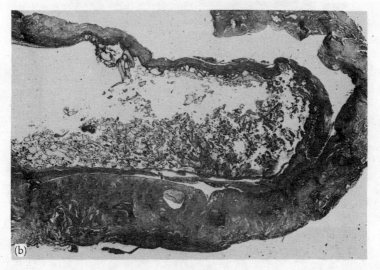

Figure 3.4 (a) an abortion specimen passed in 2 parts, embryo and placenta on the right and decidual cast without villi on the left. (b) section of a similar ovum in which the 2 parts are connected only at a few points. (From: Gruenwald, P. (1965). Decidual sloughing in abortion, premature birth, and abruptio placentae. *Bull. Johns Hopkins Hosp.*, **116**, 363, The Johns Hopkins University Press)

placenta average, according to Boyd and Hamilton[3], 22 in number, ranging from 10 to 38. The same authors have called these large units lobes or compound placentomes. They designated the smaller units within them, all

attached to one villous trunk and occupying one compartment of the intervillous space, as lobules or single placentomes. The term placentome is used
in analogy to the unit in some mammals composed of fetal cotyledon and
maternal caruncle. There is no real caruncle in primates, but a characteristic
relationship of the placental unit to maternal blood vessels exists as will soon
be described. Crawford[6] called these subunits cotyledons. It is obvious that
this term is misleading because of the variety of ways in which it has been
used, and the functional unit will therefore be termed lobule. According to
Crawford[6] the placenta near term has about 200 lobules, the bulk of the
organ consisting of about 10 large and 50 medium-sized units. The 'lobes'
visible on the maternal surface consist of interdigitating lobules. Wilkin[7]
found 20–40 villous stems in each placenta, without change from the time
when the placental disc is established until term. Large stems form up to ·5
tambours (baskets, lobules) whereas smaller branches form single ones.

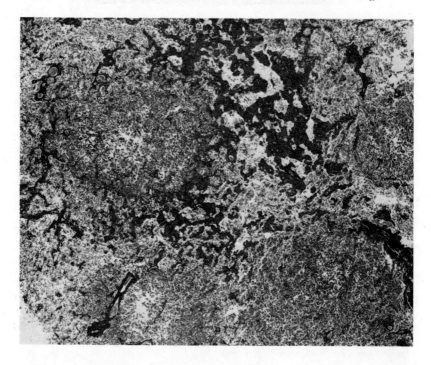

Figure 3.5 Section of part of a human placenta at term, cut parallel to chorion and
decidua. The lobules have a dense peripheral portion and a small, loose centre. The
villous stems at the borders of the lobules are accentuated in this instance by fibrin.
(From: Gruenwald, P. (1966). The lobular architecture of the human placenta. *Bull.
Johns Hopkins Hosp.*, **119**, 172, The Johns Hopkins University Press)

Growth of the base of the placenta along with that of the uterus results in pulling apart of anchoring points of villi of each lobule to form a circle, the *couronne d'implantation*. How the portions of stems about half-way between chorion and decidua move apart about 3 times as far to form the equator of the lobule, is not explained.

The principal structural features of the placental lobule are readily ascertained on microscopic sections. Individual or partially fused lobules are

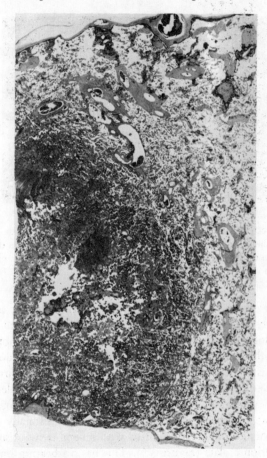

Figure 3.6 Section of a human placenta at term, cut at right angles to the chorion (top) and decidua (bottom). A dense lobule with a loose centre reaches the decidua, but is separated from the chorion and the adjacent lobule (which would be to the right beyond the edge of the field) by loosely arranged villi. (From Gruenwald, P. (1966). The lobular architecture of the human placenta. *Bull. Johns Hopkins Hosp.*, **119**, 172, The Johns Hopkins University Press)

apparent on sections taken parallel to the chorion (Figure 3.5). Each lobule consists of a dense mass of small villous branches, but mostly terminal villi which are the seat of transfer function. Many lobules have a loose, central portion of unknown origin and significance. At the periphery of the lobule bordering on the loosely textured interlobular area, are the larger villous stems forming, according to sources just mentioned, a basket and anchoring in the decidua. The loose, interlobular areas continue in man into a similarly loose

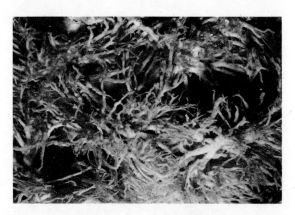

Figure 3.7 Dissected villous stems of a portion of a human placenta at term. Half the thickness near the decidua has been removed, and the small villi were dissected away. This is a view in the direction of the placental side of the chorion. The villous stems do not derive from one major stem for each lobule

subchorial area which extends between the entire chorionic plate and the lobules (Figure 3.6). Points of argument include the origin of the stems along the sides of a lobule from one larger stem attached to the chorion and, on the opposite side, the relationship of the anchoring villi to the decidua. Dissection of villous stems of formalin-fixed placentas from the base toward the chorion (Figure 3.7), and graphic reconstruction (Figure 3.8), have failed to confirm the regular connection of all the stems forming the basket around the lobule, with *one* stem of higher order[8]. While this does occasionally occur, larger villi along a lobule connect more often with several stems arising separately from the chorionic plate (Figure 3.7). This has no bearing on concepts of fetal circulation or placental function, but makes it much easier to understand the ontogenesis of the lobule as will be discussed shortly. At the basal end, where the stems attach to the decidua and perhaps turn back in the direction of the chorion, it has been said that a layer of trophoblast always separates fetal from maternal tissue, and this may bear on the immunological

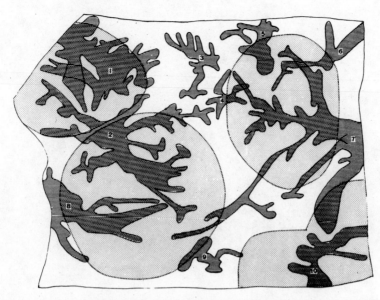

Figure 3.8 Reconstruction of lobules and major villous stems of a human placenta at term, produced by superimposing sections parallel to the chorion at regular interval from it as projected on tracing paper. Most major stems furnish branches to several lobules, and each lobule is supplied by branches of several stems. The specimen measured, after shrinkage in preparation, 35×45 mm

relationship of mother and conceptus. In the early placenta the ubiquitous trophoblast can readily be seen (Figure 3.9 (a)). Later on, however, it is the rule that villi embedded in the decidua are not covered by trophoblast (Figure 3.9 (b)), even when they appear quite viable and contain patent fetal vessels. Whether they are separated from maternal tissue by fibrinoid serving an immunological barrier function (Chapters 4, 8), is not known.

Perhaps the strongest controversy with regard to placental lobules concerns their topographic relation to the openings of maternal arteries into the intervillous space. Several workers injected the uterine arteries with the placenta *in situ*, and after hardening of the material removed the soft tissues by corrosion. They found that each lobule is supplied by one maternal artery opening below its centre and surmised, or showed to their satisfaction, that maternal blood spurts into the loose or empty central portion of the lobule and then filters toward the periphery[7, 9, 10] where it drains through the interlobular areas into maternal veins. Reynolds[11, 12] has accepted this one-to-one relationship of placental lobules of fetal origin to openings of maternal arteries in his theoretical treatises.

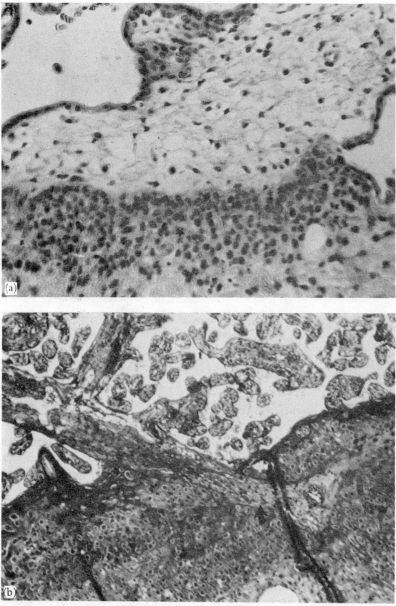

Figure 3.9 Villi of human placentas anchoring in the decidua. (a) from a pregnancy of the second month, shows an uninterrupted layer of cytotrophoblast (*) separating the villus from the decidua. (b) from a term placenta, shows the stroma of an anchoring villus (arrow) within the decidua, not completely covered by trophoblast. Whether separation is effected by fibrinoid, is undetermined

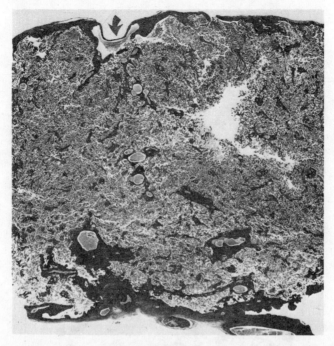

Figure 3.10 A section from a human placenta at term shows the left half occupied by a lobule with a loose centre, and a maternal artery (arrow) opening at the base of the inter-lobular area. (From Gueunwald, P. (1966). The lobular architecture of the human placenta. *Bull. Johns Hopkins Hosp.*, **119**, 172, The Johns Hopkins University Press)

On the other hand, those who examined serial sections, with or without previous injection by india ink[4, 13, 14], found arterial openings at the base of interlobular areas, often associated with slight elevations of the decidua bearing the anchoring points of large villi (Figure 3.10). The reconstruction in Figure 3.11 made from serial sections[14] shows this relationship, and Figure 3.12 gives a diagrammatic view of my concept of the relationship of lobules to villous stems on the one hand, and maternal arteries on the other. Figure 3.13, a reconstruction of a piece of a gorilla placenta, shows similar topographic relations of lobules and arteries, as is also true of other Hominoidea[15]. One special feature of Hominoidea particularly well developed in man, is the subchorial area which, like the interlobular areas, has a loose texture because of a scarcity of terminal villi between stems. There are often conspicuous deposits of fibrin, not only in the form of the well known layer underlying the chorionic plate, but also extending away from that plate. This fibrin connects with villous stems, particularly when such stems run

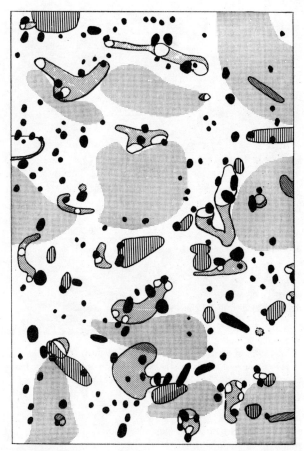

Figure 3.11 Reconstruction of part of a human term placenta. The dotted areas indicate the contact of the lobules with the decidua (not the largest diameter of the lobules); the black dots are anchoring points of large villous stems; the finely lined areas are arterial convolutes in the decidua, with openings into the intervillous space shown clear; the coarsely lined areas are openings of maternal veins. All structures are projected on a plane parallel to the decidua, from measurements on serial sections at right angles. (From Gruenwald, P. (1966). The lobular architecture of the human placenta. *Bull. Johns Hopkins Hosp.*, **119**, 172, The Johns Hopkins University Press)

nearly parallel to the chorion (Figure 3.14)[14]. How these attachments of stems to the chorion develop, and whether they serve a significant mechanical function in fixing the position of villous stems running along the chorion often for considerable distances, is not known.

Before discussing the hypotheses of maternal blood flow in the placenta,

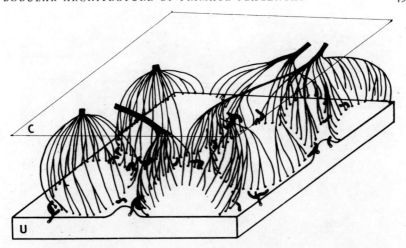

Figure 3.12 Schematic diagram of the relationship of lobules, villous stems and maternal arteries (heavy black lines near the base) in the human placenta. C, chorionic plate, U, uterine wall. On the left is a lobule with all of its villous stems derived from one major stem as postulated by most previous investigators; the rest of the lobules are shown according to information in Figures 3.7, 3.8, and 3.11

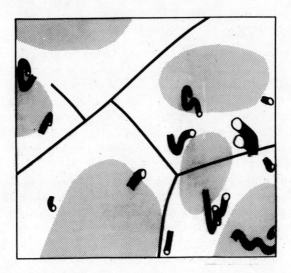

Figure 3.13 Reconstruction of a portion of a gorilla placenta at term, prepared like Figure 3.11. Only lobules and arteries are indicated. The heavy lines are intercotyledonary fissures transferred from a photograph of the block prior to embedding. One lobule seems to overly a fissure; this is due to the oblique course of the fissure. (After Gruenwald[15], by permission of Wistar Press)

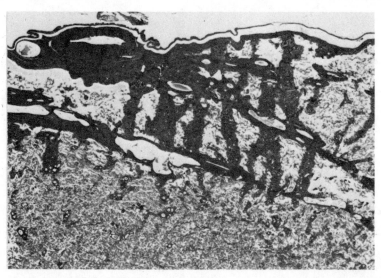

Figure 3.14 Section from a human term placenta. Villous stems running nearly parallel with the chorion are attached to it and each other by columns of fibrin. (From Gruen-wald, P. (1966). The lobular architecture of the human placenta. *Bull. Johns Hopkins Hosp.*, **119**, 172, The Johns Hopkins University Press)

we must take notice of certain features in Old World monkeys, particularly since these have repeatedly been used in studies of placental blood flow. Contrary to the 'irrigation' system of New World monkeys briefly described above, the maternal arteries of Old World monkeys such as the rhesus monkey or the baboon, open at the base of the intervillous space, but with one strange difference from the condition in man. While in both forms arterial convolutes are found in the decidua below interlobular areas, and the openings in man are right there, the arteries of Old World monkeys take a straight course to a point below the centre of the lobule and open there[15]. This would appear to agree with the opinion that arterial blood enters the centre of the lobule in a more or less solid stream[16, 17]. Actually there is, with rare exceptions, no wide open path from the mouth of the artery to the loose centre of the lobule. In the baboon, an area immediately adjacent to the arterial opening may be open, as if swept free of villi[15] (Figure 3.15) but this is always separated from the loose centre by several millimetres of densely arranged villi.

In Old World monkeys there are grooves on the fetal surface corresponding to those on the maternal side of the separated placenta, and the cotyledons thus outlined usually contain only one lobule. Venous drainage of the inter-

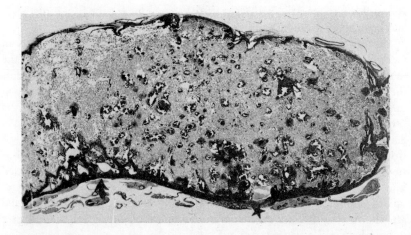

Figure 3.15 Section from a baboon placenta at term. The margin is at the right, and an interlobular area with channels draining into a maternal vein (arrow) on the left. Above the asterisk (*) is a free area of the intervillous space at the opening of a maternal artery (not seen on this section). Villus-free areas like this one were never seen to be continuous with a loose lobular centre

villous space is interlobular in all primates. In some Old World monkeys, portions of the interlobular areas are transformed into wide, fibrin-lined channels leading to the openings of maternal veins.

It has been intimated here that knowledge of circulation in the intervillous space is incomplete. In man[18] and in the rhesus monkey[19] spurts extending from the base in the direction of the chorionic plate have been demonstrated by radiography. India ink issuing from maternal arteries of resected human uteri has generally followed anchoring villi before spreading out. Just how maternal blood reaches the capillary-like spaces between terminal villi in the dense portion of the lobule, and how it leaves these areas, is not known. The idea that blood moves centrifugally from the centre of the lobule in all primates as it does in Ceboidea, is not firmly supported by the fact that in Cercopithecoidea the arterial openings lie beneath the centre of the lobules, as was just discussed. One confusing detail is that the loose centre occurs equally in these forms and in man, even though the arteries open differently. These difficulties were discussed in more detail elsewhere[15], and it was suggested that the one concept of circulation in the intervillous space which is most nearly compatible with my morphological observations, is that of Lemtis[20]. This concept has the drawback that it is based on injection of radio-opaque material into the intervillous space of delivered human placentas, but the results are, according to the author, highly reproducible.

Blood flows around the periphery of the lobule in streams forming a shell, and from there apparently infiltrates the lobule.

The ontogenesis of the placental lobule poses no difficult problems in Ceboidea where the preexisting maternal arteries apparently shape the lobules. In Cercopithecoidea the arteries come to mark the centre, and veins the periphery of the lobules. Since villous stems are distributed randomly in these placentas and no single stem must match with its ramifications the surroundings of an arterial opening, the problem is presumably again a haemodynamic one. In Hominoidea there seemed to be the problem of matching in the course of development one arterial ostium with one villous stem giving rise to the corresponding lobule. Reynolds[11,12] addressed himself to this puzzle in a speculative manner. If it is true, however, that no one-to-one relationship exists between principal villous stems and maternal arteries, and that the only significant topographic relation is that of anchoring villi with arterial ostia (Figure 3.12), then it becomes much easier to visualise how the lobules develop. The only required association of maternal and fetal components is that of arterial ostia and anchoring points of villi. It may then be supposed that when the base of the placenta enlarges as the pregnant uterus and the conceptus grow proportionately (after the above mentioned expansion of the placental site is completed), anchoring villi have developed or remain only where the arteries open. The combination of arterial ostia and anchoring villi forming the periphery of the lobule is thus the pivot of placental architecture, much as the periportal field is that of the liver. It is likely that haemodynamic forces in the intervillous space shape the intervening areas into lobules.

This is not the place to discuss in detail the relation of pathological changes to the lobules or the intervening areas. Fibrin deposition along villous stems

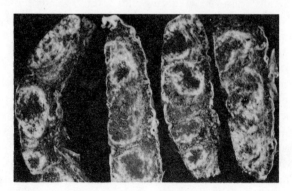

Figure 3.16 Slices of a human placenta with pale infarcts in a lobular distribution

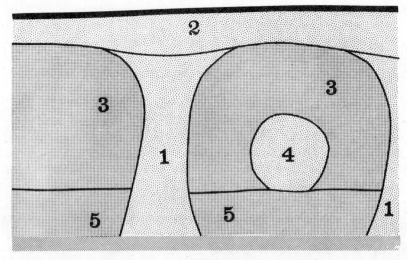

Figure 3.17 Areas in the human placenta which may differ in the appearance of terminal villi: (1) interlobular; (2) subchorial; (3–5) portions of the lobule: the dense basal part (5) may differ from the rest of the dense portion (3) under pathological circumstances; (4) loose centre of the lobule. (Slightly modified from Gruenwald, P. (1966). The lobular architecture of the human placenta. *Bull. Johns Hopkins Hosp.*, **119**, 172, The Johns Hopkins University Press)

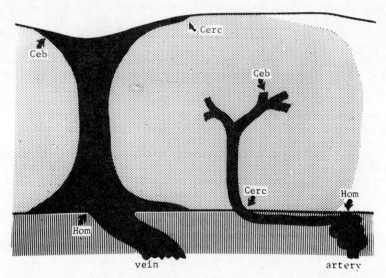

Figure 3.18 Diagram showing the differences in circulation of maternal blood between Ceboidea, Cercopithecoidea, and Hominoidea. Well defined channels in the intervillous space end at the points indicated by abbreviated names

is common in the interlobular (Figure 3.5) and subchorial areas (Figure 3.14). The shape and distribution of placental infarcts which most authors (see Chapter 12 and particularly also Carter et al.[21]) relate to disturbances of maternal blood flow, may or may not have an obvious relationship to lobules. An obvious example of infarcts involving lobules, is seen in Figure 3.16.

There is marked variation in the microscopic appearance of terminal villi in relation to their place with regard to the lobule[14]. Some of these variations indicate or simulate differences in maturation (Chapter 14). Placental pathology will not be complete until cognisance is taken of the location of changes with respect to the lobule[14] (Figure 3.17). This has been suggested, but not carried out to a significant extent.

Since certain differences between the placentas of man and monkeys used in experiments have been recognised (Figure 3.18), it is incumbent upon anyone wishing to extrapolate results from monkey to man, to determine as reliably as possible whether the feature under consideration is in fact comparable[22].

References

1. Gruenwald, P. (1972). Expansion of placental site and maternal blood supply of primate placentas. *Anat. Rec.*, **173**, 189
2. Torpin, R. (1969). *The Human Placenta: Its Shape, Form, Origin, and Development.* (Springfield: Thomas)
3. Boyd, J. D. and Hamilton, W. J. (1967). Development and structure of the human placenta from the end of the 3rd month of gestation. *J. Obst. Gynaec. Brit. Cwlth.*, **74**, 161
4. Harris, J. W. S. and Ramsey, E. M. (1966). The morphology of the human utero-placental vasculature. *Contrib. Embryol.*, **38**, 43
5. Gruenwald, P. (1965). Decidual sloughing in abortion, premature birth, and abruptio placentae. *Bull. Johns Hopkins Hosp.*, **116**, 363
6. Crawford, J. M. (1962). Vascular anatomy of the human placenta. *Am. J. Obst. Gynec.*, **84**, 1543
7. Wilkin, P. (1965). *Pathologie du placenta: étude clinique et anatomique.* (Paris: Masson)
8. Papalia-Early, A. and Gruenwald, P. (in preparation). The villous stems of the human placental lobule.
9. Arts, N. F. T. (1961). Investigations on the vascular system of the placenta. Part I: General introduction and the fetal vascular system. *Amer. J. Obst. Gynec.*, **82**, 147
10. Smart, P. J. G. (1962). Some observations on the vascular morphology of the foetal side of the human placenta. *J. Obst. Gynaec. Brit. Cwlth.*, **69**, 929
11. Reynolds, S. R. M. (1967). Derivation of the vascular elements in the fetal cotyledon of the hemochorial placenta: a contribution to the theory of placental morphogenesis. *Anat. Rec.*, **157**, 43
12. Reynolds, S. R. M. (1972). On growth and form in the hemochorial placenta: an

essay on the physical forces that shape the chorionic trophoblast. *Amer. J. Obst. Gynec.*, **114**, 115

13. Brosens, I. and Dixon, H. G. (1966). The anatomy of the maternal side of the placenta. *J. Obst. Gynaec. Brit. Cwlth.*, **73**, 357

14. Gruenwald, P. (1966). The lobular architecture of the human placenta. *Bull. Johns Hopkins Hosp.*, **119**, 172

15. Gruenwald, P. (1973). Lobular structure of hemochorial primate placentas, and its relation to maternal vessels. *Amer. J. Anat.*, **136**, 133

16. Freese, U. E. (1966). The fetal-maternal circulation of the placenta. I: Histomorphologic, plastoid injection, and x-ray cinematographic studies on human placentas. *Amer. J. Obst. Gynec.*, **94**, 354

17. Wigglesworth, J. S. (1969). Vascular anatomy of the human placenta and its significance for placental pathology. *J. Obst. Gynaec. Brit. Cwlth.*, **76**, 979

18. Borell, U., Fernström, I. and Westman, A. (1958). Eine arteriographische Studie des Plazentarkreislaufs. *Geburtsh. and Frauenheilk.*, **18**, 1

19. Ramsey, E. M. (1962). Circulation in the intervillous space of the primate placenta. *Amer. J. Obst. Gynec.*, **84**, 1649

20. Lemtis, H. (1970). Physiologie der Plazenta. *Fortschr. Geburtsh. Gynäk.*, **41**, 1

21. Carter, J. E., Vellios, F. and Huber, C. P. (1963). Circulatory factors governing the viability of the human placenta, based on a morphologic study. *Amer. J. Clin. Path.*, **40**, 363

22. Ramsey, E. M. (1972). Evaluation of *Macaca mulatta* as an experimental model for studies of primate reproduction. *Medical Primatology. 1972. Proceedings 3rd Conf. exp. Med. Surg. Primates, Lyon 1972, part I*, 308

23. Robertson, W. B., Brosens, I. and Dixon, H. G. (1967). The pathological response of the vessels of the placental bed to hypertensive pregnancy. *J. Path. Bact.*, **93**, 581

24. Sheppard, B. L. and Bonnar, J. (1974). The ultrastructure of the arterial supply of the human placenta in early and late pregnancy. *J. Obst. Gynaec. Brit. Cwlth.*, **81**, 497

25. Brosens, I., Robertson, W. B. and Dixon, H. G. (1972). The role of the spiral arteries in the pathogenesis of preeclampsia. *Obst. Gynaec. Annual*, 177

26. Moll, W. and Künzel, W. (1973). The blood pressure in arteries entering the placentae of guinea pigs, rats, rabbits, and sheep. *Pflügers Arch.*, **338**, 125

27. Moll, W., Künzel, W., Stolte, L. A. M., Kleinhout, J., DeJong, P. A. and Veth, A. F. L. (1974). The blood pressure in the decidual part of the uteroplacental arteries (spiral arteries) of the rhesus monkey. *Pflügers Arch.*, **346**, 291

CHAPTER 4

Fine Structure of the Placenta

Ralph M. Wynn

Comparative Electron Microscopy

Within the last few years reviews of placental ultrastructure[1, 2] as well as an atlas of comparative electron microscopy[3] have appeared. A major result of the ultrastructural studies of a variety of placental forms has been the provision of data indicative of functional adaptations of each of the layers of the placental membrane, especially the trophoblast. Density of the tropho-blastic nuclei, as noted with light microscopy, is explained by the high content of deoxyribonucleoprotein particles. Cytoplasmic basophilia of the physiologically active forms of trophoblast is correlated with the abundant granular endoplasmic reticulum. Deposits of glycoprotein and lipid granules are related, respectively, to the histochemically detected periodic acid-Schiff (PAS)-positive and sudanophilic materials.

Secretory cells are characterised by a well-developed system of organelles and, in many cases, by discrete granules or droplets. Since secretion is an energy-demanding process, a common feature of secretory cells is abundance of mitochondria. Active trophoblastic cells are rich in mitochondria, which generally are rod-shaped or ovoid with transverse parallel cristae. Tubular cristae, however, are occasionally encountered in connection with placental steroidogenesis.

Rough-surfaced endoplasmic reticulum is associated with protein syn-thesis. According to Björkman[4], it is extensively developed not only in trophoblast, but also in uterine epithelial cells in swine, in the cryptal syncytium of sheep, and in maternal endothelium of many endotheliochorial placentas.

Decidual cells, although often containing sparse organelles, may in certain species and certain areas develop an extensive endoplasmic reticulum[5]. Such examples are the so-called decidual giant cells of the carnivores, the basal decidua of the rabbit, and the decidual cells in the basal plates of guinea pig and man[6], where they may approach in ultrastructural complexity the trophoblastic giant cells. Prominent smooth-surfaced endoplasmic reticulum is characteristic of cells that produce substances other than proteins, such as steroids.

In general the active secretory forms of trophoblast contain well-developed, rough-surfaced endoplasmic reticulum, whereas elements such as Langhans cells, which serve basically as reserve, or stem, trophoblastic cells, contain relatively sparse endoplasmic reticulum but numerous polyribosomes. The Golgi apparatus, which is believed to be the site of formation of secretory granules, is best developed in tissues that are most active in the formation of secretory products. Such tissues include human syncytiotrophoblast, trophoblastic giant cells in rodents and ruminants, and maternal endothelium in the typical endotheliochorial labyrinth. All these tissues have well-developed Golgi membranes and vesicles.

The so-called trophoblastic brush border appears under the electron microscope as a border of inconstant microvilli. Convolutions of plasma membranes and formation of pinocytotic vesicles and vacuoles are related to the transport of water and ions. Some of the largest vacuoles, however, which can be detected with the light microscope, represent dilated cisternae of endoplasmic reticulum. In well-preserved tissues all components of the placental membrane can be shown to contribute to a virtually continuous system of channels from the free trophoblastic surface through the syncytio-plasm, basal laminae, and fetal capillary; thus a direct route for rapid transport of products of absorption and secretion is provided.

A notable feature of some placental epithelia is the system of complexly folded basal plasma membranes. This specialisation is most prominent in epithelia noted for transport of water, such as the proximal and distal convoluted tubules of the kidney and choroid plexus.

Micropinocytosis is considered an important activity of capillary endo-thelium, as well as of trophoblast. The term pinocytosis refers to the incorporation of fluid by the cell for its own use, whereas the term cytopempsis applies more accurately to the transport of vesicles and their contents across the cell. Cytopempsis may be difficult to distinguish from pinocytosis, although the occurrence of multivesicular bodies, which may possibly result from the collection of micropinocytotic vesicles, may be an indication of absorption[4].

Enders[7] has suggested an anatomical classification of haemochorial placentas based on the number of layers of trophoblast as described by electron microscopy. In the labyrinthine placentas of guinea pig and chipmunk a single complete layer of syncytial trophoblast (the haemomonochorial condition) is found. In other rodents, such as *Zapus hudsonicus* (the jumping mouse), the haemomonochorial membrane comprises exclusively giant cells rather than a true syncytium. In the villous haemomonochorial category are the placentas of man and macaque, as well as the taxonomically unrelated armadillo. In the haemomonochorial membrane in which only the syncytial layer is continuous, as in the guinea pig's labyrinth or in the mature human villus, individual cytotrophoblastic elements are occasionally

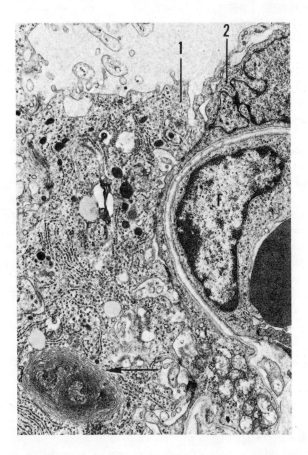

Figure 4.1 Haemodichorial placenta of the rabbit at term. Note two-layered trophoblast (1, 2), fetal capillary (F), and membranous whorl (arrow) characteristic of this species. × 8050

found and presumably represent cells that give rise to the syncytium, as described later in this chapter. In the armadillo the syncytium arises from caps of cytotrophoblast at the tips of the growing villi, for a layer of Langhans cells is absent. In the syncytiotrophoblast of the armadillo, the complexity of the microvilli and the apparent polarity of the organelles are more pronounced than in other haemochorial forms thus far studied ultrastructurally.

The true rabbit (*Oryctolagus cuniculus*) (Figure 4.1) and the cottontail rabbit (*Sylvilagus floridanus*) have haemodichorial membranes in which the outer layer is syncytial and the inner layer basically cellular. The membrane may become so thin focally that two layers cannot be resolved with the

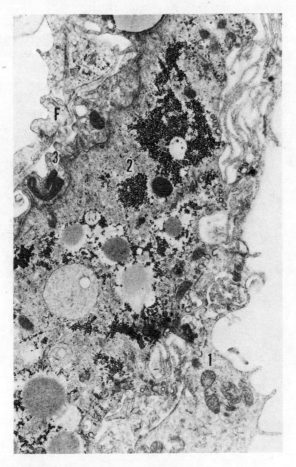

Figure 4.2 Haemotrichorial placenta of the hamster at term. Three-layered trophoblast (1, 2, 3) and fetal capillary endothelium (F) are shown. × 9520

light microscope. At times, even the entire trophoblastic covering appears absent, although normally it is always detectable with the electron microscope.

In several species the 3-layered trophoblast forms a haemotrichorial membrane, as in the laboratory rat and mouse, the hamster (Figure 4.2), the deer mouse (*Peromyscus maniculatus*), and the meadow mouse or common vole (*Microtus pennsylvanicus*)[8]. In these placentas the outer layer of trophoblast is cellular, whereas the inner 2 layers form either a true syncytium or a series of imbricated pseudosyncytial masses. The layer of trophoblast nearest the maternal blood is rich in granular endoplasmic reticulum, whereas the inner 2 layers are usually less well differentiated.

In typical endotheliochorial forms[9], the base (fetal side) of the syncytium forms podocytic processes that resemble those of the visceral epithelium of Bowman's capsule. The free surface (maternal side) is thrown up into blunt

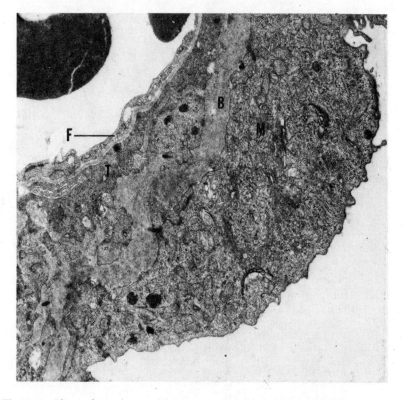

Figure 4.3 Placental membrane of dog at term, showing hypertrophied maternal endothelium (M) and basal lamina (B), trophoblast (T), and fetal endothelium (F)

microvilli, which are generally less well developed than those in the haemo-chorial forms (Figure 4.3). In the cat, for example, maternal endometrial stromal cells persist to form an essentially syndesmochorial condition.

The postulated haemoendothelial and endothelio-endothelial conditions have recently been shown by electron microscopy to be haemochorial[10] and endotheliochorial[11], respectively. In all placentas thus far subjected to electron microscopy, at least one layer of trophoblast has been shown to persist throughout gestation. The immunological significance of this persistent trophoblast is discussed later in this chapter.

Ultrastructural examination of the less intimate placental membranes has consistently revealed the epitheliochorial, rather than the syndesmochorial, condition. Electron-microscopic studies of the horse, pig, and rhinoceros and histological examination of the camel, dromedary, and llama leave little doubt that the placenta in these animals is epitheliochorial[10]. The classification of placentas of other ruminants, however, remained somewhat controversial until the demonstration of microvillous interdigitations between trophoblast and cryptal epithelium in the placentome. Björkman[3] has shown that the placentas of cow and even sheep, formerly considered prototypical syndes-mochorial organs, were actually epitheliochorial (Figure 4.4).

The equine placenta represents the typical epitheliochorial condition with its 6-layered thick membrane. Both trophoblast and endometrial epithelium are complete, and the capillaries only occasionally abut the basal surfaces of the epithelia. Other epitheliochorial placentas have thinner membranes. The porcine placenta, often considered one of the most primitive in Grosser's classification, becomes a considerably reduced barrier toward midgestation as a result of intra-epithelial capillaries on both sides. Thus fetal and maternal blood streams are separated only by endothelia and thin layers of cytoplasm of trophoblast and endometrial epithelium. According to Björkman[4], intra-epithelial capillaries also occur in ruminants, although to a lesser extent. The 'barrier', furthermore, is influenced not only by the number of layers and their permeabilities, but also by the spatial relations of the cells within each layer. The fetal tissue immediately adjacent to maternal tissue or blood forms a continuous layer, except for the external layer of trophoblast in the haemotrichorial placenta. If this tissue is cellular, the apical portions of the cells are joined by tight junctions. Extracellular spaces between the basal lamina and the trophoblast occur in many endotheliochorial and haemo-chorial placentas. Similar spaces may be found on the maternal side, as in the porcine placenta, but they are always sealed distally by tight intercellular junctions. Although such spaces may reduce the barrier to some extent, substances passing along this route must traverse the plasma membranes and cytoplasm because of the tight junctions.

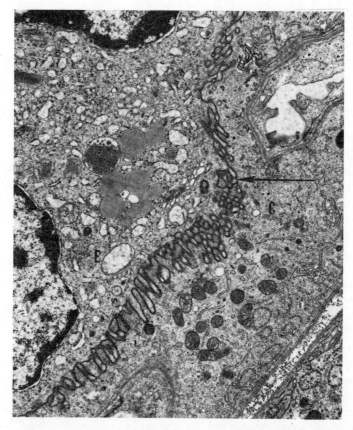

Figure 4.4 Placenta of sheep at term, showing chorionic (C) and endometrial (E) epithelia with tightly apposed plasma membranes (arrow) and absence of fibrinoid and necrosis

The Human Placenta

Histology

The human placental membrane comprises 3 layers: trophoblast, connective tissue, and capillary endothelium. The syncytial trophoblast, which is in contact with maternal blood, is relatively thick in early placental development but becomes progressively thinner throughout gestation. Toward the end of the first trimester, the Langhans cells, or villous cytotrophoblast, begin to decrease in prominence, although they persist in reduced numbers throughout gestation. The cytotrophoblast, as described later in this chapter, remains the source of all syncytium throughout gestation. In pathological states in which there is greater formation of new syncytium, perhaps as a homeostatic response to a stress, such as hypoxia, the Langhans cells assume greater prominence.

The total thickness of the placental membrane may decrease from 0·025–0·002 mm. During maturation the villus may be converted from a thick structure with an almost uninterrupted layer of cytotrophoblast (Figure 4.5)

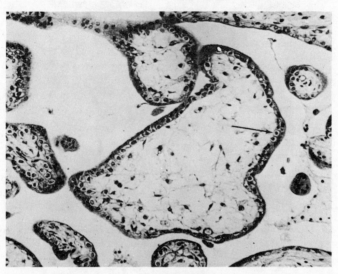

Figure 4.5 Human placenta from first trimester of pregnancy. The 2-layered trophoblast consists of outer syncytium and inner cytotrophoblast, or Langhans cells (arrow). × 70

to an extremely thin membrane that separates fetal and maternal blood streams at term (Figure 4.6). In normal placental development, however, at least syncytiotrophoblast and fetal capillary endothelium are consistently present.

As the placenta ages, its terminal villi form increasingly numerous subdivisions. The more obvious histological changes that are consistent with increased efficiency of transfer include an increase in the ratio of villous surface to volume, a decrease in thickness of the syncytium, discontinuity of the Langhans layer, and reduction in the proportion of villous connective tissue relative to the trophoblast. In the villi of the early placenta, fibrocytes with branching processes are separated by abundant, loose intercellular matrix. The core of the mature villus comprises a denser stroma with

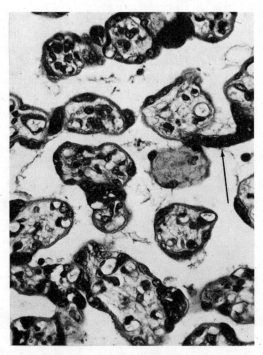

Figure 4.6 Term human placenta showing syncytial knot (arrow), and fibrinous deposits on several villi. Fetal capillaries approach the epithelium quite closely. × 140

closely packed spindly cells. The villous capillaries, moreover, increase in number and progressively approach the surface. During placental maturation the so-called Hofbauer cells are also markedly reduced in number. The origin and significance of these rounded cells with vesicular, often eccentric, nuclei and granular or vacuolated cytoplasm have been studied by Wynn[12] and more recently by Enders and King[13].

Whereas the apparent conversion of the terminal villi to delicate sacs virtually filled with thin-walled vessels may lead to increased efficiency of transfer, not all changes characteristic of placental ageing may be so directed. Thickening of the basement membranes of endothelium and trophoblast, obliteration of fetal and maternal vessels, and deposition of fibrinoid in the chorionic and basal plates, septa, and intervillous space appear incompatible with more efficient placental function. Such changes, furthermore, may be initiated as early as the first trimester. Details of the histology and histo-chemistry of the human placenta are provided in the classic papers from Wislocki's laboratory[14, 15].

Metabolic adaptations

The syncytiotrophoblast, the single most active and variable component of the human placenta, has been shown by electron microscopy to be a true syncytium, which may be constantly reorientated about the terminal villi. Formation of syncytial clumps at one pole of the villus may be associated with extreme attenuation of the trophoblast to form epithelial plaques, or maximal reduction in thickness of the placental membrane, at the other pole.

The ribonucleoprotein particles associated with the extensive ergastoplasm of the syncytium and the numerous free ribosomes create the basophilia noted in light microscopy; distension of channels of endoplasmic reticulum creates the vesicular syncytioplasm observed by conventional histological methods. The free surface of the syncytium is characterised by a microvillous border associated with pinocytotic vesicles and vacuoles. The plasma membranes abutting the basal lamina are often complexly convoluted, occasionally forming podocytic processes comparable with those of the renal glomeruli and tubules. Typical Langhans cells, however, are ultrastructurally simple, with large nuclei, prominent nucleoli, large mitochondria, and a few Golgi bodies. The cytoplasm is studded with numerous free ribosomes but is relatively devoid of well-developed endoplasmic reticulum (Figure 4.7). These ultrastructural features are common to embryonic and neoplastic cells, the primary function of which is growth and differentiation rather than elaboration of specialised endocrine or exocrine products.

The normal chorionic villus is completely covered by syncytial trophoblast, which rests in part on a basal lamina and in part on the incomplete layer of Langhans cells. Although the Langhans layer, which is more or less continuous in the early villus, usually becomes attenuated or interrupted during placental maturation, Langhans cells may be identified in the human placenta throughout gestation. Secretory granules, often bounded by membranes, are commonly found in the syncytium but only rarely in typical Langhans cells. The large mitochondria that are located between the folds of membranes are presumably related to the supply of energy for transfer against a gradient. Vacuoles and vesicles that extend throughout the trophoblast may communicate with channels of endoplasmic reticulum to form a virtually continuous conduit from maternal surface of the trophoblast through fetal capillary endothelium. Pinocytosis, furthermore, may originate in the capillary in the direction of fetus or placenta to intervillous space, in accordance with the known secretory functions of the feto-placental unit. According to Fawcett[16], after pinocytosis a compensatory synthesis of plasma membranes may occur.

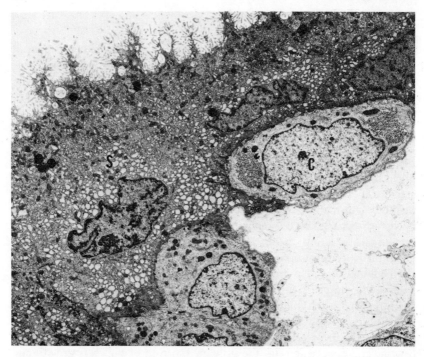

Figure 4.7 Human villus at 6 weeks. Dense syncytium (S) and ultrastructurally simple cytotrophoblast (C) are shown. × 8050 .

In classic pinocytosis, outfoldings of the plasma membrane enclose relatively large globules of fluid. In micropinocytosis of the type associated with microvilli, invaginations of the plasma membrane effect transfer of fluid-filled microvesicles across the capillary wall at a rate adequate at least for metabolism of the cell itself. Such stable differentiations as striated borders are related principally to selective absorption, whereas unstable microvilli may be associated with both absorption and secretion. Minor ultrastructural differences in the trilaminar unit membrane may explain significant differences in placental absorption, secretion, and transfer against a gradient in both directions.

During synthesis, the endoplasmic reticulum may be distended with products of varying electron density (Figure 4.8). Precursors that are synthesised in the endoplasmic reticulum are subsequently assembled into secretory granules in the Golgi complexes. Mitochondria and Golgi complexes, though numerous, may be difficult to detect in the electron-dense syncytioplasm. The smooth-surfaced endoplasmic reticulum, which functions in

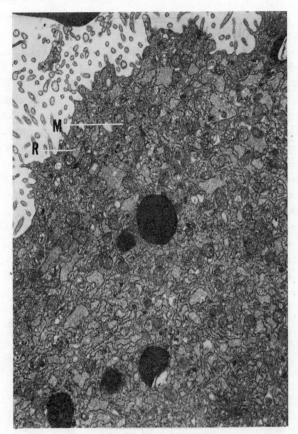

Figure 4.8 Human syncytial trophoblast at 12 weeks packed with numerous mitochondria (M) and dilated channels of endoplasmic reticulum (R). × 8050

segregation and transport of cellular products other than proteins, also is
well developed in the active syncytium. Lysosomes, which contain such
hydrolytic enzymes as acid phosphatase, are numerous in the syncytium but
not in the cytotrophoblast. Many granules in the syncytiotrophoblast are
limited by single membranes and appear proteinaceous, whereas certain
intensely osmiophilic droplets unlimited by membranes are very likely
lipids, including steroids. In some series of vacuoles there is a progressive
decrease in density of contents as the distance from the free syncytial surface
increases, a picture compatible with the gradual incorporation of metabolites
obtained through absorption from the intervillous space. Other granules
appear to maintain their membranes until they are incorporated into a

promontory of syncytium from which they are discharged into the inter-villous space, as in apocrine or merocrine secretion.

Transfer may be facilitated by the plasmodial activity of the syncytium, which minimises the thickness of the membrane in certain areas. Although classic pinocytosis may achieve the incorporation of sizable droplets of fluid by the plasma membranes and their transfer across trophoblast and endo-thelium, micropinocytosis, accompanied by submicroscopic vesiculation of the plasma membrane, may be more selective. The demonstration, par-ticularly in glutaraldehyde-fixed material, of antennulae microvillares on the syncytiotrophoblast has added another element of selectivity to the process of micropinocytosis that perhaps entails the exclusion of certain classes of proteins from the cell. Mesenchymal cells, too, may adjust their rates of synthesis and transfer to demand and thus provide an additional means of transport of metabolites. Electron microscopy has amply demon-strated the participation of all placental elements in greatly diversified but finely coordinated functions that serve to maintain fetal homeostasis, despite altering physiological conditions.

Ancillary structural adaptations, detected by electron microscopy, include gradual decrease in the mass of cytotrophoblast and possibly attenuation of basal laminae, at least of the endothelium. At all times, however, the normal minimal histological barrier comprises trophoblast, fetal capillary, and their basal laminae. The persistence of trophoblast is probably of prime significance in maintaining the immunologically crucial buffer zone, as discussed later in this chapter.

Origin of the syncytium

Elucidation of the mechanism of syncytial growth requires resolution of the discrepancy between the increase in number of nuclei in the syncytiotropho-blast and the apparent absence of intrinsic nuclear replication. Mitotic figures, though frequently observed in the cytotrophoblast (Figure 4.9), are not found in the syncytium.

The syncytium is derived from cellular elements and is itself a mitotic end stage. The electron-microscopic corroboration of the derivation of the syncytium from the cytotrophoblast has been provided by the demonstration of morphologically transitional cells in the normal placentas of man and monkey and in neoplastic human trophoblast. The absence of intratropho-blastic basement membranes separating syncytium from Langhans cells, as suspected by light microscopists, has been confirmed. The typical Langhans cell has a large nucleus with a prominent nucleolus, occasional large mito-chondria, and few Golgi bodies. The cytoplasm is studded with numerous free ribosomes but is relatively devoid of smooth and rough endoplasmic

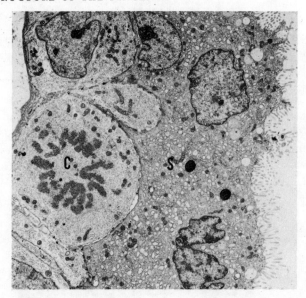

Figure 4.9 Early (6 weeks) villus showing cytotrophoblast (Langhans cell) in mitosis (C), as well as syncytium (S) to which it gives rise. × 000

reticulum. Such an ultrastructural pattern is common to many poorly differentiated tumours and is characteristic of those cells the primary function of which is growth and differentiation, rather than elaboration of specialised exocrine or endocrine products. In the transitional, or intermediate, cells, the nucleocytoplasmic ratio decreases and the intranuclear deoxyribonucleoprotein (DNP) granules become more numerous and less evenly distributed, whereas within the cytoplasm both smooth and rough forms of endoplasmic reticulum increase. Mature syncytial trophoblast characteristically has well-developed ergastoplasm and Golgi bodies, the organelles necessary for production of protein. Both nuclear and cytoplasmic transitions occur as cytotrophoblast differentiates into syncytium, the ultrastructurally mature form of trophoblast. Residual plasma membranes with attached desmosomes in well-fixed syncytium provide additional evidence of incorporation of the cytotrophoblast into syncytium. The demonstration of well-preserved organelles in areas between the membranes decreases the likelihood of artifact and suggests that plasma membranes gradually disappear as syncytium evolves from cellular trophoblast, to which it may remain attached by desmosomes.

The significance of these findings lies in the capacity of the placenta to form new syncytiotrophoblast throughout its life from the cellular reserve elements. In conditions of stress, such as hypoxia, new syncytium may form more rapidly to meet the needs of the fetus. The evidence bearing on the cytotrophoblastic contribution to the syncytium has been summarised by Boyd and Hamilton[17].

Nonvillous trophoblast

Wynn[18] has recently directed attention to the ultrastructure of types of trophoblast other than the villous syncytium and Langhans cells (Figure 4.10).

The primitive cytotrophoblast forms all trophoblastic derivatives, cellular and syncytial. The villous cytotrophoblast (Langhans layer) is continuous

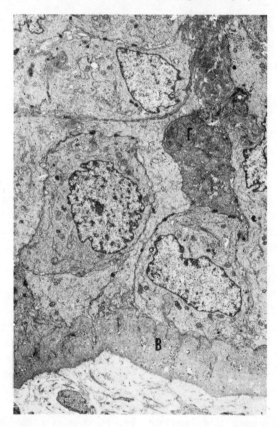

Figure 4.10 Anchoring villus from 12 weeks' gestation, showing an exceedingly thick basal lamina (B). This clump of cytotrophoblast comprises elements that are slightly more complex than typical Langhans cells. A few of them appear to be transitional. Fibrinoid (F) is interspersed among the trophoblastic elements. × 4200

with the cytotrophoblast of the chorionic plate, which in turn merges into that of the chorion laeve. Elements of the cytotrophoblastic shell later become part of the boundary zone at the basal plate and contribute to the placental septa and probably to the cell islands[6].

Ultrastructurally these cytotrophoblastic variants are more complex than Langhans cells. Like the intermediate cells in the villi, they may approach or equal the mature syncytial trophoblast in ultrastructural complexity. The specialised cytotrophoblast of the basal plate, cell islands, and septa may be difficult to distinguish, even ultrastructurally, from the complex decidual elements with which they may be intimately related in those areas.

Specialised syncytial areas that require further study include, in the terminology of Hamilton and Boyd[19], syncytial sprouts, stromal trophoblastic buds, syncytial knots, multinuclear giant cells, syncytiotrophoblast of the chorion laeve, and the epithelial plaques described earlier in this chapter. In regions where the fetal capillary is very close to the overlying trophoblast, the two basal laminae may be so intimately related as to appear confluent. These regions form so-called vasculo-syncytial membranes, or junctions, the minimal anatomical separation between intervillous space and fetal blood.

The villous mesenchyme

The villous core, which comprises fetal capillaries, fibroblasts, Hofbauer cells, and other mesenchymal elements, has been less extensively studied by electron microscopy than has the trophoblast. Ultrastructural alterations in these elements, however, may affect placental transfer and metabolism significantly. During placental development the lumen of the capillary may widen and the endothelial lining may thin to adapt to increased efficiency of transfer. Fenestrations in the endothelium, moreover, have been shown to represent not pores but sites for active exchange. To minimise the histological barrier, the pericytes surrounding the capillaries and the endothelial basal lamina may thin or disappear, and outpouchings of the endothelium toward the trophoblastic basal lamina may bring the capillary and trophoblast virtually into contact. On the luminal side of the capillary, large projections may be found, particularly near the junction of two endothelial cells. These structures are associated with classic pinocytosis. Micropinocytotic vacuoles are also prominent elsewhere near the capillary endothelial surface to assist in more selective transfer. This micropinocytosis may be important in meeting metabolic requirements of the placenta itself. Another possible ultrastructural adaptation to the needs of the placenta is the development of a variety of mesenchymal cellular vacuoles, which may be vehicles of transport for metabolism of the villus.

The origin and function of the Hofbauer cells continue to generate speculation. Wynn[12] studied their sex chromatin, histochemistry, and ultrastructure
in an attempt to ascertain their immunological and metabolic significance,
if any, in human placentation. Hofbauer cells are characterised by vacuolar
cytoplasm, scant endoplasmic reticulum, and relative paucity of other
organelles (Figure 4.11). The cells may be distinguished by both histo-
chemistry and electron microscopy from typical fibroblasts and plasma cells,

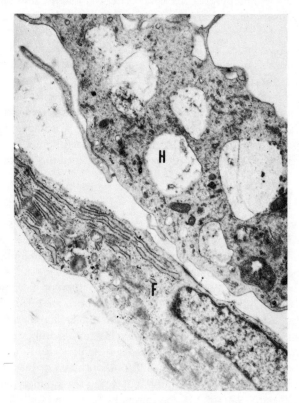

Figure 4.11 Human placenta at term. Hofbauer cell (H) and fibrocyte (F) within core of
villus are shown. × 6300

although degenerating fibroblasts and Hofbauer cells may be indistinguishable. It is, however, most unlikely that the rare plasma cells in the placenta
give rise to the numerous Hofbauer cells. The relation of fibrocytes to
Hofbauer cells is complicated by the finding of primitive mesenchymal
elements that may differentiate in either direction and by the common

vacuoles and irregular outlines of older fibrocytes, which make them quite similar to Hofbauer cells.

Enders and King[13] recently examined human placentas at various stages of gestation and showed that the Hofbauer cells are ultrastructurally similar to ordinary macrophages except for unusually large cytoplasmic flanges and inclusion vacuoles. They believe that the vacuoles result from macropinocytosis. In addition, these investigators found micropinocytotic vesicles coated with a layer of moderately dense filamentous material and presumably related to uptake of protein. The present consensus is that the typical Hofbauer cell is most likely a macrophage with an unusual capacity for ingestion of fluid.

Endocrine adaptations

Although the principal ultrastructural adaptations to formation of steroid and peptide hormones apply to the placenta, as well as to other endocrine organs, special features unique to a tissue that produces both types require further comment. A detailed modern account of the ultrastructural features of endocrinologically active cells is provided by Fawcett and co-workers[20]. According to them, stimulation of a particular cell is attended by marked increase in the endoplasmic reticulum and enlargement of the Golgi complex. In many endocrine organs, and presumably in the trophoblast as well, certain granules not released or needed, as well as excess membranes and ribosomes of the endoplasmic reticulum, may be incorporated into autophagic vacuoles and digested by lysosomal enzymes. Lysosomes with cytochemically demonstrable acid phosphatase are numerous in syncytiotrophoblast.

Release of a hormone, according to Fawcett and co-workers[20], involves movement of membrane-bound dense granules to the cell surface followed by a fusion of their limiting membrane with the plasma membrane. Because intermediate stages of extrusion of granules are rare, it is assumed that fusion of the secretory vesicles with the cell membrane is rapid and that solubilisation of the extruded granule is almost immediate. The bulk of ultrastructural evidence favours a process involving coalescence of membrane-limited vesicles, with the cell membrane extruding intact secretory granules that undergo dissolution extracellularly. At high rates of secretion the cell product may not be concentrated into granules before release, but the same mode of discharge is believed to apply to the pale vesicles, the contents of which may be fluid under these conditions. In the placenta the hormones are released into the maternal blood (intervillous space) rather than the fetal capillaries.

The ultrastructural features of typical steroid-producing cells, such as those of testis, ovary, and adrenal, differ from those of protein-secreting cells. The organelles associated with protein synthesis are relatively inconspicuous in steroid cells, and there are no demonstrable granules or vacuoles of stored secretory product. The most distinctive ultrastructural features of steroid-secreting cells are an extensive smooth-surfaced endoplasmic reticulum, very prominent Golgi complexes, mitochondria of highly variable size and often of unusual internal structure, numerous lysosomes and accumulations of lipochrome pigment, and lipid droplets. In steroid cells there may be a large juxtanuclear Golgi complex without a clearly defined boundary between the Golgi tubules and the smooth endoplasmic reticulum. In protein-secreting cells, however, the two organelles are believed to be morphologically distinct but functionally interrelated by way of small vesicles that arise from the granular endoplasmic reticulum and migrate to the Golgi complex, where they coalesce with the membranes of its outermost cisternae[20]. The mitochondrial cristae of steroid-secreting cells are thought to be tubular extensions of the inner membrane rather than flat folds or lamellae (Figure 4.12). In the placenta the steroid cells usually have conventional, rather than tubular, cristae, although in first-trimester trophoblast both varieties are observed[18]. Throughout placental development, membrane-limited dense bodies of diverse internal structure, usually

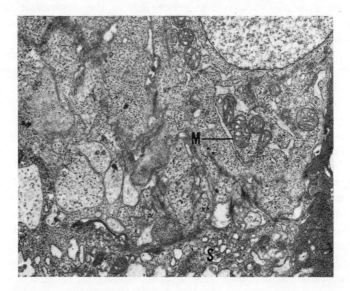

Figure 4.12 Cell column at 12 weeks, showing moderately well-differentiated cellular trophoblast. The mitochondria (M) in these cells have characteristic tubular cristae. Attached syncytium (S) has a vesicular endoplasmic reticulum. × 8750

interpreted as representing various stages in transition from lysosomes to lipofuscin pigment, are found. These bodies may be spherical with a homogeneous, finely granular content of moderate density, or they may have extremely dense osmiophilic granules of varying size and shape scattered throughout the less dense granular matrix. According to Fawcett and co-workers[20], these irregular, heterogeneous structures are often regarded as lipofuscin pigment and represent accumulated undigestible residues of autophagic activity.

Lipid droplets often appear black after fixation in osmium tetroxide and pale gray after fixation in glutaraldehyde. The agranular endoplasmic reticulum in the trophoblast may be difficult to distinguish in the electron-dense syncytium but may comprise randomly orientated tubules or concentric systems of fenestrated cisternae. The number of lipid droplets tends to be low when steroid secretion is maximal. Steroid-secreting cells, however, show no recognisable accumulation of secretory materials in the Golgi complex or elsewhere, nor can morphological evidence of release of hormones be detected at the cell surface.

Because the human syncytiotrophoblast is believed to produce both peptide and steroid hormones, all the ultrastructural specialisations just described may be found in that tissue. The evidence is strong that the endocrinologically active tissue of the human placenta is the syncytiotrophoblast, with possible small contributions from other well-differentiated specialised forms of trophoblast.

In their classic histological description of the human placenta, Wislocki and Bennett[14] attributed to the syncytium the production of the steroids estrogen and progesterone, which were considered the basis for the phenyl-hydrazone reaction demonstrated histochemically. Positive staining of the Langhans cells with the periodic acid-Schiff reagent was considered suggestive of localisation of chorionic gonadotropin, which was known to be a glycoprotein, in the cellular trophoblast. Their suggestion was supported by circumstantial evidence of the association of high levels of chorionic gonadotropin with clinical situations in which there are increased numbers of Langhans cells, such as early pregnancy, chorionic neoplasia, and plural gestations. Nevertheless, to students of placental ultrastructure the simplicity of the villous cytotrophoblast was inconsistent with that of other tissues known to produce proteins, as previously described. In the syncytium were found all the subcellular organelles required for this function, especially abundant rough-surfaced endoplasmic reticulum, Golgi complexes, and numerous mitochondria, which provide the enzymes. Immunofluorescent localisation of chorionic gonadotropin in trophoblast[21] has supported the concept that both steroids and proteins are produced by the syncytium.

Furthermore, many so-called cytotrophoblastic elements that appear to localise chorionic gonadotropin under the light microscope are ultrastructurally transitional, a phenomenon suggesting simultaneous maturation of endocrine activity during morphological evolution of Langhans cells to syncytium. Human chorionic somatomammotropin (placental lactogen) similarly has been localised in syncytiotrophoblast but not in Langhans cells[22]. It is reasonable to predict that the third postulated protein hormone of the placenta, chorionic thyrotropin, will also be localised to the syncytiotrophoblast. The syncytium may thus be regarded as the endocrinologically and morphologically mature form of trophoblast, whereas the Langhans cells are reserve, or stem, elements, the main function of which is to form new syncytium. The temporal coexistence of maximal cytotrophoblastic proliferation with high titres of chorionic gonadotropin in urine and serum has often been quoted. The lower titres of the hormone late in gestation, however, may reflect decrease not in mass of cytotrophoblast but in production by the multifunctional syncytium.

Although there is impressive evidence from several laboratories that the placental syncytium is the source of these protein hormones, the anatomical localisation of a hormone cannot necessarily be equated with its origin at a particular site. In simplest terms, the more complex the trophoblast, the more capable it is of producing hormones. As Langhans cells differentiate ultrastructurally, their endocrine potential increases simultaneously. Although the typical Langhans cell in the mature chorionic villus is an unlikely source of protein hormones, transitional villous trophoblast and ultrastructurally complex forms of cytotrophoblast elsewhere in the normal placenta and in chorionic neoplasms may be endocrinologically active.

Although there has never been serious doubt that the syncytium produces the steroid hormones, correlation of blood levels of hormonal steroids with ultrastructural identification of lipid is impractical. For example, lack of increase in syncytial lipid granules, despite elevated blood levels of steroidal hormones, may well reflect increased excretion by the syncytium rather than decreased production.

In conclusion, the syncytium appears to be the differentiated form of trophoblast, capable of synthesis of steroids and peptides, and primarily responsible for the production of all placental hormones.

Immunological Considerations

Attempted explanations for the retention of the placental homograft have been provided in detail elsewhere[23, 24]. In short, comparative electron microscopy of the placenta has supported the concept of the prime role of the trophoblast in maintaining the immunological barrier. In all placentas examined with the electron microscope, at least one layer of trophoblast persists throughout gestation in the major portion of the placenta. If the trophoblast lacks or fails to express histocompatibility antigens, an immunological barrier would be created. The suggestion by Kirby and co-workers[25] that an extracellular peritrophoblastic deposit, rather than a relative lack of histocompatibility antigens in the trophoblast, was the basis of the barrier rekindled interest in so-called fibrinoids as a general phenomenon of mammalian placentation. I have employed the term fibrinoid, however, in the restricted conventional sense of the histopathologist to refer to a group of substances recognised with the light microscope. Although fibrinoids are not demonstrable in all mammalian placentas, a submicroscopic glycocalyx may be found with the aid of the electron microscope on most trophoblastic plasma membranes. It is still not clear, however, to what extent these extracellular polysaccharides, which often form incomplete coverings, serve as mechanical barriers to the passage of transplantation antigens from fetus to mother.

The deposition of fibrinoids and related non-cellular components at the surfaces of contiguous fetal and maternal tissues could theoretically inhibit the immune response. A second important factor may be the passage of fetal blood or trophoblastic sprouts into the maternal circulation, thereby saturating the maternal antibody-producing system. A third factor, at least in certain species, could be relative deficiency of endometrial lymphatics, which theoretically confers a degree of immunological protection to the placenta in those animals. A fourth potentially significant factor may be immunological enhancement.

Ultrastructural examination of the placenta has elucidated several immunological factors. Because the highly invasive trophoblast of the guinea pig is purely syncytial but that of the mouse is cellular, syncytial transformation is not prerequisite to immunological protection. In many haemochorial placentas the pericellular decidual capsules may provide some protection through formation of mechanical barriers, but these materials are not found in placentas of all types or in ectopic human pregnancies. In the floor of the human placenta, for example, ultrastructurally well-preserved trophoblast and decidua are rarely in direct contact but remain separated by regressing tissues of fetal and maternal origins, by fibrinoid, or by both. This fibrinoid may arise from degeneration of decidual or trophoblastic cytoplasm or through transformation of the ground substance surrounding these cells. In the human basal plate the apparently viable giant cells are essentially syncytiotrophoblastic and represent either derivatives of the peripheral syncytium or results of differentiation *in situ* of cytotrophoblast. Studies by Kirby and co-workers[25] indicated that the fibrinoid in the mouse placenta was of trophoblastic origin, whereas ultrastructural examination of the human basal plate by Wynn[6] suggested that there is a contribution by decidua also. Fibrinoids and similar acellular barriers have been described in the decidual capsule and between the decidua and fetal giant cells of the rat's placenta, as well as in the guinea pig's junctional zone. In the cat's placenta, for example, the terminal web of the trophoblast may be mistaken for extracellular 'basement membrane-like' material[9]. Although histologically demonstrable fibrinoids are absent from the epitheliochorial placentas of the sow, cow, mare, and sheep, mucopolysaccharides may be found by electron microscopy on the interdigitating microvilli of chorionic and endometrial epithelia.

On the one hand, the fibrinoids that are recognised by conventional histochemical techniques appear to reflect the cellular interplay of trophoblast and endometrium. On the other hand, the ultrastructurally demonstrable mucopolysaccharides (glycocalyces) may play important roles in immunological protection of the placental homograft. Perhaps the most interesting current development along these lines concerns the role of human chorionic gonadotropin. Adcock and co-workers[26] recently reported that this glycoprotein inhibits the response of lymphocytes to phytohaemagglutinin. Their observations support the hypothesis that the fetus is accepted because HCG represents trophoblastic surface antigen and blocks the action of maternal lymphocytes.

References

1. Wynn, R. M. (1973). Placental ultrastructure. In: *Obstetrics and Gynecology Annual*, Vol. 3, p. 1. (R. M. Wynn, editor) (New York: Appleton–Century–Crofts.)
2. Wynn, R. M. (1973). Fine structure of the placenta. In: *Handbook of Physiology*, Section 7: Endocrinology, Vol. II: Female Reproductive System, Part 2, p. 261. (R. O. Greep, editor) (Washington, D.C.: American Physiological Society)
3. Björkman, N. (1970). *An Atlas of Placental Fine Structure*. (London: Ballière, Tindall and Cassell)
4. Björkman, N. (1968). Contributions of electron microscopy in elucidating placental structure and function. *Internat. Rev. Gen. Exptal. Zool.*, **3**, 309
5. Wynn, R. M. (1974). Ultrastructural development of the human decidua. *Amer. J. Obstet. Gynec.*, **118**, 652
6. Wynn, R. M. (1967). Fetomaternal cellular relations in the human basal plate: An ultrastructural study of the placenta. *Amer. J. Obstet. Gynec.*, **97**, 832
7. Enders, A. C. (1965). A comparative study of the fine structure of the trophoblast in several hemochorial placentas. *Amer. J. Anat.*, **116**, 29
8. Mossman, H. W. (1967). Comparative biology of the placenta and fetal membranes. In: *Fetal Homeostasis*, Vol. II, p. 13. (R. M. Wynn, editor) (New York: New York Academy of Science)

9. Wynn, R. M. and Björkman, N. (1968). Ultrastructure of the feline placental membrane. *Amer. J. Obstet. Gynec.*, **102**, 34

10. Wynn, R. M. (1968). Morphology of the placenta. In: *Biology of Gestation*, Vol. I, p. 93. (N. S. Assali, editor) (New York: Academic Press)

11. Wimsatt, W. A., Enders, A. C., and Mossman, H. W. (1973). A reexamination of the chorioallantoic placental membrane of a shrew, *Blarina brevicauda*: resolution of a controversy. *Amer. J. Anat.*, **138**, 207

12. Wynn, R. M. (1967). Derivation and ultrastructure of the so-called Hofbauer cell. *Amer. J. Obstet. Gynec.*, **97**, 235

13. Enders, A. C. and King, B. F. (1970). The cytology of Hofbauer cells. *Anat. Rec.*, **167**, 231

14. Wislocki, G. B. and Bennett, H. S. (1943). Histology and cytology of the human and monkey placenta with special reference to the trophoblast. *Amer. J. Anat.*, **73**, 335

15. Wislocki, G. B. and Dempsey, E. W. (1948). The chemical histology of the human placenta and decidua with reference to mucoproteins, glycogen, lipins, and acid phosphatase. *Amer. J. Anat.*, **83**, 1

16. Fawcett, D. W. (1965). Surface specializations of absorbing cells. *J. Histochem. Cytochem.*, **13**, 75

17. Boyd, J. D. and Hamilton, W. J. (1970). *The Human Placenta.* (Cambridge: Heffer)

18. Wynn, R. M. (1972). Cytotrophoblastic specializations: an ultrastructural study of the human placenta. *Amer. J. Obstet. Gynec.*, **114**, 339

19. Hamilton, W. J. and Boyd, J. D. (1966). Specializations of the syncytium of the human chorion. *Brit. Med. J.*, **1**, 1501

20. Fawcett, D. W., Long, J. A. and Jones, A. L. (1969). The ultrastructure of endocrine glands. *Recent Progr. Hormone Res.*, **25**, 315

21. Midgley, A. R., Jr. and Pierce, G. B., Jr. (1962). Immunohistochemical localization of human chorionic gonadotropin. *J. Exper. Med.*, **115**, 289

22. Sciarra, J. J., Kaplan, S. L., and Grumbach, M. M. (1963). Localization of anti-human growth hormone serum within the human placenta: evidence for a human chorionic 'growth hormone-prolactin'. *Nature* (London), **199**, 1005

23. Wynn, R. M. (1969). Noncellular components of the placenta. *Amer. J. Obstet. Gynec.*, **103**, 723

24. Wynn, R. M. (1971). Immunological implications of comparative placental ultra-structure. In: *The Biology of the Blastocyst*, p. 495. (R. J. Blandau, editor) (Chicago: University of Chicago Press)

25. Kirby, D. R. S., Billington, W. D., Bradbury, S. and Goldstein, D. J. (1964). Antigen barrier of the mouse placenta. *Nature* (London), **204**, 548

26. Adcock, E. W. III, Teasdale, F., August, C. S., Cox, S., Meschia, G., Battaglia, F. C., and Naughton M. A. (1973). Human chorionic gonadotropin: its possible role in maternal lymphocyte suppression. *Science*, **181**, 845

CHAPTER 5

Morphometry

W. Aherne

The placenta is perhaps the most underrated of organs. It is inevitably over-shadowed by the birth of a healthy infant, and commonly blamed when the fetus is stillborn. With rather more justice it is occasionally implicated in serious obstetrical difficulties, when its attachment to the uterus is either insecure or too secure. And it has an unpleasant shape and feel. Yet, it is remarkably versatile. It acts as a respiratory and an alimentary organ, it manufactures essential hormones, and it takes in its stride functions which are later performed by the infant's biliary and urinary systems.

In this chapter we shall be concerned with one aspect of its many structural adaptations to efficient function. As a respiratory organ, like the lung in postnatal life, it must expose as large a surface as is appropriate to the uptake of oxygen and the excretion of carbon dioxide at an efficient rate. The same elaboration of a large absorbing surface is necessary to its function as an alimentary organ, though here the mechanisms of absorption are different. In this chapter we take a small step towards understanding these two functions by estimating the surface area of the chorionic villi and of the fetal capillaries they enclose. We shall consider also some other morphometric aspects, such as the volumes of both fetal and material vascular beds, and the adaptive placing of fetal vessels. Finally, we shall consider relationships between fetal weight and placental weight.

Material

The morphometric results are based on a study of 44 placentas[1]. Clearly, it is important to establish what may be regarded as normal, and here we are immediately faced with a problem. If a woman goes into spontaneous labour at (say) 28 weeks may we justly regard her placenta as representative of the class of all normal placentas at that point in pregnancy? In the following account we shall *assume* that we may; but I emphasise that this is an assumption forced upon us. Similar considerations apply to non-normal pre-term placentas; we cannot disentangle age effects from disease effects, except (as in the present study) by excluding placentas with any clear histological evidence of disease.

Of the 44 placentas 21 will be regarded as representative of the normal organ over at least the last trimester of pregnancy. The abnormal ones comprise 13 from pregnancies complicated by hypertension* and 10 associated with fetuses that were small-for-dates†. The remaining 6 form a miscellaneous group. Placentas showing more than a minimal peripheral infarction were excluded. Each placenta was weighed with its membranes trimmed off and its umbilical cord cut to within 2 cm of its insertion. This practice is strongly recommended; labour ward weights commonly include an indeterminate mass of membranes, cord, blood clot and amniotic debris.

Methods

For those who may wish to extend the modest investigations described in this chapter there follows a brief account of the morphometric principles involved. First, an estimate of the volume of the placenta, trimmed as described above, is made. This should be done directly, rather than by calculation from the placental weight and the specific gravity of placental tissue. It may be done by displacement of water, and a series of readings should be taken. For this purpose the appropriate device is a container with a siphon, so that water displaced by the placenta can be run off into a measuring cylinder. The siphon ensures that the run-off will stop abruptly when the water level falls to the pre-set value at which it stood before the placenta was immersed.

Unfortunately, the volume of the delivered placenta is an underestimate of the true, *in situ* volume, since blood is readily lost from the intervillous space during delivery. The significance of this error in the morphometric work-up will be discussed presently.

As in any aspect of histology adequate fixation is important. The whole placenta fixes well in about 14 days in 10% formol-saline. It can then be cut into 10–15 transections, each about 1 cm thick. Shrinkage during this phase of the investigation is negligible; the significance of this too will be explained presently.

* Diastolic pressure > 100 mmHg.
† Birth weight below the appropriate mean by 2 SD or more.

Morphometric techniques

It is convenient to interrupt the description of the macroscopic study of the placenta at this stage, since some knowledge of morphometry is necessary if the reader is to understand the next few steps. Our particular need at this stage is for some convenient method of estimating the relative volumes of the various components visible on the cut surfaces.

The estimation of volume proportions—A variety of empirical methods of making this estimation exist but we shall confine our attention to a technique based on concepts of geometrical probability. The key concept is the so-called theorem of Delesse[2] which is more properly called a *conjecture* since Delesse was never able to prove it. He was a geologist and his problem was to quantify the component materials of heterogeneous rocks. His insight was this: the area occupied by any given mineral seen on the polished surface of a heterogeneous rock is proportional to the volume of that mineral in the rock as a whole.

In terms of the placenta, if the areal extent of the chorionic tissue visible on a set of cut surfaces is (say) a_C, that of the decidual plate is a_D, and that of the parenchyma (villi and intervillous space) is a_P, it can be shown that

$$a_C/(a_C + a_D + a_P) = v_C/(v_C + v_D + v_P) = v_C/V$$

and, of course, similarly for v_D/V and v_P/V, where the lower case v's are volume proportions and the capital V is the overall volume of the placenta. Thus, having measured the relative areas a_C, a_D, and a_P, preferably on 10–15 cut surfaces, we can calculate v_C, v_D, and v_P relatively; and if in addition we know V we can calculate these volume components absolutely. The significance of the fact that V underestimates the overall volume of the placenta is now clear; it leads to an underestimate of the volume of the parenchymal part of the organ, and hence (as we shall see) to an underestimate of both the intervillous maternal space and the surface area of fetal villi and capillaries. It is probably not a serious underestimate, and is of little consequence in *comparative* studies.

To return to the macroscopic examination of fixed placental transections: we now need a way of applying the principle of Delesse, so that the relative areas—and hence the relative volumes—of a_C, a_D and a_P can be estimated. Ordinarily we group the placental components into two categories only, namely parenchyma (P) and non-parenchyma (non-P). Delesse used pieces of tin-foil cut to the various sizes of the components he was interested in; the relative weights of these were, of course, proportional to (and therefore indicative of) their relative areas and thus their relative volumes. One still encounters variants of this method; for example, the practice of cutting out areas of interest from photo-micrographs and weighing them as Delesse weighed his tin foil. This tedious method should be dismissed from morphometry and replaced by the technique of point-counting.

The theory of point-counting is easily understood without recourse to formal mathematics. Imagine a square containing a large number (N) of dots, distributed regularly or at random—the former is more easily conceived but no more accurate in the long run. If we now draw a diagonal we shall have two equal triangles, each containing (to a sufficient degree of accuracy) $N/2$ dots. Here we have used area to estimate a number of dots. The converse operation is equally valid; we may use the number of dots to define an area. In practice, when we wish to quantify the respective areas of parenchymal tissue and non-parenchymal tissue we superimpose on the placental slices a grid of dots drawn on transparent plastic sheeting, and estimate the relative areas of P and non-P by counting the relative number of dots falling on these structures respectively. We may then argue

$$a_P/A \to v_P/V, \text{ and } a_{non-P}/A \to v_{non-P}/V,$$

where A is the total count of points, and V is the overall volume of the trimmed placenta.

The next step is to prepare blocks for histological processing. These may be taken in a stratified random manner, i.e. each transection of the placenta should be represented but the site from which the block is taken from any particular transection may be randomly chosen. Full thickness blocks, or at least an equal sampling of the fetal and the maternal zones is desirable. Each block should be carefully measured in two dimensions, so that a correction can be made in due course for the inevitable shrinkage that occurs during passage through the alcohols prior to embedding in wax. The significance of this step will become apparent when we come to estimate the surface area of the feto-maternal interface.

The technique of point-counting may be applied without significant modification at microscopical level by means of a suitable eyepiece graticule such as the Weibel multipurpose test system. This is marketed by Messrs. Wild Heerbrugg Ltd. It provides a grid of points which can be superimposed on the components of the tissue under examination. We thus estimate the relative volume proportions of villous tissue, intervillous space and any other feature of interest (e.g. fibrinoid in certain cases).

The estimation of surface area—This technique we apply at microscopical level only. The principle is this: a graticule line of measured length, projected repeatedly and randomly on a set of histological sections, will intersect the boundaries of the component whose surface area we wish to measure. It will thus be divided up into a number of line segments whose mean length is a quantity termed 'the mean linear intercept'. This we shall symbolise as λ. The surface area in question can be shown[3] to be inversely proportional to the mean linear intercept. This is not an obvious concept and does need formal mathematical demonstration, which would not be appropriate here. The reader may see intuitively that the more villi, for example, in a given volume of placental parenchyma, the more intersections there will be and therefore the smaller the mean linear intercept. The computing formula for surface area is

$$S = 2V/\lambda$$

We now see why the underestimate of V, due to loss of blood from the intervillous space during delivery of the placenta, leads to an underestimate of villous (and likewise of fetal capillary) surface area. Fortunately, our concern is primarily with *comparative* studies.

This, then, is a sketch of the morphometric methods used to establish the relative quantities of placental components, and the surface areas of chorionic villous tissue and fetal capillaries. The details may be filled in by recourse to some of the many publications now available in this field; for example: Weibel[4], Freere and Weibel[5], Dunnill[6], Aherne[7].

Results of Morphometric Estimates

These are displayed in Tables 5.1–5.6. Taking the relative volume studies first we note the following conclusions in particular.

(1) Assuming that pre-term placentas are normal the overall volume of the trimmed normal placenta increases from 170 ml at 28 weeks of gestation to 723 ml at term (39–42 weeks). As usual the range is a poor statistic, and the latter figure is misleading. The mean placental volume at term ($n = 10$) is 488 ml, with a standard *error* of 31·4 ml. The mean volume of placentas associated with hypertensive pregnancies at term is 363 ml, which is significantly lower than normal ($t = 2·76$; $0·01 < P < 0·02$). The mean volume of placentas at term associated with small-for-dates babies, 350 ml, is also significantly lower than normal ($t = 3·22$; $0·001 < P < 0·01$). The reader should note that the placentas associated with small-for-dates babies came from normotensive women. In other words, we must seek some factor other than hypertension to account for this reduction in size.

(2) The mean values for the volume proportions of chorionic tissue and intervillous space (approximately 60% and 40% respectively) do not differ significantly as between the three categories. This is a reflection of the choice

Table 5.1 Macroscopic features of placentas, and fetal weights, from normal pregnancies

Gestational age (wks)	*Volume of fresh placenta (ml)	Percentage volume proportions		Infant birth weight (kg)
		Parenchyma	Non-parenchyma	
28	170	80	20	0·88
28	285	80	20	1·23
32	235	64	36	1·50
33	387	80	20	2·35
34	246	74	26	1·59
34	270	79	21	3·18
34	327	72	28	2·16
36	358	77	23	2·38
37	290	78	22	2·50
38	455	78	22	3·60
39	450	80	20	3·96
40	391	76	24	3·32
40	403	80	20	3·43
40	430	82	18	3·26
40	432	87	13	3·57
40	466	76	24	3·10
40	492	80	20	3·83
40	518	75	25	3·23
40	575	75	25	3·35
40	723	80	20	3·94
42	637	76	24	3·77

* 1. This may be converted to weight in grams by using the factor × 1·04

 2. The percentage volume proportion of infarcted tissue was noted in three cases: the greatest was 7%. These figures are not included in the table.

of placentas free from secondary changes such as infarction. Moreover, the quantity of non-parenchymal tissue does not differ either; the absolute quantity in normal placentas is 106·8 ml, in placentas associated with hypertension 97·4 ml, and in the small-for-dates syndrome 100·9 ml.

(3) The clearest result is a deficit of *parenchyma* in both hypertensive and small-for-dates syndromes. In the hypertensive case the mean proportion of parenchyma is 72·52% which differs from normal at the 0·05 level of significance ($t = 2·38$; $0·02 < P < 0·05$). The deficit of parenchyma in the small-for-dates case is more striking: the proportion of parenchyma is 67·23%, which is highly significantly different from the normal value of 77·66% ($t = 4·107$; $P < 0·001$). Since the parenchymal tissues in placentas from each of these syndromes appeared normal (at least in the light microscope) we

Table 5.2 Macroscopic features of placentas from pregnancies complicated by hypertension (diastolic pressure > 100 mmHg)

Gestational age (wks)	Volume of fresh placenta (ml)	Percentage volume proportions		Infant birth weight (kg)
		Parenchyma	Non-parenchyma	
30	267	67	29	1·02
34	145	68	30	1·35
36	372	73	27	2·16
37	345	60	40	2·21
38	293	74	26	1·47
39	250	79	21	→ 1·95
39	292	77	23	2·64
39	328	76	24	→ 2·22
39	430	82	18	3·26
39	470	78	22	2·84
40	380	57	43	→ 1·93
40	395	79	21	2·46
42	380	73	27	3·00

The arrows indicate cases small-for-date at term (39–42 weeks).

Table 5.3 Macroscopic features of placentas associated with normotensive pregnancies but infants small-for-dates (mean − 2 SD, or less)

Gestational age (wks)	*Volume of fresh placenta (ml)	Percentage volume proportions		Infant birth weight (kg)
		Parenchyma	Non-parenchyma	
37	125	76	24	1·25
37	232	68	32	1·95
38	410	69	31	2·16
40	261	78	22	2·15
40	361	68	32	2·27
40	315	64	36	2·20
40	400	67	33*	2·15
40	420	61	39	2·38
41	410	46	54†	2·40
42	285	75	25	2·16

* This includes 11% of solid material which microscopy revealed to be intervillous fibrinoid.
† This includes a quantity of intervillous fibrinoid which could not be accurately quantified.

may conclude provisionally that there was no loss of villi but rather a primary failure of growth.

We turn now to the estimates of villous and fetal capillary surface areas, made by the mean linear intercept technique. These are displayed in Tables 5.4, 5.5, and 5.6.

Table 5.4 Microscopic features of placentas from normal pregnancies

	Percentage volume proportions			Surface area	
Gestational age (wks)	Intervillous space	Villous tissue	Villous fetal capillaries	Villi (m²)	Villous capillaries (m²)
28	40	46	14	3·4	3·1
28	42	58	—	6·6	—
32	41	59	—	4·4	—
33	40	49	11	9·8	9·4
34	36	64	—	6·1	—
34	39	50	11	6·0	5·4
34	34	53	13	8·1	5·4
36	42	43	15	7·7	8·8
37	37	47	16	7·2	6·4
38	36	46	18	10·6	14·0
39	34	66	—	11·6	—
40	33	56	11	10·0	8·6
40	38	48	14	9·8	7·4
40	39	51	10	9·2	8·8
40	35	58	7	11·6	—
40	42	58	—	9·1	—
40	34	66	—	11·8	—
40	32	53	15	12·2	10·2
40	38	53	9	11·9	20·3
40	34	50	16	12·6	16·9
42	40	48	12	14·7	13·5

1. Where not specifically quoted the proportion of villous fetal capillaries are included with 'villous tissue'.

2. The percentage volume proportion of fibrinoid material is included with 'villous tissue'. The largest percentage observed was 8·7% (at term).

(1) The area of the *normal* feto-maternal interface, i.e. the extent of chorionic villous surface presented to maternal blood ranges from 3·4 m² at 28 weeks gestation to 12·6 m² at term. The mean villous surface area of the 10 *normal* placentas at term is 11·0 m² (SD 1·3 m²; SE 0·41 m²) and the mean surface area of the fetal vessels in the villi is 12·2 m² (SD 4·85 m²; SE 1·83 m²; $n = 7$).

(2) The mean villous surface area of the placenta associated with *hypertension* is 7·4 m² at term (SD 2·01; SE 0·71; $n = 8$) which is significantly lower than normal ($t = 4·37$; $0·001 < P < 0·01$). The mean area of the fetal vascular bed is 10·2 m² (SD 2·65 m²; SE 1·08; $n = 6$).

Table 5.5 Microscopic features of placentas from pregnancies complicated by hypertension 4 (diastolic pressure > 100 mmHg)

| Gestational age (wks) | Percentage volume proportions | | | Surface area | |
	Intervillous space	Villous tissue	Villous fetal capillaries	Villi (m²)	Villous capillaries (m²)
30	46	54	—	4·5	—
34	48	52	—	2·8	—
36	34	50	16	8·3	6·7
37	32	42	26	6·6	10·4
38	65	35	—	6·6	—
39	46	54	—	→ 5·9	—
39	40	50	10	7·6	6·0
39	33	39	28	→ 4·51	8·8
39	37	43	20	10·5	13·6
39	33	37	30	→ 7·5	11·7
40	47	53	—	5·5	—
40	37	47	16	8·9	11·4
42	37	48	15	8·9	9·7

The arrows indicate small-for-date at term (39-42 weeks).

Table 5.6 Microscopic features of placentas associated with normotensive pregnancies but infants small-for-dates (mean − 2 SD, or less)

| Gestational age (wks) | Percentage volume proportions | | | Surface area | |
	Intervillous space	Villous tissue	Villous fetal capillaries	Villi (m²)	Villous capillaries (m²)
37	37	63	—	2·3	—
37	40	33	27	4·4	4·8
38	36	45	19	9·2	9·0
40	38	41	21	5·5	5·6
40	30	51	19	7·5	6·9
40	42	50	8	4·8	4·8
40	40	35	25	8·0	9·4
40	33	40	27	7·8	8·8
41	29	59	12	5·9	6·3
42	38	50	12	9·2	9·0

(3) The mean villous surface area in the *small-for-dates* syndrome at term is 6·9 m² (SD 1·58; SE 0·59; $n = 7$) which, of course, is also significantly lower than normal. The mean area of the fetal vascular bed is 7·2 m² (SD 1·82; SE 0·68; $n = 7$).

The relationship between villous surface area and gestational age, in the abnormal cases, is shown in Figure 5.1.

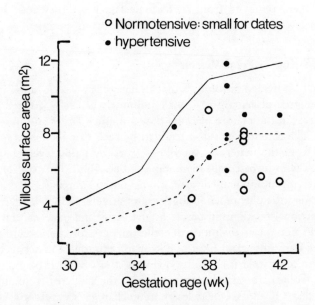

Figure 5.1 The figure shows the relationship between gestational age and placental villous surface area in twelve pregnancies complicated by hypertension (diastolic pressure >100 mmHg) and ten pregnancies that issued in babies who were small-for-dates. The continuous line is the mean value of placental weight, based indirectly on the 1958 British Perinatal Mortality Survey. The dashed line lies two standard deviations below the mean. Note that the placentas from three of the hypertensive patients fall into the small-for-dates region, and two from infants who were small-for-dates fall above the critical mean − 2 SD boundary.

Comment on Morphometric Results

The application of quantitative methods in biology differs profoundly from the application of essentially similar quantitative methods in geology or material science. For the biologist's specimen is a plastic object, constantly changing its shape and size (though not its topological species), whereas the objects which metallurgists and geologists study are absolutely static. Again, the biologist's sample is a 3-dimensional one, examined by transmitted light, while that of the metallurgist and the geologist is 2-dimensional, i.e. a polished surface, usually examined by incident light.

For reasons such as these the quantitative results presented here must be interpreted in two ways. As estimates of the parameters of living plastic

organs they are approximate. As estimates of these parameters in a given
fixed specimen, removed from its biological context, they may be made
exact as one wishes, but only for that particular fixed specimen.

Optimal Siting of Fetal Vessels

It is well known to histologists that fetal capillary vessels (sinusoids) tend
in the immature placenta, to be small and nearly centrally situated in most
villi, whereas in the mature placenta they are much larger and much more
eccentric. The eccentric position tends to be such that the fetal capillary is
separated from the maternal intervillous space by a thin layer of syncytial
trophoblast with its basement membrane and possibly a little collagen. Such
regions are commonly named 'vasculosyncytial' membranes.

This maturation phenomenon suggests, intuitively, an increasing efficiency
in the functional relationship between fetal vessel and maternal intervillous
space. I do not mean to imply that the thickness of the vasculosyncytial
membrane is an important limiting factor in diffusion of materials between
mother and fetus; that is an outmoded idea. But even if it be granted that
most metabolites are actively transported by the syncytial trophoblast it is
still true that O_2 and CO_2 (at least) are exchanged by diffusion, and that
some molecules must traverse villous mesenchyme at points away from the
vasculosyncytial membrane.

Theoretically one envisages streams of 'flux', Ψ, entering the villous
surface at right angles and curving to enter the fetal capillary also at right
angles. The O_2 or other molecules presumably descend (or ascend) a concentration gradient, crossing a sequence of 'equipotential curves' (Figure
5.2) as they go. The question now arises: is it possible to quantify the increase
in exchange efficiency which results from this margination and enlargement
of fetal vessels?

An analytical solution is rendered difficult by the very phenomenon we
wish to study, i.e. the *eccentric* position of the vessels, and even more by the
fact that each villus contains more than one vessel, so that the flux pattern is
determined by a complicated interaction of the flow lines and equipotential
lines appropriate to each vessel. However, there is a graphical procedure,
much used in heat flow engineering, which can be adapted to our purpose.
Figure 5.3 shows an idealised villus, containing one 'capillary', which is
central at first but later moves into progressively more eccentric positions.
The first step in constructing a so-called 'flux-plot' is to draw a set of equipotential lines along which the concentration of some substance may be
supposed constant. The next step is to draw a set of flow lines orthogonal
to the equipotential lines in such a way that a set of approximate, 'curvilinear'

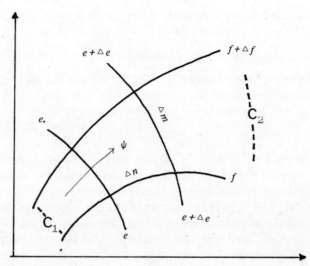

Figure 5.2 A 'flow tube', bounded by flow lines across which two 'equipotential lines' (e, e) and ($e + \Delta e$, $e + \Delta e$) are drawn. Streams of flux (Ψ) move from C_1 to C_2. The size of the curvilinear square Δm. Δn may be used as an indicator of flux velocity

squares results. As the capillary enlarges and moves to an eccentric position the equipotential lines are necessarily crowded together, indicating that the concentration gradient of the substance in question is growing steeper. We find, *pari passu*, that the number of curvilinear squares increases. Each sequence of curvilinear squares constitutes a 'flow tube' and the efficiency of exchange between the fetal capillary and the maternal intervillous space is directly proportional to the number of flow tubes. Figure 5.2 shows that the concentration gradient is $-\Delta C/\Delta n$, where n is a distance. Clearly, the

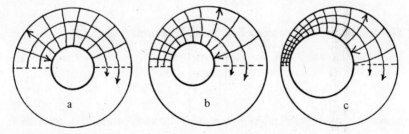

Figure 5.3 An idealised villus, with a single fetal vessel. As the vessel moves to an eccentric position, and increases in diameter (a→b→c), the number of flow tubes across the 3 equipotential lines increases from 9 (in a) to 18 (in c), indicating a theoretical doubling in diffusion efficiency

flux velocity $\Psi' = \Delta\Psi'/\Delta m$ is proportional to the concentration gradient, i.e. $\Psi' = k_0 \left(-\Delta C/\Delta n \right)$. It follows that

$$\Psi' = k_1(1/\Delta m) = k_2(1/\Delta n),$$

i.e. the smaller the space elements Δm and Δn become the greater the flux velocity. But smaller Δm and Δn, with $\Delta m \sim \Delta n$, implies that a given absolute unit of space will contain a larger number of squares. Therefore

$$\Psi' \sim N$$

where N is the total number of squares on the flux plot, provided the (arbitrary) number of equipotential lines is constant from plot to plot.

Table 5.7 shows data from five placentas at successive stages in gestation. It is evident that (a) the mean diameter of the chorionic villus diminishes with time, (b) the mean diameter of the fetal capillary increases with time, although the final fixed state does rather depend upon the vagaries of delivery, and (c) the capillary moves outward during maturation of the placenta, so that eventually it comes to lie under the syncytial trophoblast. The reduction in villous diameter is roughly $\times 0.5$, the increase in capillary diameter roughly $\times 1.5$ and the minimal distance from capillary to inter-villous space is reduced by roughly $\times 0.25$. A flux-plot based on these findings, and interpreted in a comparative way, shows that the efficiency rating for the villus increases from 90 units (curvilinear squares) at 16 weeks to 198 units at term. Part of this plot is shown in Figure 5.4(a), (b). If this is combined with the increase in the number of villi in the latter half of gestation, which is roughly threefold, the efficiency rating of *normal* chorionic tissue increases to within a few units of 600, i.e. by a factor of 6 to 7 times. We have as yet no information about the efficiency rating of abnormal placentas. It would be particularly interesting to examine the small-for-dates placenta in this way.

The Relationship between Fetal and Placental Mass

Since the placenta is, for the most part, a fetal organ the formal mass relationship which comes naturally to mind is the allometric equation

$$m = aM^b$$

where m is the mass of the placenta, M is the mass of the fetus and a, b are constants. In a previous publication[8] I proposed an equation in which $a = 2.1$ and $b = 0.67$. This was based on a series of 'normal' products of conception. Since then the series has been extended and I would now revise the equation to read

Table 5.7 Mean comparative size, position and number of villous capillaries in placentas of different gestational stages

Case and its gestational stage	Mean diameter of villus (arbitrary units)	Mean diameter of capillaries (arbitrary units)*	Mean number of capillaries per villus	Mean minimal distance capillary to intervillous space (arbitrary units)†	Number of villi and (in brackets) number of capillaries measured
(1) at 16 weeks	816·4	72·0	3·1	77·8	15 (50)
(2) at 28 weeks	422·1	98·1	4·7	21·5	15 (71)
(3) at 34 weeks	523·4	117·3	4·0	38·8	15 (60)
(4) at 37 weeks	466·3	143·0	3·7	33·0	15 (57)
(5) at 40 weeks	386·9	105·5	3·3	20·2	10 (33)

* The diameter of villous capillaries depends a good deal on how much fetal blood is allowed to remain in the placenta.
† In the less mature placentas this is the distance from the capillary endothelium to the outer aspect of the syncytial trophoblast. In the more mature cases it is the thickness of the vasculosyncytial membrane.

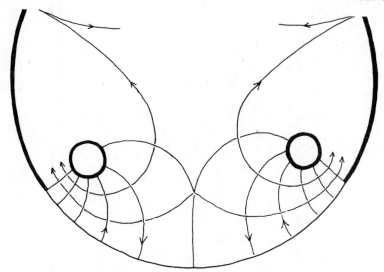

Figure 5.4(a) This diagram, representing an early phase in gestation, is based on the measurements recorded in Table 5.7. Two fetal capillaries are shown, with associated equipotential lines and flow tubes. Ten of the possible 20 flow tubes are indicated; the addition of the third capillary (which is out of sight above the diagram) would increase the number of flow tubes to 30

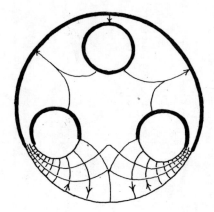

Figure 5.4(b) This diagram is also based on the data of Table 5.7 and represents the mature villus. It is drawn to the same scale as the villus in Figure 5.4(a). 22 of the possible 66 flow tubes are indicated. This, together with the three-fold increase in the number of villi as gestation proceeds, leads to a six-fold increase in diffusion efficiency

$$m = 2 \cdot 17 \ M^{0 \cdot 67};$$
$$\text{standard error of ‘}a\text{’: } 0 \cdot 087;$$
$$\text{standard error of ‘}b\text{’: } 0 \cdot 058;$$

and I would add the proviso that it applies only to the second half of gestation. Indeed, it is not surprising that the relationship is not stable between the 12th and the 20th week of gestation; for the placenta does not begin to appear in definitive form until the beginning of this period. Between the 12th and the 20th week the main feature of the relationship is a falling value of the parameter ‘a’ from about $5 \cdot 6$ to a mean value of $2 \cdot 17$. From this stage onwards to 40 weeks ‘a’ may reasonably be called a constant. The extra data has also shown that ‘b’ is not as stable as it first appeared. Critics of the ‘2/3 power law’ of metabolic rate may find significance in this, though I would suggest that the evidence has not demolished the hypothesis that a mean value $b = 0 \cdot 67$ is compatible with the notion that placental mass is adapted to fetal weight-specific metabolic rate, as defined by Brody and Proctor[9], Smith[10], and Bertalanffy[11], in the context of which thermoregulation is irrelevant. I do, however, subscribe to the warning issued by Sholl[12] against the danger of drawing facile but unwarranted biological conclusions from double-logarithmic graphs. Mainly for this reason, and also because one's material is not yet adequate, I believe the time is not yet ripe for assessing the fetoplacental allometric relationship in abnormal pregnancies. Suffice it to say, in this small study, that the relation $m = 2 \cdot 17^{0 \cdot 67}$ held fairly well (Normal, term; $m = 508$ g, $aM^b = 514$: hypertensive, term; $m = 380$ g, $aM^b = 415$: small-for-dates, term; $m = 372$ g, $aM^b = 380$). There was no clear deviation in the case of abnormal placentas, and in particular there was no clear distinction between (a) placentas from hypertensive pregnancies with infants whose weights were normal for their gestational ages, (b) placentas from hypertensive pregnancies with infants small-for-dates and (c) placentas from normotensive pregnancies with infants small-for-dates. The relationship between villous surface area and infant birth weight seemed independent of such categorisation.

The main problem in studies of the delivered placenta is, of course, that one has access to only half of the functional uteroplacental unit; the ramifications of the maternal supply vessels and any pathological changes that may have occurred in them remain hidden from us in all but a few exceptional cases. This is a further reason for caution in interpreting morphometric results such as I have presented in this chapter.

It is interesting that the total surface area of fetal vessels is very close to the surface area of the villi that house them. The tissues of the villi provide protection for the delicate fetal capillaries, as well as a repertoire of active transport systems, without diminishing the area of contact with maternal blood.

The estimates of villous surface area and volume proportions of parenchymal components presented here are similar to those published by Wilkin[13], who arrived at his conclusions by planimetry. Though the morphometric methods described above are much more rapid and convenient than planimetry they are nevertheless too demanding for routine use. If we believe it desirable to include morphometric estimates as part of the routine examination of the placenta, and if we are *prepared to sacrifice technical rigour* in that endeavour, we have motives for some rules-of-thumb. The following rules are suggested.

Approximate Methods for Routine Use

(1) The placenta should be trimmed, as described above, and fixed for at least 14 days, after which its volume V (ml) can be established.

(2) It should then be cut into 10–15 slices. The 'length' of each slice should be measured, together with the 'length' of any infarcted or otherwise abnormal parenchymal tissue. The volume proportion (v) of infarcts or other lesions can then be estimated as $\Sigma l/\Sigma L$, where Σl is the summed lengths of lesions and ΣL is the summed lengths of the 10–15 slices.

(3) The volume of healthy parenchyma is thus either V or $(V - v)$ ml. We may roughly estimate the volume proportion of chorionic tissue as $0.6 \, V$ ml [or $0.6 \, (V - v)$] ml, and that of the intervillous space as $0.4 \, V$ ml [or $0.4 \, (V - v)$] ml.

(4) Taking account of average values[14] for the mean linear intercept (λ) and the factor for converting processed to 'fresh' dimensions, we may estimate the villous and fetal vascular surface areas as $S = 0.234 \, V$ m², or $S = 0.234 \, (V - v)$ m² each.

(5) The volume of the trimmed placenta at term should lie between 430 ml and 550 ml in all but about 5% of cases.

(6) In the rough estimates outlined above it may be more convenient to use the mass (weight) of the placenta than its volume. Mass and volume are related by the equation mass $= 1.04 \, V$.

(7) The mass of the trimmed placenta (m) should, in general, be related to the mass of the fetus (M), at least approximately, by the equation

$$\log_{10} m = b \, \log_{10} M + 0.3$$

where b lies between 0.60 and 0.80 in all but about 5% of cases.

References

1. Aherne, W. and Dunnill, M. S. (1966). Quantitative aspects of placental structure. *J. Path. Bact.*, **91**, 123
2. Delesse, M. A. (1847). Procédé méchanique pour determiner la composition des roches. *C. R. Acad. Sci. (Par.)*, **25**, 544
3. Rogers, C. A. (1950–51). Quoted by Short, R. H. D., Alveolar Epithelium in relation to Growth of the Lung. *Phil. Trans. B*, **235**, 35
4. Weibel, E. R. (1963). Principles and Methods for the Morphometric Study of the Lung and Other Organs. *Lab. Invest.*, **12**, 131
5. Freere, R. H. and Weibel, E. R. (1966). Stereological techniques in microscopy. *J. Roy. Micro. Soc.*, **87**, 25
6. Dunnill, M. S. (1968). Quantitative methods in Histology. In: *Recent Advances in Clinical Pathology*. (S. C. Dyke, editor) (London: Churchill)
7. Aherne, W. (1970). Quantitative Methods in Histology. *J. Med. Lab. Technol.*, **27**, 160
8. Aherne, W. (1966). A Weight Relationship between the Human Fetus and Placenta. *Biol, Neonat.*, **10**, 113
9. Brody, S. and Proctor, R. C. (1932). *Univ. Missouri Agr. Exp. Sta. Res. Bull.*, **166**, 89
10. Smith, R. E. (1956). Quantitative relation between liver mitochondria metabolism and total body weight in mammals. *Ann. N.Y. Acad. Sci.*, **62**, 403
11. Bertalanffy, L. (1960). In: *Fundamental Aspects of Normal and Malignant Growth* (W. W. Nowinski, editor) (New York: Elsevier Publishing Co.)
12. Sholl, D. A. (1954). In: *Dynamics of Growth Processes*. (E. J. Boell, editor) (Princeton University Press)
13. Wilkin, P. (1960). In: *The Placenta and Fetal Membranes*. (C. A. Villce, editor) (Baltimore: University Park Press)
14. Aherne, W. Unpublished observations

CHAPTER 6

Physiology: Transfer and Barrier Function

Joseph Dancis and Henning Schneider

Introduction

The placenta in the human arises as a specialised organ from the chorion supplied by allantoic vessels. It retains throughout pregnancy the primary role of membranes, that is a selective permeability of materials. With particulate matter, such as blood cells, transfer is severely restricted, a function aptly described as the 'placental barrier'. At the other end of the spectrum, the transfer of many essential nutrients is accelerated by a variety of transport mechanisms. Although the placenta shares basic functions with even simple cell membranes, it must be assumed that modifications have been introduced to make it more effective in its specialised role in pregnancy and caution must be exercised in extrapolating to the placenta from results obtained in the study of other membranes. There are, in fact, a series of membranes interposed between the maternal and fetal circulations, beginning with the capillary membranes.

It is even hazardous to generalise concerning transport among placentas of different species. There are easily visible anatomical differences between the placentas of the ungulates and of the human, for example, and there are also functional differences. And yet, because of technical advantages offered to the experimentalist, the sheep has become a particularly useful animal for the study of placental function and fetal physiology. Because of an understandable reluctance to subject the pregnant human to investigative studies, much of the information concerning placental transfer derives from animal experiments. Similarities do abound in mammalian physiology, and many of the observations in animals undoubtedly are pertinent to the human.

However, identity of function must not be assumed.

In this chapter, we shall be primarily concerned with the physiological transfer of materials normally found in maternal or fetal blood. The role of the placenta will be emphasised. The importance of the maternal supply line will be considered in Chapter 10.

The Placental Barrier

The concept of a placental barrier has changed over the years. Ancient anatomists believed that the maternal and fetal circulations were continuous with each other, and that there was no barrier. The early efforts of modern physiologists were directed towards demonstrating that the maternal and fetal circulations were completely independent. More recently the stress has been on defining the imperfections of the barrier.

The possibility that fetal red blood cells may, on occasion, enter the maternal circulation was first suggested by clinical observations related to erythroblastosis fetalis. Direct evidence became available with the development of histochemical methods for the identification of fetal haemoglobin. Leakage of fetal erythrocytes into the maternal circulation could be detected in almost half the investigated cases, the incidence increasing progressively throughout pregnancy[1]. Transfer of red blood cells in the reverse direction was considerably less frequent (less than 4%)[2, 3].

It has been generally assumed that the leakage of fetal erythrocytes occurs through minute ruptures of delicate villous vessels. The frequent detection of trophoblast cells in the maternal circulation lent support to this hypothesis[4]. However, it is also possible that bulk flow of fetal blood across the placenta follows transient increases in intravascular pressure within chorionic capillaries, such as might be produced by a temporary increase in resistance in the venous circuit. The plausibility of this mechanism has been demonstrated in the guinea pig[5]. Progressively increasing the pressure in the umbilical vein produced a transfer across the placenta of water and plasma proteins followed by blood cells. When the pressure was returned to normal, evidence of leak disappeared. The anatomical arrangement in the human of unsupported chorionic villi suspended in the maternal placental lake would seem to favour such a mechanism, with the direction of flow predominantly from fetus to mother. Increases in pressure in the intervillous space would tend to collapse the chorionic vessels.

The emphasis on the imperfections of the barrier must not obscure the fact that it is generally very effective. Estimates of the amount of cells transferred are very small, of the order of a fraction of millilitre per day. Such events may be of considerable significance immunologically, but not nutritionally. Other mechanisms of placental transfer are necessary to meet the nutritional requirements of the fetus.

Gas Transport

The placenta has been described as the 'fetal lung'. As an organ for gas exchange, it is far less efficient than the lung[6]. The diffusion rate for gases per unit weight of placenta is approximately one fiftieth that of lung. The multiple functions of the placenta have required the sacrifice of efficiency of gas transfer. However, many of the fundamental principles that are pertinent to pulmonary respiration are also applicable to the placenta, with one major difference. The exchange of gases across the placenta is between two blood circulations.

It is generally believed that gases cross the placenta by *simple diffusion*. Fick's law★ describes the factors that influence the rate of diffusion. The driving force is the concentration difference on both sides of the membrane, in the present instance the difference in partial pressures of the physically dissolved gas in the maternal and fetal circulations. The ease with which a particular compound diffuses through a membrane is defined by its diffusion coefficient and is related to its physico–chemical characteristics. In general, the larger the molecular size, the more polar and the more highly charged the molecule, the more slowly it will diffuse through a membrane. And finally, the rate of transfer will be influenced by the thickness of the membrane and the area of the membrane available for exchange.

The essentials of Fick's law are classically simple and easy to grasp. Application to placental transfer is commonly complicated by circulatory factors controlling the rate of delivery and removal from the placenta. Furthermore

★ Fick's diffusion equation may be stated as follows:

$$\frac{dm}{dt} = \frac{DF}{b}(C_1 - C_2)$$

$\dfrac{dm}{dt}$ = amount transferred per unit time

D = diffusion coefficient

F = area of exchange

b = thickness of membrane

$C_1 - C_2$ = concentration gradient

As applied to gases: D = diffusion coefficient × solubility coefficient

$C_1 - C_2$ = partial pressure gradient

$\dfrac{DF}{b}$ = diffusion capacity: amount of gas which diffuses through the membrane per unit time per unit partial pressure gradient

Diffusion resistance is $\dfrac{1}{\text{diffusion capacity}}$ [7]

circulating materials are often protein-bound, and that may also affect transfer rates. Despite these limitations and the frequent lack of basic data required for accurate application of Fick's equation, the principles offer a useful structure for discussion.

Oxygen transfer

Attempts to apply Fick's equation to oxygen transfer will illustrate some of the inherent difficulties.*

The diffusion capacity (see footnote on Fick's equation, p. 100) is commonly used to evaluate membrane permeability. In order to determine placental diffusion capacity for oxygen the mean partial pressure gradient is necessary. It has not been possible to obtain accurate measurements of the partial pressure of oxygen on both sides of the placental membrane in the area of gas exchange, and so the pressure gradient is generally estimated from measurements made in the uterine and umbilical vein. The mean pressure gradient for oxygen across the placenta has been reported to be 19–24 mmHg[8]. This relatively large oxygen partial pressure gradient would indicate a low diffusion capacity suggesting that oxygen delivery to the fetus is partially limited by diffusion resistance of the membrane.

There is, however, reason to question this. The presence of 'shunting' in maternal and fetal circulations could introduce sizable errors (Figure 6.1).

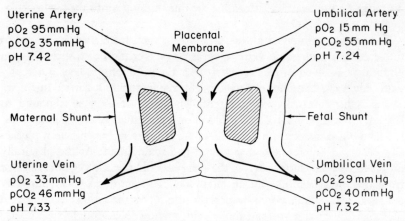

Uterine Artery
pO_2 95 mm Hg
pCO_2 35 mmHg
pH 7.42

Placental Membrane

Umbilical Artery
pO_2 15 mm Hg
pCO_2 55 mmHg
pH 7.24

Maternal Shunt →

← Fetal Shunt

Uterine Vein
pO_2 33 mm Hg
pCO_2 46 mm Hg
pH 7.33

Umbilical Vein
pO_2 29 mm Hg
pCO_2 40 mm Hg
pH 7.32

Figure 6.1 Schematic representation of placental gas exchange (modified from Bartels et al.[1]). Blood values in the human from Bartels[12]. 'Shunts' represent blood flows that are not exposed to the membrane for exchange. Uterine and umbilical veins contain a mixture of blood from the shunts and of blood exposed to exchange at the membrane

* It has recently been reported that cytochrome P450 functions as a carrier for the transfer of oxygen across the placenta[9], which could make the laws of diffusion inapplicable. The study has yet to be confirmed.

In the human, it is possible that not all of the maternal blood that enters the intervillous space is exposed to the placental membrane. Some investigators believe that there is also shunting in the fetal circulation, but that is more controversial. The effect of shunting would be to give a falsely high estimate of the transplacental gradient, when deduced from measurements in the uterine and umbilical veins.

A second complicating feature in the interpretation of the transplacental gradient is oxygen consumption by the placenta. The placenta is a large, metabolically active organ which appears to require for itself as much as 10–30% of the oxygen delivered to it[10]. Fick's equation makes no allowance for the effect of this factor on the transplacental gradient.

Longo and co-workers[6] studied the diffusion characteristics of carbon monoxide in sheep placenta. With this information, they estimated the diffusion capacity for oxygen and concluded that diffusion resistance of the membrane was not limiting for oxygen transfer. The diffusion capacity was four times that previously estimated from the partial pressure gradients in uterine and umbilical veins indicating that a significant error had been introduced into the calculations.

More significant to the delivery of oxygen to the fetus are the circulatory factors. The amount of oxygen delivered to the placenta depends on the concentration in the maternal blood and the flow rate, and similar factors operative on the fetal side determine the rate of uptake into the fetal circulation.

The processes involved in the release of oxygen from maternal blood to the placenta are the same as those effecting oxygenation of tissues. Oxygen physically dissolved in plasma determines the diffusion gradient but represents only a small amount of oxygen delivered (0·30 ml O_2 carried in 100 ml plasma when normally oxygenated). The bulk of oxygen is bound to haemoglobin (15·8 ml/100 ml of blood under normal conditions).

The oxygen dissociation curve describes the equilibrium between physically dissolved oxygen and that bound to haemoglobin. As the physically dissolved oxygen diffuses across the placenta, additional oxygen is released from maternal haemoglobin. In fetal blood, oxygen uptake is favoured by a higher haemoglobin concentration (ca 10 gm% in the mother as compared to 12 gm% in the fetus) and more avid binding to haemoglobin, i.e. at a given partial pressure more oxygen is bound in fetal than in maternal blood (Figure 6.2).

The difference in the oxygen dissociation curves between maternal and fetal blood is the result of the interaction of adult and fetal haemoglobin with 2,3 diphosphoglycerate. The effect of 2,3 diphosphoglycerate is to release oxygen from haemoglobin. The concentration of this compound is

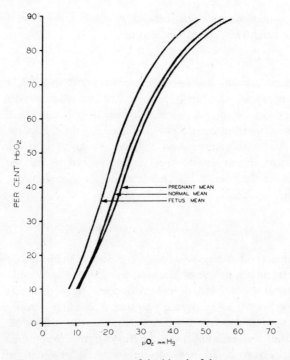

Figure 6.2 Oxygen dissociation curves of the blood of the non-pregnant and pregnant woman and the human fetus. (From Reid, Ryan, and Benirschke[122] as adapted from the article by Darling, Smith, et al.[123])

about the same in fetal and maternal erythrocytes but the effectiveness in releasing oxygen is greater with adult haemoglobin[11]. The transfer of oxygen to the fetus is also favoured by the transfer of carbon dioxide in the reverse direction (Bohr effect).

Efficiency of exchange is influenced by the relation of the maternal and fetal circulations to each other. The sheep placenta, with concurrent flow (the direction of blood flow in maternal and fetal capillaries of the placenta is in parallel) has the least efficient design, and the rabbit with countercurrent flow has the most efficient[12]. The human placenta lies somewhere in between[13].

The older literature contains considerable discussion and some controversy concerning the relative efficiency of the various placentas: the 'thick' v. the 'thin' placentas and countercurrent v. concurrent circulations[14]. Some of the controversy arose from confusion between efficiency and effectiveness. The sheep placenta which is both thick and has concurrent circulations is still capable of nourishing the relatively large lamb fetus even though not designed as efficiently as the rabbit placenta.

Carbon dioxide transfer

The transfer of carbon dioxide from the fetal to maternal circulations is affected primarily by circulating factors. The diffusion constant is twenty times higher than for oxygen, so that membrane resistance is clearly not a factor. Carbon dioxide is carried in blood in three forms, physically dissolved (about 8%), as bicarbonate (about 62%), and bound to haemoglobin (30%). The three forms are in equilibrium. Release of carbon dioxide from fetal haemoglobin at the placenta is facilitated by the simultaneous uptake of oxygen (Haldane effect).

Water

The introduction of isotopes to medical research made possible new approaches to the investigation of placental transfer. An early and provocative study was the measurement of the exchange rate of deuteriated water[15]. The rate rose progressively during pregnancy reaching a peak of 3·5 litres per hour at 35 weeks, and then fell towards term to 1·5 litres per hour. The medical world was unfamiliar at the time with concepts of molecular exchange and was confused by visions of great tides of water gushing across the placenta. It was, however, clear to all that water could pass readily across the placenta and that maximal efficiency was reached a few weeks before birth. The latter aspect attracted considerable attention providing support for the emerging concept of postmaturity and placental insufficiency.

The clinician was more interested in the net transfer of water than in exchange rates. The response to osmotic forces was first demonstrated in the rabbit[16]. A hypertonic solution of sucrose was infused into the pregnant doe raising the maternal osmotic pressure approximately 30 milliosmoles. Within 30 minutes, the osmotic pressure of the fetal plasma had risen to levels equivalent to the mother as a result of rapid movement of water into the maternal circulation with accompanying dehydration of the fetus[17]. Similar observations were soon made in other species including man[18-20].

Although these experimental observations demonstrated that water crosses the placenta in response to an osmotic gradient, it has not been possible to obtain evidence that this is the mechanism for the net transfer of water to the fetus required for its growth. Attempts to demonstrate the existence of a physiological gradient in osmotic pressure across the placenta have been generally unsuccessful. However, the rapidity with which water responds to osmotic forces may be expected to prevent the development of a detectable gradient. The most reasonable explanation of the accumulation of water in the fetal compartment is the creation of osmotic forces as a result of synthesis of fetal tissues containing macromolecules and electrolytes.

Haemodynamic gradients may also produce a net transfer of water across the placenta. These observations were first made in the guinea pig[5] but similar observations have been made in the isolated, perfused human placenta[21]. As explained above (see Placental Barrier) the direction of flow is more likely to be towards the maternal circulation.

Electrolytes

Sodium

The exchange rate of sodium across the human placenta has been measured, with results similar to those obtained with deuterium[22]. There is an increase in the efficiency of exchange as pregnancy progresses, reaching a peak at 35 weeks gestation, and then a rapid fall towards term (Figure 6.3). Anatomical correlations have been suggested in efforts to explain the functional

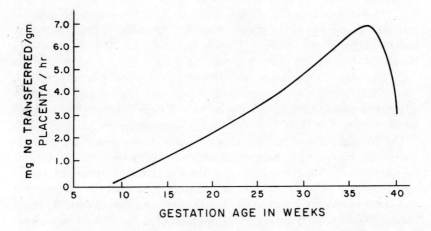

Figure 6.3 Sodium exchange rate as related to gestational age (from Flexner *et al.*[22]). The efficiency of exchange across the placenta reaches a peak about 35 weeks gestation and then falls towards term

changes. The progressive vascularisation and thinning of the barrier between the maternal and fetal circulations that occurs during the course of gestation increase the area of the membrane and reduce the distance required for sodium to diffuse. Towards term, the deposition of fibrinoid on the surface of the villi may contribute towards lowering the efficiency of exchange, though this is probably not the only factor.

A comparative study of placental transfer among several species yielded results that were consistent with this interpretation[23]. The ungulate has a 'thick' placenta, i.e. there are several cellular layers interposed between the maternal and fetal circulations. In contrast, in the guinea pig and human placentas, erosion of the endometrium overlying the maternal capillaries has produced 'thin' placentas. The exchange rate for sodium in the latter is considerably faster than it is in the ungulate.

Flexner and his colleagues were also responsible for introducing the concept of 'safety factor', expressed as the ratio of placental transfer to fetal requirements. The safety factor for sodium at term was calculated to be over 1000 because the exchange rate was 1000 times the rate of accumulation of sodium by the fetus. The concept attracted immediate interest and the determination of the safety factor of a series of materials followed. There are limitations and potential pitfalls in this approach.

(1) Fetal requirements are often difficult to estimate. Materials that can be synthesised or degraded present a complex problem. Even substances that are not metabolically altered, like sodium, may enter into essential reactions in addition to the requirements for deposition in fetal tissue, e.g. sodium exchange appears to play a role in the transfer of amino acids and glucose across a variety of membranes.

(2) Exchange rates may not be indicative of the capacity for net transfer.

(3) Transfer rate may be controlled by fetal need. This would automatically yield a safety factor of one, but it does not mean that transfer could not be increased to keep pace with increased fetal requirements.

The transfer rates of sodium and antipyrine across guinea pig placenta have been compared[24]. Antipyrine diffuses very rapidly across organic membranes including the placenta. The decisive factors in the rate of transfer are the rates of delivery and removal of antipyrine from the placenta, the flow-rates exerting a major influence. Transfer of antipyrine has therefore been described as 'flow-limited'. The diffusion of sodium across the placenta is considerably slower. Although major changes in flow-rate alter the transfer rate of sodium, the decisive factors are generally the nature and condition of the membrane. The transfer of sodium has therefore been characterised as 'membrane-limited'. Similar observations have been made in the subhuman primate[25].

Potassium

Relatively little effort has been expended on the study of potassium transfer. The older literature had reported that fetal levels were higher than maternal.

The studies were repeated when flame photometer techniques became available with the conclusion that maternal and fetal levels closely approximated to each other[26]. However, an observation made originally by Stewart and Welt[27], and confirmed in our laboratory, made it clear that factors other than diffusion control the fetal level. Fetal potassium levels in the rat remained normal in spite of sizable reductions in the mother induced by potassium-poor diets. It was noted that the potassium concentration in the placenta fell only slightly, and it was suggested that this may have served to maintain the fetal blood level[28]. It is clear, however, that simple diffusion is not adequate to explain the relation of maternal and fetal levels.

In contrast to the effect of potassium deprivation, raising the maternal level acutely with infusions produced an increase in fetal concentration[28].

Anion transfer

Chloride exchange rate in the subhuman primate approximates that of sodium[25]. The levels in the maternal and fetal circulations are normally about equal. *Iodide* levels are higher in fetal than maternal blood in the guinea pig and rabbit. The gradient is maintained by a transport mechanism that is inhibited by thiocyanate[29]. A gradient is also maintained for phosphate in the guinea pig, with higher levels in the fetus. The 'safety factor' has been estimated as one[30, 31].

Divalent cations

The transfer of *iron* has been studied extensively in the rabbit[32]. Iron circulates in the plasma partially bound to a specific protein, transferrin. Maternal iron is released from transferrin at the placenta[33] by an active metabolic process[34] similar to that described for the reticulocyte. Fetal requirements for iron in the last trimester are great. By term, over 90% of the iron turned over in the maternal plasma is directed towards the fetus[32] and there is no transfer in the reverse direction. Fetal blood levels are higher than maternal so that transfer is against a gradient. Changes in maternal metabolism induced by such factors as infection may alter the delivery of iron to the fetus[32].

The importance of the placenta in extracting iron from maternal plasma was clearly demonstrated by experiments in which the fetuses were removed. The placenta concentrated within itself an amount of iron equivalent to that normally found in both the placenta and fetus. The factors controlling release to the fetus have not been defined.

The placental transfer of *zinc* has been studied in the rabbit[35]. As with iron, there is a sharp increase in transfer rate about the 21st day of gestation, but the transfer rate is slower and is bi-directional. Following fetectomy, the placenta removes as much zinc from the maternal circulation as does the intact feto-placental unit.

Calcium concentration in the human is higher in the fetal blood than it is in the maternal circulation[36]. The gradient includes both the protein-bound and ultrafiltrable fractions. In the guinea pig, net transfer of calcium to the fetus continues against very high gradients, experimentally induced[37]. Exchange across the placenta is bi-directional with a calculated safety factor in the subhuman primate of 6–10[38].

The net transfer of *magnesium* in the guinea pig is also against a concentration gradient of the ultrafiltrable fraction[39]. An active transport mechanism is assumed. There is no consistent gradient in the human[40].

Carbohydrates

Glucose is the major metabolic fuel for the fetus. Its molecular weight and high polarity suggest that diffusion rate across the placenta would be slow, possibly inadequate to meet fetal requirements. Widdas, from his analysis of the kinetics of glucose transfer in the sheep, has concluded that the diffusion is 'facilitated' by a transport mechanism[41]. Facilitated diffusion is visualised as involving a carrier molecule that shuttles back and forth across the membrane, speeding the rate of transfer in either direction, and yet not requiring the expenditure of energy. In this last respect, it differs from 'active transfer' as defined by the physiologists. It is resistant to metabolic poisons, and is incapable of transfer against a gradient or 'uphill'.

The placental transfer of glucose is stereospecific, a common characteristic of carrier mechanisms. Fructose, a ketohexose with the same molecular weight as glucose, is transferred at a much slower rate than glucose in several animals including the human[42–45]. A particularly convincing demonstration of stereospecifity was provided in the guinea pig with xylose[46]. D-xylose, a pentose which appears to use the same transport mechanism as glucose, was transferred about three times as fast as its stereoisomer, L-xylose. Competitive inhibition among hexoses has been demonstrated[47, 48], even though the capacity of the transport mechanism appears to be much larger than that for amino acids (Figure 6.4)[49]. The transfer rate of glucose across human placenta is extremely rapid, approaching that of antipyrine, and is about equivalent in both directions[50].

The maternal level of glucose in the human is consistently higher than in the fetus, approximately 96 and 75 mg% respectively as measured at term. The gradient *in utero* may actually be higher, because the stress of delivery may raise the fetal concentration[51]. Net transfer to the fetus is therefore 'downhill.' The factors that maintain the gradient may be similar to those

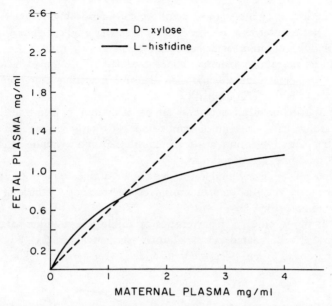

Figure 6.4 Placental transfer of carbohydrate and amino acid (from Dancis, J. *et al.*[49]). Histidine and xylose were infused into pregnant guinea pigs for 30 minutes and then fetal and maternal plasma concentrations were determined. The straight line relation for D-xylose, which was maintained with maternal concentrations as high as 10 mg/ml, indicates large capacity of transport mechanism and contrasts with histidine

discussed for oxygen:arterio-venous shunts, placental metabolism, and possibly fetal consumption. Diffusion resistance appears to be very small.

An interesting species peculiarity is found in the ungulate. The placenta has an efficient mechanism for converting maternal glucose into fructose which is secreted into the fetal circulation. Although the same capability exists in the human, the amount of fructose that is synthesised is negligible[52].

Amino Acids

Amino acids are delivered to the fetus for protein synthesis, and apparently contribute to requirements for fetal energy[53]. A mechanism has been developed to accelerate placental transport which shares many of the operational features described for glucose (facilitated diffusion) but differs in two important respects typical of active transport: energy is expended in transport and transfer can occur against a gradient.

The evidence for specific transport mechanisms for amino acids is simply enumerated:

(1) Fetal levels for most amino acids are consistently higher than maternal[54-57]. Net transfer towards the fetus is against a gradient. The gradient varies for different amino acids between 1·2 and 4·0[57].

(2) With increasing maternal concentrations of an amino acid, the transfer rate increases initially and then plateaus, indicating saturation of the transport mechanism (Figure 6.4)[49].

(3) Simultaneous infusion of two amino acids may reduce transfer rate of each amino acid as a result of competition for transport sites[58].

(4) The natural L-amino acids are transferred more rapidly than the D-form, indicating stereospecificity[59-61].

(5) Metabolic poisons inhibit the uptake of amino acids by placental slices, probably the first step in transplacental transport, indicating a dependence on energy[62, 63].

Two of the significant characteristics of amino acid transfer have been demonstrated with isolated, perfused human placenta (Figure 6.5). Equivalent concentrations of D- and L-leucine were added to the perfusates. The transfer

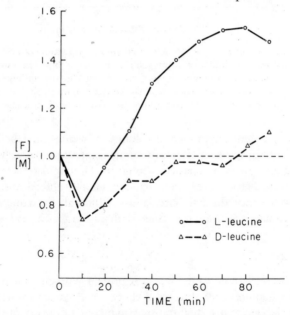

Figure 6.5 Stereospecificity of placental transfer of leucine (from Schneider, H. and Dancis, J.[124]). An isolated cotyledon from human placenta was perfused *in vitro*. D- and L-leucine were added in equal concentration to maternal and fetal perfusates. Following an initial drop in level in the fetal circulation because of dilution with buffer retained within the placenta, L-leucine concentration increases rapidly and a gradient is established (Fetal: Maternal concentration $> 1 : 0$)

rate of L-leucine was considerably faster than its stereoisomer, and a gradient was established with the concentration of the natural amino acid higher in the fetal circulation.

There are many individual differences among the amino acids. The transfer rate of cysteine–cystine is slow and no gradient is established[64]. Rates of uptake by placental slices and the intracellular:extracellular ratios achieved by a series of amino acids suggest different transport systems[21]. These require further investigation.

Plasma Proteins

Maternal plasma proteins, in spite of their large molecular size, are transferred to the fetus. Such transfer has been demonstrated for several plasma protein fractions in the human[65] and, given sufficiently sensitive techniques, could probably be demonstrated for all. However, the transfer rate is considerably slower than for amino acids from which the fetus synthesises most of its proteins[66].

Route of transfer—There are interesting species differences. In the human and subhuman primate, transfer is across the chorioallantoic placenta[67, 68]. In the rabbit and guinea pig, maternal plasma proteins are secreted into the uterine cavity and then absorbed by the splanchnopleure, a fetal membrane derived from the yolk sac[69]. There appears to be only minimal protein transfer to the fetus of the ungulate, a deficit that is compensated for by intestinal absorption of proteins from maternal colostrum during the first days of life.

Mechanism—Proteins are believed to pass through membranes by pinocytosis, which is visualised as an engulfment process somewhat analogous to the better known phagocytosis by macrophages. The transport process appears to be less efficient early in pregnancy than towards term[70–72]. Differences in transfer rates among proteins cannot be explained by molecular weight. For example, IgG gamma globulin is over twice the size of albumin but is transferred to the fetus at a faster rate[67, 68]. This selectivity appears to depend on specific receptors on the placental surface[73].

Significance to the fetus—The human infant is born with an IgG level approximately that of the mother. The fetus *in utero* is exposed to few antigens, so that circulating antibodies are derived transplacentally from the mother. The delivery of maternal IgG to the fetus is of major importance to survival. Two factors make it possible; the selective mechanism that leads to a more rapid transfer rate than for other plasma proteins and the relatively low utilisation rate by the fetus of IgG. The latter has not, in fact, been measured, but the long half-life of IgG after birth ($T\frac{1}{2} = ca$ 20–30 days) makes it a reasonable presumption.

Of all plasma protein fractions for which we have information, only IgG is known to fulfil this role towards the fetus. Serum albumin also has a long half-life, and the transfer rate, though slower than for IgG, is probably sufficiently rapid to provide a significant amount of albumin to the fetus. However, the fetal liver is capable of synthesising albumin from early gestation[74] so that the fetus is not dependent on maternal supplies. The half-lives of other plasma proteins are considerably shorter so that it is unlikely that maternal contributions play a significant role. Insignificant amounts of immunoglobulins, other than IgG, reach the fetus.

Polypeptide Hormones and Thyroxin

The placental transfer of these endocrines is generally too slow to affect the fetus significantly. It appears that the fetal endocrine system matures early and functions autonomously. With sufficiently sensitive techniques, transfer of maternal endocrines can usually be demonstrated, as it has been with radioactive insulin[75], thyroxin and tri-iodothyronine[76]. However, clinical and experimental situations indicate the inadequacy of such transfer.

Acute changes induced in maternal glucose levels result in insulin responses in maternal and fetal circulations that show no correlation[77]. Anencephalic monsters have low circulating levels of growth hormone[78] and hypoplastic adrenals[79] due to lack of ACTH stimulation indicating the inability of maternal pituitary hormones to compensate for fetal insufficiency. Athyreotic cretins have signs of thyroid deficiency at birth. Hypophysectomy in fetal sheep causes a fall in thyroid stimulating hormone and thyroxine[80]. The fetus also synthesises its own parathyroid hormone[81].

The relative impermeability of the placenta to the protein hormones is clearly demonstrated by chorionic gonadotropin and placental lactogen. Both are synthesised in the placenta and secreted into the maternal circulation where the levels are considerably higher than in fetal blood. Thus, the serum level in the mother of the latter is 5–10 μg/ml and only ·02 μg/ml in the fetus[82].

From the standpoint of placental function, it would be of interest to know the mechanism by which the limited transfer of polypeptides does occur, whether by pinocytosis or some other means, and whether molecular size speeds or retards transfer. Such investigations have not been undertaken.

Lipids

Many of the processes involved in the transfer of lipid-soluble or hydrophobic materials are analogous to those discussed under oxygen transfer. The physically dissolved lipids, representing only a small fraction of the total amount delivered to the placenta, produce the diffusion pressure across the placenta. The protein-bound lipids in the plasma (similar to the oxygen carried by haemoglobin) provide a reservoir of additional materials that, in theory, may be released into the plasma or directly to the placenta for transport. Within the placenta, the rate of movement is determined by the diffusion resistance without apparent intervention of specialised transport mechanisms.

Free fatty acids circulate in plasma bound to albumin. The levels are low but the turn-over rate is fast so that large amounts of free fatty acids are potentially available for transfer to the fetus. The amounts actually transferred appear to vary considerably among the species: they are high in the guinea pig[83, 84] and rabbit[85] and low in the sheep[86] and human[87]. Analyses of subcutaneous fat of the human fetus and newborn suggest that during the second trimester of pregnancy the transfer of fatty acids from the mother keeps pace with fetal requirements for the synthesis of adipose tissue. However, the very rapid deposition of fat towards term exceeds the capacity for placental transfer and *de novo* synthesis by the fetus accounts for most of the fat[87, 88].

Phospholipids and cholesterol are transported in plasma in more complex association in the lipoprotein fraction. In the rabbit, the phospholipids are released from the plasma proteins, and hydrolysed in the placenta. The lipids are resynthesised into phospholipids, by fetal liver[89, 90] and possibly by placenta. The amount of lipids made available to the fetus by this mechanism is small. The transfer rate for cholesterol is also slow, but the utilisation rate by the fetus is low so that significant amounts of fetal cholesterol in the rat[91], guinea pig[84], and monkey[92] are derived from the mother. There is little information concerning the transfer rate of neutral triglycerides but it also appears to be very slow[84].

Steroids—The placental transfer of *estrogens* and their conjugates has been carefully studied in the guinea pig and human[93, 94]. The unconjugated estrogens are transferred very rapidly in both directions, contrasting sharply with the restricted transfer of the polar conjugates, the sulphates and glucosiduronates. Sulphatases in the placenta cleave the sulphates to the unconjugated form facilitating their transfer. There are no hydrolases in placenta for the glucosiduronates. *Progesterone* and *testosterone*[95] are also transferred rapidly across guinea pig placenta. Only the former has been studied in the human[96], with similar results. Diffusion of *cortisol* across sheep placenta is limited[97]. In the human fetus at term, cortisone is primarily of maternal origin whereas only 25% of the cortisol is derived from the mother[98]. These observations do not provide direct information on transport rates or mechanisms.

Bilirubin—The transfer of bilirubin adheres to the same basic principles described for the estrogens. Unconjugated bilirubin is rapidly transferred across the placenta whereas the glucosiduronate is not[99, 100]. The suppression of glucosiduronation in the fetus prior to birth facilitates the transplacental excretion of bilirubin, and explains the absence of jaundice at birth in the infant affected with congenital haemolytic disease[101] (Figure 6.6). The

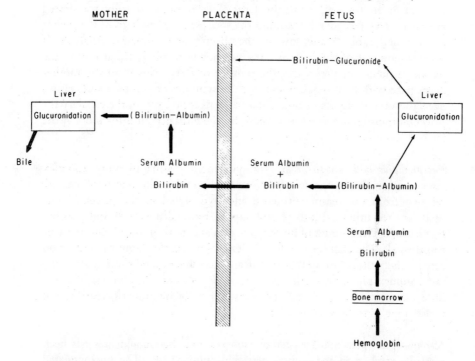

Figure 6.6 Antepartum excretion of bilirubin (from Dancis, J.[125]). Fetal bilirubin is transferred from fetal serum albumin through the placenta to the maternal circulation, then conjugated by maternal liver and excreted into bile. Fetal synthesis of poorly trans ferred glucuronides is suppressed

placental transfer of bilirubin and the glucosiduronate in the reverse direction shows the same selectivity. A case has been reported in which the mother was intensely jaundiced for 3 weeks prior to delivery[102]. At birth, the level of indirect bilirubin in the infant was equivalent to that in the mother, but the direct bilirubin was much lower.

Vitamins

Fat-soluble vitamins

The transfer of the fat-soluble vitamins (A, D, E, and K) are assumed to resemble in mechanism those described for lipids. The vitamins are transported in plasma bound to proteins, sometimes in lipoprotein complexes. The mechanisms and ease of release to the placenta have not been defined. Placental transfer is believed to be by simple diffusion. The levels in the fetal circulation are generally lower than in the maternal. It has been assumed that transfer rates are low, but there is little supporting evidence.

Vitamin A circulates in plasma as the vitamin, retinol, and as the pro-vitamin, carotene. The maternal and fetal concentrations of carotene vary in parallel, with the fetal concentrations maintained at about one-tenth the maternal level. The fetal concentration of retinol appears to vary independently of the maternal, although it also remains generally lower [103, 104]. The observations have been interpreted as indicating that maternal carotene is transferred to the fetus which converts it to the relatively poorly transferred retinol. Studies of *vitamin D* transfer have been hampered by inadequate analytical methods. Placental transfer of *vitamins E*[105] and *K*[106] has been demonstrated in rats using radioactive materials, but the design of the experiments permits no conclusions concerning rates or mechanisms of transfer. Cord blood levels of vitamin E, in the human, are lower than in the mother[107].

The fetal blood levels of *water-soluble vitamins* are higher than the maternal suggesting active transport processes, and differing in this respect from the lipid-soluble vitamins. The vitamins commonly circulate in the blood in more than one form, making uncertain the interpretation of transplacental equilibria.

Vitamin C is found in blood as reduced L-ascorbic acid and as oxidised dehydroascorbic acid. In the human, the levels of the latter are approximately equivalent in maternal and fetal blood, whereas the ascorbic acid concentration is higher in cord blood[108]. The mechanisms of placental transport have been explored in the guinea pig. Dehydroascorbic acid is transferred far more rapidly than L-ascorbic acid leading to the reasonable deduction that the oxidised vitamin is preferentially transferred across the placenta, then reduced to the slowly transferred L-ascorbic acid by the fetal liver, thus establishing a gradient in the fetal circulation. However, the isolated, perfused human placenta is capable of independently establishing a gradient with L-ascorbic acid[109].

Vitamin B_1 (thiamine) is almost twice as high in cord blood, in the human, than in the mother[110]. In the guinea pig, a gradient exists for free thiamine but placental transfer is slow[111].

Vitamin B_2 (riboflavin) measured as free riboflavin, is approximately four times higher in cord blood than maternal blood, whereas flavin adenine dinucleotide (FAD) is twice as high in maternal blood[112]. The placenta can convert FAD to riboflavin. Based on these observations, it was suggested that the placenta is relatively impermeable to both forms of the vitamin, that FAD is taken up by placenta from maternal blood, converted to ribo-flavin and released to the fetus.

Vitamin B_6 (pyridoxol) blood levels are lower in the pregnant woman than in the non-pregnant, and fetal levels are about three times higher than maternal[113]. Administration of pyridoxol to the mother increases fetal blood levels of pyridoxol and pyriodoxol phosphate. The observations have been interpreted as a diversion of the vitamin from maternal to fetal needs.

Vitamin B_{12} studies have yielded similar results. Maternal blood levels are reduced during pregnancy, and fetal levels exceed maternal[114, 115]. Intestinal absorption of the vitamin increases during pregnancy, most of which is transferred to the fetus[116].

Folic and folinic acid as measured by microbiological assays, are both higher in cord blood than in maternal blood[117].

Nucleic Acids

Nucleic acids are necessary for such fundamental life processes as the genera-tion of energy and the control of protein synthesis. The ability to synthesise nucleic acids from small molecules is widely distributed in living cells. It was therefore not surprising when it was reported that the fetal rat synthe-sised the great bulk of its nucleic acids *de novo*[118]. It was noted that the observations did not exclude the possibility that the acid-soluble fraction (purine bases, nucleosides and nucleotides) might cross the placenta. Hayashi *et al.*[119] have since shown that such transfer can take place but its role in the fetal economy remains undefined.

Fetal to Maternal Transfer

Most placental transport mechanisms are bidirectional; however, under normal circumstances, it would be expected that the fetus would transfer to the mother only the end products of fetal metabolism, namely, carbon dioxide and water, and the nitrogenous products, urea, uric acid, creatinine, and bilirubin. Of these, carbon dioxide and bilirubin transfer have already been discussed. The metabolic production of water has been estimated to be less than that needed for growth, so that net transfer would be towards the fetus.

Of the nitrogenous end products, other than bilirubin, only urea has been adequately studied. The placenta, like other membranes, is easily permeable to urea[25, 120]. The clearance in monkeys is 15 ml per minute per kilogram fetal weight. Transfer is probably by simple diffusion.

Defects in Placental Transport

It is not too difficult to envisage intrinsic defects in placental transport. Reduction in the area of exchange such as occurs in separations of the placenta or in infarcts must certainly reduce the potential for transfer. Relatively gross alterations in the membrane such as deposition of fibrinoid, edema and thickening of the basement membrane may be expected to change the diffusion characteristics of the placenta. Possibly more subtle modifications in placental composition are also operative. Active transport mechanisms are believed to involve specific proteins, the synthesis of which is under genetic control. Genetic diseases of transport involving the kidney and the intestine have been described, and it is possible that the placenta may suffer from similar defects.

Although it is perfectly reasonable to assume that such defects in placental transport do occur, and probably many more, there is virtually a complete absence of supporting data. Without clinical methods for measuring the efficiency of placental transport, the physician is forced to make crude guesses from pathological observations concerning the magnitude of physiological deficiencies. Flexner's observations[22] on the reduction in sodium and water exchange after the 35th week of gestation remains almost unique in the attempt to correlate function with anatomical changes. Somewhat more information is available on the effect on placental transfer of disturbances in maternal supply (see Chapter 10).

Table 6.1 Relative Levels of Some Constituents of Maternal and Cord Blood

	About equal	Lower in fetus	Higher in fetus
Amino acids			+
Urea	+		
Uric acid	+		
Creatinine	+		
Inorganic P			+
Free fatty acids		+	
Cholesterol		+	
Glucose		+	
Lactic acid			+
Calcium			+
Magnesium	+		
Chloride	+		
Sodium	+		
Potassium	+		
Iron			+
Vitamins			
fat-soluble		+	
water-soluble			+
Chorionic gonadotrophin		+	
Placental lactagen		+	
Growth hormone			+

References

1. Cohen, F., Zuelzer, W. W., Gustafson, D. C. and Evans, M. M. (1964). Mechanisms of isoimmunization. 1: The transplacental passage of fetal erythrocytes in homospecific pregnancies. *Blood*, **23**, 621
2. Cohen, F. and Zuelzer, W. W. (1964). Identification of blood group antigens by immunofluorescence and its application to the detection of the transplacental passage of erythrocytes in mother and child. *Vox Sang.*, **9**, 75
3. Cohen, F. and Zuelzer, W. W. (1965). The transplacental passage of maternal erythrocytes into the fetus. *Amer. J. Obstet. Gynec.*, **93**, 566
4. Thomas, L., Douglas, G. W. and Carr, M. C. (1959). The continual migration of syncytical trophoblasts from the fetal placenta into the maternal circulation. *Trans. Assn. Amer. Phys.*, **72**, 140
5. Dancis, J., Brenner, M. and Money, W. L. (1962). Some factors affecting the permeability of guinea pig placenta. *Amer. J. Obstet. Gynec.*, **84**, 570
6. Longo, L. D., Power, G. G. and Foster, R. E., II. (1967). Respiratory function of the placenta as determined with carbon monoxide in sheep and dogs. *J. Clin. Invest.*, **46**, 812
7. Bartels, H., Moll, W. and Metcalfe, J. (1962). Physiology of gas exchange in the human placenta. *Amer. J. Obstet. Gynec.*, **84**, 1714

8. Barran, D. H. (1952). Calculation of mean materials to fetal PO_2 differences from measurements to the O_2 tension in uterine and umbilical arterial and venous blood. *Yale J. Biol. Med.*, **24**, 169

9. Gurtner, G. H. and Burns, B. (1972). Possible facilitated transport of oxygen across the placenta. *Nature (London)*, **240**, 473

10. Campbell, A. G. M., Dawes, G. S., Fishman, A. P., Kyman, A. I. and James, G. B. (1966). The oxygen consumption of the placenta and fetal membranes in the sheep. *J. Physiol. (London)*, **182**, 439

11. Bauer, C., Ludwig, I. and Ludwig, M. (1968). Different effects of 2,3-diphosphoglycerate and adenosine triphosphate on the oxygen affinity of adult and foetal human haemoglobin. *Life Sci.*, **7**, 1339

12. Meschia, G., Battaglia, F. C. and Bruns, P. D. (1967). Theoretical and experimental study of transplacental diffusion. *J. Appl. Physiol.*, **22**, 1171

13. Bartels, H. and Moll, W. (1964). Passage of inert substances and oxygen in the human placenta. *Pflueger Arch. Ges. Physiol.*, **280**, 165

14. Flexner, L. B., editor (1955). *Gestation, Transaction of First Conference.* (New York: Corlies, Macy and Company, Inc.)

15. Hellman, L. M., Flexner, L. B., Wilde, W. S., Vosburgh, G. J. and Proctor, N. K. (1948). The permeability of the human placenta to water and the supply of water to the human fetus as determined with deuterium oxide. *Amer. J. Obstet. Gynec.*, **56**, 861

16. Dancis, J., Worth, M., Jr. and Schneidau, P. B. (1957). Effect of electrolyte disturbance in the pregnant rabbit on the fetus. *Amer. J. Physiol.*, **188.**, 535

17. Bruns, P. D., Linder, R. O., Drose, V. E. and Battaglia, F. (1963). The placental transfer of water from fetus to mother following the intravenous infusion of hypertonic mannitol to the maternal rabbit. *Amer. J. Obstet. Gynec.*, **86**, 160

18. Adolph, E. F. and Hoy, P. A. (1963). Regulation of electrolyte composition of fetal rat plasma. *Amer. J. Physiol.*, **204**, 392

19. Battaglia, F., Prystowsky, H., Smisson, C., Hellegers, A. E. and Bruns, P. (1960). Fetal blood studies. XIII: The effect of the administration of fluids intravenously to mothers upon the concentrations of water and electrolytes in plasma of human fetuses. *Pediatrics*, **25**, 2

20. Bruns, P. D., Hellegers, A. E., Seeds, A. E., Jr., Behrman, R. E. and Battaglia, F. C. (1964). Effects of osmotic gradients across the primate placenta upon fetal and placental water contents. *Pediatrics*, **34**, 407

21. Schneider, H., and Dancis J. (Unpublished observations)

22. Flexner, L. B., Cowie, D. B., Hellman, L. M., Wilde, W. S. and Vosburgh, G. J. (1948). The permeability of the human placenta to sodium in normal and abnormal pregnancies and the supply of sodium to the human fetus as determined with radioactive sodium. *Amer. J. Obstet. Gynec.*, **55**, 469

23. Flexner, L. B. and Gellhorn, A. (1942). The comparative physiology of placental tranfer. *Amer. J. Obstet. Gynec.*, **43**, 965

24. Dancis, J. and Money, W. L. (1960). Transfer of sodium and iodo-antipyrine across guinea pig placenta using an in situ perfusion technique. *Amer. J. Obstet. Gynec.*, **80**, 215

25. Battaglia, F. C., Behrman, R. E., Meschia, G., Seeds, A. E. and Bruns, P. D. (1968). Clearance of inert molecules, Na and Cl ions across the primate placenta. *Amer. J. Obstet. Gynec.*, **102**, 1135

26. Earle, D. P., Bakwin, H. and Hirsch, D. (1951). Plasma potassium level in newborn. *Proc. Soc. Exper. Biol. Med.*, **76**, 756

27. Stewart, E. L. and Welt, L. G. (1961). Protection of the fetus in experimental potassium depletion. *Amer. J. Physiol.*, **200**, 824

28. Dancis, J. and Springer, D. (1970). Fetal homeostasis in maternal malnutrition: Potassium and sodium deficiency. *Pediat. Res.*, **4**, 345

29. Logothetopoulos, J. H. and Scott, R. F. (1956). Active iodide transport across the placenta of the guinea pig, rabbit and rat. *J. Physiol.*, **132**, 365

30. Fuchs, F. and Fuchs, A. R. (1956). Studies in the placental transfer of phosphate in the guinea pig. *Acta Physiol. Scand.*, **38**, 379

31. Wilde, W. S., Cowie, D. B. and Flexner, L. B. (1946). Permeability of the placenta of the guinea pig to organic phosphate and its relation to fetal growth. *Amer. J. Physiol.*, **147**, 360

32. Bothwell, T. H., Pribella, W. F., Mebust, W. and Finch, C. A. (1958). Iron metabolism in the pregnant rabbit: Iron transport across the placenta. *Amer. J. Physiol.*, **193**, 615

33. Larkin, E. C., Weintraub, L. R. and Crosby, W. H. (1970). Iron transport across rabbit allantonic placenta. *Amer. J. Physiol.*, **218**, 7

34. Laurell, C. B. and Morgan, E. (1964). Iron exchange between transferrin and the placenta in the rat. *Acta Physiol. Scand.*, **62**, 271

35. Terry, C. W., Terry, B. E. and Davies, J. (1960). Transfer of zinc across the placenta and fetal membranes of the rabbit. *Amer. J. Physiol.*, **198**, 303

36. Delivoria-Papadopoulos, M., Battaglia, F. C., Bruns, P. D. and Meschia, G. (1967). Total protein-bound and ultrafiltrable calcium in maternal and fetal plasmas. *Amer. J. Physiol.*, **213**, 363

37. Twardock, A. R. and Austin, M. K. (1970). Calcium transfer in perfused guinea pig placenta. *Amer. J. Physiol.*, **219**, 540

38. MacDonald, N. S., Hutchinson, D. L., Hepler, M. and Flynn, E. (1965). Movement of calcium in both directions across the primate placenta. *Proc. Soc. Exper. Biol. Med.*, **119**, 476

39. Dancis, J., Springer, D. and Cohlan, S. Q. (1971). Fetal homeostasis in maternal malnutrition. II. Magnesium deprivation. *Pediat. Res.*, **5**, 131

40. Lipsitz, P. J. (1971). The clinical and biochemical effects of excess magnesium in the newborn. *Pediat.*, **47**, 501

41. Widdas, W. F. (1952). Inability of diffusion to account for placental glucose transfer in the sheep and consideration of the kinetics of a possible carrier transfer. *J. Physiol. (London)*, **118**, 23

42. Davies, J. (1955). Permeability of the rabbit placenta to glucose and fructose. *Amer. J. Physiol.*, **181**, 532

43. Holmberg, N. G., Kaplan, B., Karvonen, M. J., Lind, J. and Malm, M. (1956). Permeability of human placenta to glucose, fructose and xylose. *Acta Physiol. Scand.*, **36**, 291

44. Karvonen, M. J. (1949). Fructose of sheep fetal blood. *Ann. med. exper. et biol. Fenniae*, **27**, 197

45. Karvonen, M. J. and Räihä, N. (1954). Permeability of placenta of the guinea pig to glucose and fructose. *Acta Physiol. Scand.*, **31**, 194

46. Folkart, G. R., Dancis, J. and Money, W. L. (1960). Transfer of carbohydrates across guinea pig placenta. *Amer. J. Obstet. Gynec.*, **80**, 221

47. Colbert, R. M., Calton, F. M., Dinda, R. E. and Davies, J. (1958). Competitive transfer of sorbose and glucose in placenta of rabbit. *Proc. Soc. Exper. Biol. Med.*, **97**, 867

48. Ely, P. A. (1966). The placental transfer of hexoses and polyols in the guinea pig as shown by umbilical perfusion of the placenta. *J. Physiol. (London)*, **184**, 255

49. Dancis, J., Olsen, G., and Folkart G. (1958). Transfer of histidine and xylose across the placenta and into the red blood cell and amniotic fluids. *Amer. J. Physiol.*, **194**, 44

50. Challier, J. C., Schneider, H. and Dancis, J. (Unpublished observations)

51. Dawes, G. S. (1968). Carbohydrate Metabolism in the Fetus and Newborn. In: *Carbohydrate Metabolism*, Vol. 2 (F. Dickens, editor) (New York: Academic Press)

52. Hagerman, D. D. and Villee, C. A. (1952). Transport of fructose by human placenta. *J. Clin. Invest.*, **31**, 911

53. Gresham, E. L., Simons, P. S. and Battaglia, F. C. (1971). Maternal-fetal urea concentration difference in man: Metabolic significance. *J. Pediat.*, **79**, 809

54. Ghadimi, H. and Pecora, P. (1964). Free amino acids of cord plasma as compared with maternal plasma during pregnancy. *Pediatrics*, **33**, 500

55. Glendening, M. B., Margolis, A. J. and Page, E. W. (1961). Amino acid concentrations in fetal and maternal plasma. *Amer. J. Obstet. Gynec.*, **81**, 591

56. Van Slyke, D. D. and Meyer, G. M. (1913). The fate of protein digestion products in the body. III. The absorption of amino acids from the blood by the tissues. *J. Biol. Chem.*, **16**, 197

57. Young, M. and Prenton, M. A. (1969). Maternal and fetal plasma amino acid concentrations during gestation and in retarded fetal growth. *J. Obstet. Gynec. Brit. Comm.*, **76**, 333

58. Christensen, H. N., and Streicher, J. A. (1948). Association between rapid growth and elevated cell concentrations of amino acids. I: In fetal tissues. *J. Biol. Chem.*, **175**, 95

59. Mischel, W. (1963). Diaplacental transfer of stereoisomeric amino acids. *Arch. Gynaek.*, **198**, 181

60. Page, E. W., Glendening, M. B., Margolis, A. and Harper, H. A. (1957). Transfer of D- and L-histidine across the human placenta. *Amer. J. Obstet. Gynec.*, **73**, 589

61. Reynolds, M. L. and Young, M. (1971). The transfer of free alpha-amino nitrogen across the placental membrane in the guinea-pig. *J. Physiol. (London)*, **214**, 583

62. Longo, L. D., Yuen, P. and Gusseck, D. J. (1973). Anaerobic glycogen-dependent transport of amino acids by the placenta. *Nature (London)*, **243**, 531

63. Smith, C. H., Adcock, E. W., Teasdale, F., Meschia, G. and Battaglia, F. C. (1973). Placental amino acid uptake: Tissue preparation, kinetics, and pre-incubation effect. *Amer. J. Physiol.*, **224**, 558

64. Gaull, G. E., Räihä, N. C. R., Saarikoski, S. and Sturman, J. A. (1973). Transfer of cyst(e)ine and methionine across the human placenta. *Pediat. Res.*, **7**, 908

65. Gitlin, D., Kumate, J., Urrusti, J. *et al.* (1964). The selectivity of the human placenta in the transfer of plasma proteins from mother to fetus. *J. Clin. Invest.*, **43**, 1938

66. Dancis, J. and Shafran, M. (1958). The origin of plasma proteins in the guinea pig fetus. *J. Clin. Invest.*, **37**, 1093

67. Baugham, D. R., Hobbs, K. R. and Terry, R. J. (1958). Selective placental transfer of serum-proteins in the rhesus. *Lancet*, **ii**, 351

68. Dancis, J., Lind, J., Oratiz, M., Smolens, J. and Vara, P. (1961). Placental transfer of proteins in human gestation. *Amer. J. Obstet. Gynec.*, **82**, 167

69. Brambell, F. W. R., Hemming, W. A. and Henderson, M. (1951). *Antibodies and Embryos*. (London: Athlone Press)

70. Karte, H. (1969). The development of immunoproteins in the pre- and postnatal time. *Klin. Chem.*, **7**, 204

71. Kohler, P. F. and Farr, R. S. (1966). Elevation of cord over maternal IgG immunoglobulin: Evidence for an active placental IgG transport. *Nature (London)*, **210**, 1070

72. Morphis, L. G. and Gitlin, D. (1970). Maturation of the maternofoetal transport system for human gamma-globulin in the mouse. *Nature (London)*, **228**, 573

73. Gitlin, J. D. and Gitlin, D. (1973). Cell receptors and the selective transfer of proteins from mother to young across tissue barriers. *Pediat. Res.*, **7**, 290

74. Dancis, J., Braverman, N. and Lind, J. (1957). Plasma protein synthesis in the human fetus and placenta. *J. Clin. Invest.*, **36**, 398

75. Gitlin, D., Kumate, J. and Morales, C. (1965). On the transport of insulin across the human placenta. *Pediatrics*, **35**, 65

76. Myant, N. B. (1958). Passage of thyroxine and tri-iodo-thyronine from mother to foetus in pregnant women. *Clin. Sci. (London)*, **17**, 75

77. Paterson, P., Page, D., Taft, P. *et al.* (1968). Study of fetal and maternal insulin levels during labor. *J. Obstet. Gynaec. Brit. Comm.*, **75**, 917

78. Grumbach, M. M. and Kaplan, S. L. (1973). Ontogenesis of growth hormone, insulin, prolactin and gonadotropin secretion in the human foetus. In: *Foetal and Neonatal Physiology*. (Cambridge: Cambridge University Press)

79. Jost, A. and Picon, L. (1970). Hormonal control of fetal development and metabolism. *Adv. Metab. Dis.*, **4**, 123

80. Thoburn, G. D. and Hopkins, P. S. (1973). Thyroid function of the foetal lamb. In: *Foetal and Neonatal Physiology*, p. 488. (Cambridge: Cambridge University Press)

81. Smith, G. F. (1972). Parathyroid hormone in fetal and adult sheep. The effect of hypocalcaemia. *J. Endocr.*, **53**, 339

82. Kaplan, S. L., and Grumbach, M. M. (1965). Serum choronic 'growth-hormone prolactin' and serum pituitary growth hormone in mother and fetus at term. *J. Clin. Endocrinol. Metabol.*, **25**, 1370

83. Hershfield, M. S. and Nemeth, A. M. (1968). Placental transport of free palmitic and lineolic acids in the guinea pig. *J. Lipid Res.*, **9**, 460

84. Kayden, H. J., Dancis, J. and Money, W. L. (1969). Transfer of lipids across the guinea pig placenta. *Amer. J. Obstet. Gynec.*, **104**, 564

85. Van Duyne, C. M., Havel, R. J. and Felts, J. M. (1962). Placental transfer of palmitic acid-1-^{14}C in rabbits. *Amer. J. Obstet. Gynec.*, **84**, 1069

86. James, E., Meschia, G. and Battaglia, F. C. (1971). A-V differences of free fatty acids and glycerol in the ovine umbilical circulation. *Proc. Soc. Exper. Biol. Med.*, **138**, 823

87. Dancis, J. Jansen, V., Kayden, H. J., Schneider, H. and Levitz, M. (1973). Transfer across perfused human placenta. II: Free fatty acids. *Pediat. Res.*, **7**, 192

88. Hirsch, J., Farquhar, J., Ahrens, E. H., Jr., Peterson, M. L. and Stoffel, W. (1960). Studies of adipose tissue in man. A microtechnic for sampling and analysis. *Amer. J. Clin. Nutr.*, **8**, 499

89. Biezenski, J. J. (1969). Role of placenta in fetal lipid metabolism. I: Injection of phospholipids double layered with C^{14} glycerol and P^{32} into pregnant rabbits. *Amer. J. Obstet. Gynec.*, **104**, 1177

90. Popják, G. (1954). The origin of fetal lipids. *Cold Spring Harbor Symp. Quant. Biol.*, **19**, 200

91. Goldwater, W. H. and Stetten, DeW., Jr., (1947). Studies in fetal metabolism. *J. Biol. Chem.*, **169**, 722

92. Pitkin, R. M., Connor, W. E. and Lin, D. S. (1972). Cholesterol metabolism and placental transfer in the pregnant Rhesus monkey. *J. Clin. Invest.*, **51**, 2584

93. Levitz, M., Condon, G. P., Dancis, J., Goebelsmann, U., Eriksson, G. and Diczfalusy, E. (1967). Transfer of estriol and estriol conjugates across the human placenta perfused in situ at midpregnancy. *J. Clin. Endocr. Metabol.*, **27**, 1723

94. Levitz, M. and Dancis, J. (1963). Transfer of steroids between mother and fetus. *Clin. Obstet. Gynec.*, **6**, 62

95. Levitz, M., Money, W. L. and Dancis J. (Unpublished observations)

96. Haskins, A. L., and Soiva, K. U. (1960). The placental transfer of progesterone-4-C^{14} in human term pregnancy. *Amer. J. Obstet. Gynec.*, **79**, 674

97. Beitins, I. Z., Kowarski, A., Shermeta, D. W., DeLemos, R. A. and Migeon, C. J. (1970). Fetal and maternal secretion rate of cortisol in sheep. Diffusion resistance of the placenta. *Pediat. Res.*, **4**, 129

98. Beitins, I. Z., Bayard, F., Ances, I. G., Kowarski, A. and Migeon, C. J. (1973). The metabolic clearance rate, blood production, interconversion and transplacental passage of cortisol and cortisone in pregnancy near term. *Pediat. Res.*, **7**, 509

99. Bashore, R. A., Smith, F. and Schenker, S. (1969). Placental transfer and disposition of bilirubin in the pregnant monkey. *Amer. J. Obstet. Gynec.*, **103**, 950

100. Schenker, S., Dawber, N. H. and Schmid, R. (1964). Bilirubin metabolism in the fetus. *J. Clin. Invest.*, **43**, 32

101. Dancis, J. (1959). Aspects of bilirubin metabolism before and after birth. *Pediatrics*, **24**, 980

102. Lipsitz, P. J., Flaxman, L. M., Tartow, L. R. and Malek, B. K. (1973). Maternal hyperbilirubinemia and the newborn. *Amer. J. Dis. Child.*, **126**, 525

103. Barnes, A. C. (1951). The placental metabolism of vitamin A. *Amer. J. Obstet. Gynec.*, **61**, 368

104. Lund, C. J., and Kimble, M. S. (1943). Plasma vitamin A and carotene of the newborn infant; with consideration of fetal-maternal relationships. *Amer. J. Obstet. Gynec.*, **46**, 207

105. Sternberg, J. and Pascoe-Dawson, E. (1959). Metabolic studies in artherosclerosis. 1: Metabolic pathway of C^{14} labelled alpha-tocopherol. *Canad. M.A. J.*, **80**, 266

106. Taylor, J. D., Millar, G. J. and Wood, R. J. (1957). A comparison of the concentration of C^{14} in the tissues of pregnant and nonpregnant female rats following the intravenous administration of vitamin K_1-C^{14} and vitamin K_3-C^{14}. *Canad. J. Biochem. Physiol.*, **35**, 691

107. Straumfjord, J. V. and Quaife, M. L. (1946). Vitamin E levels in maternal and fetal blood plasma. *Proc. Soc. Exper. Biol. Med.*, **61**, 369

108. Räihä, N. (1959). On the placental transfer of vitamin C. An experimental study on guinea pigs and human subjects. *Acta Physiol. Scand.*, **45**, suppl. 155, 1

109. Hensleigh, P. A. and Krantz, K. E. (1966). Extracorporeal perfusion of the human placenta. 1: Placental transfer of ascorbic acid. *Amer. J. Obstet. Gynec.*, **96**, 5

110. Slobody, L. B., Willner, M. M. and Mestern, J. (1949). Comparison of vitamin B_1 levels in mothers and their newborn infants. *Amer. J. Dis., Child.*, **77**, 736

111. Brink, C., Esila, P., Karvonen, M. J. and Laamanen, A. (1959). Transfer of thiamine across the placenta of guinea pig. *Acta Physiol. Scand.*, **47**, 375

112. Lust, J. E., Hagerman, D. D. and Villee, C. A. (1953). The transport of riboflavin by human placenta. *J. Clin. Invest.*, **33**, 38

113. Contractor, S. F. and Shane, B. (1970). Blood and urine levels of vitamin B_6 in the mother and fetus before and after loading of the mother with vitamin B_6. *Amer. J. Obstet. Gynec.*, **107**, 635

114. Boger, W. P., Bayne, G. M., Wright, L. D. and Beck, G. D. (1957). Differential serum vitamin B_{12} concentrations in mothers and infants. *New Eng. J. Med.*, **256**, 1085

115. Killander, A. and Vahlquist, B. (1954). B_{12} vitamin concentration in serum of full-term and premature infants. *Nord. Med.*, **51**, 777

116. Hellegers, A., Okuda, K., Nesbitt, R. E. L., Jr., Smith, D. W. and Chow, B. F. (1957). Vitamin B_{12} absorption in pregnancy and in the newborn. *Amer. J. Clin. Nutr.*, **5**, 327

117. Grossowicz, N., Aronovitch, J., Rachmilewitz, M., Izak, G., Sadovsky, A. and Bercovici, B. (1960). Folic and folinic acid in maternal and foetal blood. *Brit. J. Haematol.*, **6**, 296

118. Dancis, J. and Balis, M. E. (1954). The reutilization of nucleic acid catabolites. *J. Biol. Chem.*, **207**, 367

119. Hayashi, T. T., Shin, D. H. and Wiand, S. (1968). Placental transfer of orotic acid, uridine, and UMP. 1: Comparison of acid-soluble and acid-unsoluble counts. *Amer. J. Obstet. Gynec.*, **102**, 1144

120. Faber, J. J. and Hart, F. M. (1967). Transfer of charged and uncharged molecules in the placenta of the rabbit. *Amer. J. Physiol.*, **213**, 890

121. Bartels, H. (1970). 'Prenatal Respiration'. In: *Frontiers of Biology*, Vol. 17 (London: North-Holland Publishing Company)

122. Reid, D. E., Ryan, K. J. and Benirschke, K. (1972). *Principles and Management of Human Reproduction* (Philadelphia: W. B. Saunders Company)

123. Darling, R. C., Smith, C. A., Rasmussen, E. and Cohen, F. M. (1941). Some properties of human fetal and maternal blood. *J. Clin. Invest.*, **20**, 739

124. Schneider, H., Panigel, M. and Dancis, J. (1969). *Transactions of the Fifth Rochester Trophoblast Conference* (Lund, C. J. and Choate, J. W., editors)

125. Dancis, J. Feto-maternal interaction. In: *Neonatology* (G. B. Avery, editor) (Philadelphia: J. P. Lippincott Company). (In press)

CHAPTER 7

Endocrinological Aspects of Placental Function

R. B. Thau and J. T. Lanman

Introduction

The placenta, in addition to its recognised role in gas exchange and fetal nutrition and excretion, is also an endocrine organ. This function has been demonstrated in a variety of animals and is probably present in most, if not all, mammals. The placenta is unique among endocrine organs in its capability to synthesise a diversity of hormones. As with all aspects of reproductive physiology, the endocrine functions of the placenta are highly variable among different species; the full range of its synthesising capabilities includes the production of a variety of both steroid and protein hormones. Human placenta is capable of synthesising estrogens and progesterone, and the polypeptides chorionic gonadotropin (HCG) and chorionic somatomammotropin (HCS). In addition, the production of a number of polypeptide hormones has been attributed to the placenta: human chorionic thyrotropin, adrenocorticotropic hormone, melanocyte-stimulating hormone, oxytocin, insulin, relaxin and various pressor factors. Although these hormones have been found in placental extracts, evidence that they are synthesised in the placenta is inconclusive. This latter group will not be discussed in this chapter; it has been reviewed by Saxena[1].

In animals with short gestation times, removal of the ovaries during pregnancy leads to abortion. In some animals, however, usually those with longer gestation periods, the endocrine functions of the placenta are sufficiently well-developed at some time after the beginning of pregnancy to permit maintenance of gestation after removal of the ovaries. The earliest time at which this can be done varies among different species; in the human it is about 5 weeks after conception. While the endocrine capabilities of the placenta are adequate to maintain pregnancy in the absence of maternal ovaries, and in some animals also after removal of the maternal pituitary, it is difficult to show that the placental hormones are essential for the maintenance of a normal pregnancy in animals with intact ovaries. In the human, impaired production of any of the proven placental hormones has been associated with abortion, but no cause-and-effect relationship can be established because the endocrine aspects of placental function are inextricably involved with other aspects of feto-placental physiology. The definitive experiment to show whether gestation can be maintained in the absence of the placenta and its hormones cannot be performed at this time, although molecular diseases involving a defect in the synthesis of specific hormones may offer valuable insights. In spite of these difficulties, the widespread development of the capability to synthesise a variety of placental hormones suggests that these hormones may play some role in the maintenance of gestation, in the growth and development of the fetus, or in the termination of pregnancy at the appropriate time.

Steroid Hormones

ESTROGENS

Physiology

Estrogens in the non-pregnant, sexually mature female are secreted almost exclusively by the ovarian follicle. They have numerous physiological effects; most importantly, they act as specialised growth hormones for the female reproductive organs: fallopian tubes, uterus, cervix, vagina, and breasts.

During estrus in mammals, including non-human primates, estrogens induce the production of characteristic odours, changes in skin colour, genital swelling and psychic changes with heightened sexual receptivity. These effects are minimal or absent in the human female.

Estrogens also cause changes in the cervical mucus, effected largely by alterations in its electrolyte concentration. These changes have been interpreted as facilitating the passage of sperm. In the vagina, estrogens cause squamous transformation and glycogen storage in the epithelium. They are also responsible for growth of the breasts and nipples, but lactation is complex and requires participation of other hormones. Recent evidence indicates that placental growth is also influenced by estrogens[2]. Increases in placental weight following ovariectomy in rats and rabbits and elimination of the increase by estrogen treatment suggest that estrogens inhibit placental growth and thereby fetal growth as well in these species.

Under the combined influence of estrogens and progesterone, the endometrium proliferates and the endometrial glands grow, providing a suitable medium for the maintenance of the fertilised egg before nidation and an appropriate surface for blastocyst implantation. Estrogen-induced hyperplasia and hypertrophy of the uterus provide at least initially for the accommodation of the growing fetus. Ultimately, fetal growth and the consequent stretching of the myometrium exert a stimulus for myometrial growth which is probably adequate even in the absence of estrogens. Stretching also increases myometrial excitability and becomes important in preparing the uterus for parturition, and estrogens appear to help in effecting a prompt and appropriately-timed delivery[3].

A number of more generalised metabolic effects of estrogens are less clearly related to reproduction; they include increased levels of blood cholesterol and other lipids and increased coagulability of blood, a relatively minor effect, but one that has caused some increased morbidity among women taking contraceptives containing estrogens.

The mechanisms by which estrogens act on their target cells is now known in some detail. Estrogen-sensitive cells have specific membrane receptor sites which bind estrogens; the bound steroids are transferred to a cytoplasmic transport protein which carries them to the nucleus; there, transfer to a nuclear transport protein occurs. In the nucleus, estrogens mediate the synthesis of DNA-dependent RNA, which in turn, via the usual pathways of protein synthesis, leads to the appearance of a large number of estrogen-induced enzymes and structural proteins[4]. The concept that estrogens act by inducing the synthesis of specific RNA is supported by the demonstration that estrogen-induced RNA is capable of mediating characteristic estrogen effects in what appears to be total absence of estrogen.

Quantitative aspects during pregnancy

Significant increases in estrogen synthesis and maternal excretion during pregnancy have been observed in several species: the human[5], the rhesus monkey[6], the cow[7], the horse[8] and the pig[9]. In most, if not all mammals, the placenta serves as an additional source of estrogens. In humans, the placental contribution is particularly large, and is reflected in maternal urinary estrogen values which rise progressively during pregnancy from usually well under 100 μg/day in non-pregnant women to a daily output of up to 330 mg/day near term[10]. At this time, maternal peripheral plasma levels will have reached about 150 ng/ml (Figure 7.1)[11]. Estrogens formed in the placenta are secreted into the maternal blood stream in the free form. Before urinary excretion, they are conjugated to glucuronides and, to a lesser extent, to sulphates by the maternal liver (Figure 7.2).

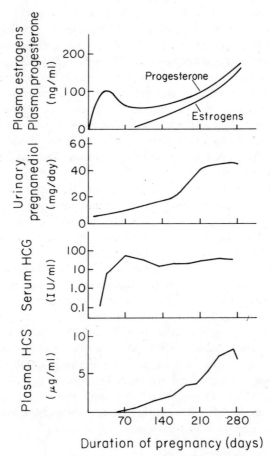

Figure 7.1 Hormone levels during human pregnancy

Conjugation diminishes the biological activity of the estrogens but increases their solubility in aqueous medium, permitting their excretion in urine, where transport proteins are not available. Most animals excrete estrogens as conjugates of estrone or estradiol, but in the human, the large and progressive rise during pregnancy reflects a feto-placental contribution largely of estriol. Like the other estrogens, estriol is conjugated in the maternal liver before excretion. It accounts for 80–95% of estrogens excreted in the human in late pregnancy[12]. No other known animal follows this pattern; the macaque makes little or none of this estrogen. Since estriol has relatively modest estrogenic activity and its conjugates still less, the excretion

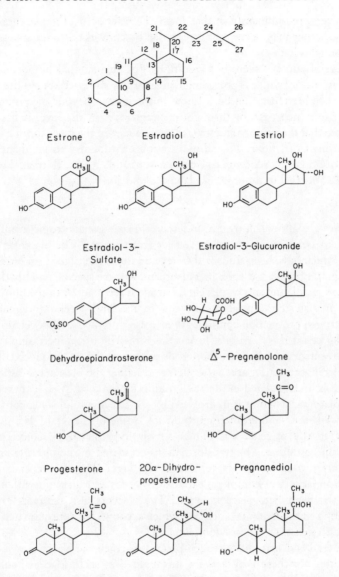

Figure 7.2 Chemical formulas of some steroids. The top formula, cholestane, shows the proper number for each carbon atom

of large amounts of estrogens during human pregnancy has less biological significance than the total numerical value would imply. Placental estrogens also pass to the fetus, again in the free form, but there they are sulfated and transported predominantly in that form. Transfer across the placenta from fetus to mother may occur, but is preceded by conversion to the free steroid by placental sulfatase.

In several animals there is a significant rise in maternal blood estrogen levels for one or two days preceding delivery. The rise is striking in the ewe[11] but no such increment has been found in the human beyond a continuation of the rise which extends throughout pregnancy. In the ewe, it has been suggested that the prepartum estrogen rise is a part of the mechanism triggering the onset of labour. The administration of stilbestrol to pregnant ewes has been shown to induce uterine contractions and, in animals treated within 10 days of normal term, to induce labour and delivery.

Biosynthesis

The mature mammalian ovary, under appropriate gonadotropic stimulus, is capable of synthesising estrogens *de novo* from acetate. The placentas of all species which have been studied also develop the capacity to form estrogens, although not from a 2-carbon precursor, and in some species, notably the rat, only very small amounts of placental estrogens are made[13]. In the human, in whom ovarian steroid production wanes by the ninth week of pregnancy[14], total estrogen production continues to increase, and the placenta becomes the main source for this hormone. It depends primarily on an increasing supply of the precursor dehydroepiandrosterone sulphate (DHEAS) produced mainly by the fetal adrenal (Figure 7.3)[15]. Before reaching the placenta, most of the DHEAS is hydroxylated in the 16α position by the fetal liver. It then passes to the placenta, where it is hydrolysed by the enzyme sulphatase, converted to a Δ^4-3-ketone and aromatised to estriol. Some of the fetal DHEAS goes directly to the placenta without 16α hydroxylation and is converted to estrone and estradiol. The transformations occurring in the placenta are not effectively carried out by the fetus, and vice versa. The interdependence of fetus and placenta in completing the pathway for estrogen biosynthesis has led to the term 'feto-placental unit'. The placenta also receives DHEAS originating in the maternal adrenal[16] which accounts for approximately 10% of the estrogen excreted in late pregnancy.

Both fetal and maternal estrogen precursors reach the placenta as sulfated conjugates, but there they are not metabolised as such. Placental sulfatase first converts them to free steroids. The importance of this step in the pathway of estrogen synthesis has been emphasised by one interesting clinical observation. France and Liggins[17] have reported the case of a woman with placental sulfatase deficiency and severely impaired estrogen production. This deficiency was associated with fetal death and abortion in 3 out of 7 pregnancies. Studies in 2 subsequent pregnancies revealed maternal urinary

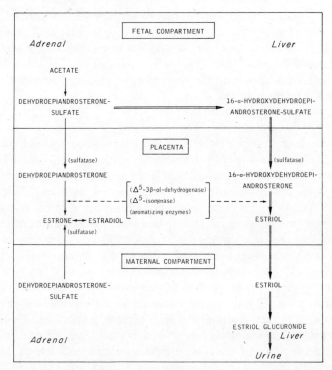

Figure 7.3 Main pathways of estrogen metabolism in human pregnancy

estriol excretion of only about 5% of that in a normal pregnancy. These observations indicate that the placenta, utilising sulfated precursors, supplied the major part of estrogens excreted during pregnancy. Both of these pregnancies were terminated by Caesarean section at 38 weeks: the 2 male infants were normal and subsequently did well, indicating that placental estrogens were not necessary for fetal growth and development, but leaving unanswered their possible role in the termination of gestation at normal term.

The extraordinary rise in total estrogen production during human pregnancy reflects increasing production of DHEAS by the fetal adrenal. In the human, though not in most animals, the fetal adrenal is strikingly hypertrophied. Its enlargement appears to reflect fetal pituitary ACTH stimulation, occasioned probably by a feedback mechanism activated by loss of fetal adrenal glucocorticoids. Loss occurs by metabolism in the fetal liver and by transfer across the placenta to the mother[10]; transcortin levels rise progressively in the maternal circulation during pregnancy[18], creating a transplacental gradient across which fetal corticosteroids are lost. Further maternal-fetal disparity is created by the competition of progesterone for cortisol binding sites[19], with relatively higher levels of progesterone in the fetal circulation[20]. As in other situations with increased ACTH stimulation of the adrenal, the production of adrenal C-19 compounds, in this case predominantly DHEAS, is also increased, providing the precursor for the large amounts of estriol synthesised by the placenta.

Clinical aspects

Because estriol has its origin predominantly in the feto-placental unit, maternal estriol assays afford a clinical index for the condition of the fetus and placenta, and are useful particularly in situations of increased hazards, such as fetal growth retardation, toxaemia and prolonged pregnancy. Wide variations of estriol values occur normally among individuals, so that serial determinations are necessary, with falling values indicating increasing feto-placental impairment. Fetal death is accompanied by a sharp drop in urinary estriol[21]. Also in pregnancies with anencephalic fetuses having defective pituitaries and secondarily hypoplastic adrenals, urinary estrogen values, particularly estriol, are reduced, usually to about one-tenth of those found in normal pregnancies[22]; these low values reflect the relative lack of estrogen precursors from the unstimulated fetal adrenals and are usually observed concurrently with diminished peripheral plasma levels. Decreased urinary estrogen excretion without changes in plasma estrogen levels can be due to impaired renal function, hypertension or toxaemia of the mother.

PROGESTERONE

Physiology

Progesterone is a secretory end product of steroid metabolism in corpora lutea and in the placenta. In the cycling human female, its synthesis is restricted predominantly to the post-ovulatory phase when, together with estrogens, it induces the secretory phase of the uterine glands in preparation for ovum implantation. Progesterone suppresses estrus and the release of pituitary luteinising hormone. In preventing the requisite ovulatory surge of luteinising hormone, it is also effective in inhibiting ovulation, and one basis for the usefulness of progesterone and other progestational steroids as contraceptive agents is based on this activity. During pregnancy, progesterone is necessary for maintenance of a quiescent, non-contractile uterus. After conception has occurred, pregnancy maintenance is initially dependent on ovarian hormones in all mammals. But, in those in which ovariectomy ultimately becomes possible without inducing abortion, the placenta, at times varying with the species, becomes capable of producing sufficient progesterone to maintain gestation even after ovariectomy.

Progesterone acts in some way to prevent abortion induced by premature uterine contractions. The mechanism by which it acts is not clear. It has been postulated that it acts on the myometrium to inhibit the spread of the contractile wave, thereby preventing coordinated and forceful uterine contractions and creating what has been termed the progesterone block[23]. There are serious theoretical objections to the progesterone block theory[24]. Effects on myometrial contractility attributed to the action of progesterone are demonstrable in certain lower animals, notably the rabbit, but the phenomena are less clear in humans and in certain other animals with long gestation periods. Unlike the situation in the rabbit, uterine contractions at term in the human are not associated with falling blood progesterone levels[25], nor does progesterone administration, even at high doses[26], inhibit labour. However, proponents of the progesterone block theory point out that blood levels in the human do not accurately reflect the local level of progesterone, which is synthesised in the placenta and transmitted to the subjacent myometrium. Parenterally-administered progesterone, even at high doses, may not reach the myometrium to afford levels comparable with those supplied locally by the placenta.

Progesterone is also involved in some aspects of maternal behaviour, such as hair pulling, nest building, and mothering. Species variability is striking. In the mouse, progesterone induces or stimulates such behaviour[27], whereas in the pregnant and pseudopregnant rabbit, the plucking of fur occurs in association with the cessation of progesterone secretion[28].

Quantitative aspects

In the human, the placenta is recognised as an important site of progesterone production during pregnancy. At term, the placenta secretes approximately 250 mg of progesterone per day[29] estimated from direct measurements of progesterone in umbilical and uterine veins. The progesterone concentration in maternal peripheral plasma is elevated during pregnancy and rises as gestation progresses (Figure 7.1), reaching values ranging from 11 to 32 μg/100 ml of plasma[30], as compared with non-pregnancy levels varying from 0·1 to 2 μg/100 ml of plasma[31] at different times in the menstrual cycle. The increase in plasma progesterone levels during pregnancy is reflected in increasing maternal urinary excretion of pregnanediol, one of its major metabolites. From amounts averaging about 10 mg/24 hours at the end of the first trimester, pregnanediol excretion rises to an average of about 45 mg/24 hours at the 36th week, after which it remains relatively constant[29]. Wide variations occur, both among individuals and from day-to-day in the same individual.

An early peak in plasma progesterone concentration at 5 weeks of pregnancy, attributed to corpus luteum secretion, is followed by a short decline interpreted as reflecting diminished corpus luteum function. Increasing placental synthesis is believed to be responsible for a second gradual increase from the tenth to approximately the 37th week of pregnancy, after which the level remains constant until delivery. Recent studies suggest that while the ovary becomes dispensable after the fifth week of human pregnancy, the corpus luteum during normal gestation continues to produce progesterone throughout gestation[30].

The myometrial progesterone concentration is highest subjacent to the placenta and falls in the more peripheral areas[32]. Absolute concentrations vary greatly among individuals, and no significant changes have been found in association with the onset of labour. The situation in humans contrasts with that in rats, in which the myometrial progesterone concentration declines during the latter part of gestation, with no corresponding change in the plasma concentration[33]. However, in all animals, both tissue and plasma concentrations are influenced by the availability of binding and transport proteins, so that concentrations expressed without knowledge of these factors are not readily interpretable. Much current research is directed toward this problem.

Metabolism

In the human trophoblast, cholesterol from the maternal compartment is the main substrate for progesterone synthesis[34] (Figure 7.4), and fetal precursors are not important. Placental conversion of acetate to progesterone is quantitatively insignificant[35]. $\Delta 5$-3β-hydroxysteroid dehydrogenase and $\Delta 5$-isomerase, enzymes capable of converting pregnenolone to progesterone, have been found in the human trophoblast, but not in the rabbit placenta, in which no detectable progesterone synthesis occurs. Placental progesterone production evidenced by elevated maternal pregnanediol excretion can persist in the human for up to several weeks following intrauterine fetal death[36] or in the presence of an anencephalic fetus with hypoplastic adrenals[37] or following removal of the fetus with the placenta left *in situ*, as has occurred in cases or ectopic pregnancy. The intervillous circulation appears capable of maintaining the trophoblast, which it directly bathes. Few progesterone metabolites are found in the human placenta. The major metabolite in the perfused midterm[38] and term[39] placenta is 20α-dihydroprogesterone (Figure 7.4). Some C_6-hydroxylation of progesterone occurs, but no C_{11}, C_{16} or C_{21} hydroxylation has been detected. Some $C_{11}\alpha$-hydroxylation and C_{22} side-chain cleavage occurs *in vitro*, but these reactions are not physiologically significant. In the absence of these transformations, the placenta produces no glucocorticoids and only insignificant amounts of androgens or estrogens from

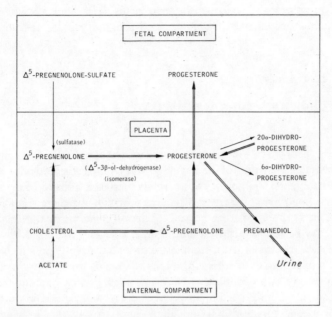

Figure 7.4 Main pathways of progesterone metabolism in human pregnancy

progesterone. Placental progesterone passes both to the mother and the fetus. In the mother, pregnanediol glucuronide is formed in the liver and excreted in the maternal urine. Although this is the principal maternal metabolite, its excretion accounts for less than 4% of the total progesterone produced. Of the remainder, a large, but not precisely measured, fraction passes to the fetus, where it is metabolised in the fetal adrenal and liver. In the adrenal, hydroxylation in the 11, 17, and 21 positions and sulphation lead to the production of a variety of corticosteroid sulfates; 6α and 16-OH-progesterone sulfates are also formed. In the liver, the principal metabolic product is 20α-dihydroprogesterone which occurs also predominantly as sulfate.

Clinical aspects

Measurement of maternal urinary pregnanediol excretion has been used clinically to assess feto-placental well-being. The test should reflect placental progesterone production which should, in turn, be influenced by the condition of the fetus and placenta. Clinical usefulness has been limited, however, probably because significant maternal ovarian production persists and because placental progesterone production can continue even after fetal death.

Pre-term birth has, in some studies, been associated statistically with lower maternal progesterone levels than in term births. In individual cases, how-ever, maternal progesterone levels have no prognostic value for pre-term birth[40].

Protein Hormones

HUMAN CHORIONIC GONADOTROPIN

Physiology

Placental gonadotropins originating in the trophoblast have been found in several primates: human, 3 of the 4 apes (gorilla, chimpanzee, and orangutan), and a monkey, the macaque. The mare synthesises a gonadotropin in the uterine endometrial cups, a tissue of maternal origin, and there is suggestive evidence, but not proof, that gonadotropins originating in the uterus or placenta may be found in the rat and in other species.

The gonadotropins of man, monkey, and chimpanzee appear to be bio-chemically related to each other, although the time course during pregnancy of their presence and quantitative aspects of their urinary excretion differ. The macaque, with a gestation period of about 167 days, excretes monkey chorionic gonadotropin (MCG) from about day 14 to day 31 of pregnancy[41]. The corresponding period of excretion for the chimpanzee, with a gestation period of about 230 days, is from about day 61 to day 90 of gestation with considerably longer periods in some individuals. In the human female, urinary excretion of human chorionic gonadotropin (HCG) as usually measured clinically becomes detectable at about four weeks after conception and rises to a maximum at about 60 days; the rise is followed by a decline to a lower level maintained throughout the second and third trimesters of pregnancy[1].

HCG was first discovered in 1927 in the urine of pregnant women[42], and its detection in urine has been used as a clinical test for pregnancy, originally employing a bioassay in toads or rabbits, and presently a simpler and more rapid complement fixation test[43]. Since the development of radio-immuno-assays, blood levels during pregnancy can also be assayed, and with the most sensitive techniques, not presently generally available, the diagnosis of pregnancy can be made within a few days of conception. This capability should prove important in the accurate selection of cases for early abortion. Maternal serum HCG levels show a pattern similar to that of urinary excre-tion[44] (Figure 7.1). Fetal plasma contains only about 1/500 of the concentra-tion found in maternal plasma, despite the fact that HCG is synthesised in the trophoblast[45], a tissue of fetal origin. Except for rare ovarian and testicular tumours, and rarer tumours not of endocrine origin, HCG synthesis is unique to the placenta and to tumours derived from trophoblast: hydatidiform mole and choriocarcinoma.

The action of HCG is generally regarded as similar to that of luteinising hormone (LH). This view is from the period when the functions of LH were regarded more simplistically than recent evidence permits, and it is unlikely that HCG can mimic the diverse roles of LH now recognised. LH has different effects in different species and, in the rabbit, may be either luteolytic or luteotropic, depending on dosage[46]. In the human and in the monkey, their respective CGs are luteotropic. Their stimulatory effect on the early corpus luteum may be needed to maintain function until the time when the corpus luteum is no longer essential for the maintenance of pregnancy. Hodgen and coworkers[41] have shown in the monkey that the production of MCG begins during a time of falling maternal progesterone levels reflecting declining corpus luteum function. The subsequent rise in progesterone levels presumably is related first to the stimulatory effect of HCG on the corpus luteum and later to placental progesterone production. MCG then disappears from the urine at about the end of the first month of pregnancy, and the corpus luteum becomes smaller. Recent evidence suggests, however, that it continues to produce progesterone and that its size and function increase in the final weeks of pregnancy, thus far without a recognised recurrence of placental gonadotropin production[47].

HCG is an effective antigen, and anti-HCG antibodies are readily made in rabbits in response to HCG administration even without the use of adjuvants. It is perhaps surprising that the human female, who for many years prior to her first pregnancy is not exposed to HCG, should not respond immunologically to this placental protein. While her exposure to HCG during her own fetal life might, at that time, have induced tolerance, the persistence of tolerance is usually regarded as requiring the persistence of antigen.

It has recently been found that HCG inhibits the *in vitro* lymphocyte stimulating effect of phytohaemagglutinin[48]. This finding has been interpreted by some as indicating a partial suppression of immunity and as affording a means by which the human fetus, which is immunologically foreign to the mother because of inherited paternal antigens, avoids rejection as a foreign graft. There is at present little other supporting evidence for these speculations, and an immunosuppressive action by a hormone found only in primates affords little insight into the control of maternal–fetal immunological incompatibility in other placental animals.

Although HCG is not normally present in the male, its administration in a variety of animals influences testicular interstitial cells in the same way as does LH, producing differentiation, hypertrophy and increased androgen secretion. Effects of HCG on the adrenal glands have been repeatedly sought.

Adrenotropic effects reflected in adrenal size have been reported, but no convincing effects on adrenal steroidogenesis have been found[49].

Biochemical aspects

HCG is a glycoprotein. The carbohydrate portion represents approximately 30% of the molecule[50]. Each molecule contains 20 sialic acid residues, glycosidically linked to the carbohydrate chain and biologic activity is lost when sialic acid is removed with neuraminidase[51]. The sequence of amino acids in the protein portion[52] and of monosaccharides in the oligocarbohydrate portion[53] has been determined. As with follicle-stimulating hormone (FSH) and LH, HCG consists of two non-covalently bonded subunits, α and β[54] with molecular weights of approximately 18 000 and 28 000, respectively[50]. The α-subunit of HCG is interchangeable with the α-subunits of bovine thyrotropin and bovine LH with no loss in biological or immunological activity[55]. The β-subunit is specific to HCG, and the preparation of antibodies to the β-subunit is the basis for the radio-immunoassay specific for HCG. The disappearance rates of HCG and its α- and β-subunits from the human circulation are exponential; the rates for each of the two subunits are more than 10 times faster than that of the whole molecule[56]. The subunits appear to lack biological activity, either because of their short circulatory half-life or because they fail to bind to receptors specific for HCG.

Clinical aspects

The detection of HCG in the urine is useful in the diagnosis of pregnancy. Serial urinary HCG determinations afford a clinical index in the management of threatened abortion; patients with an unphysiological decline or with consistently low urinary HCG levels are more likely to abort. However, missed abortion cannot be reliably diagnosed by HCG assay; following fetal death, trophoblastic tissue may survive for long periods of time in sufficient amounts to maintain detectable HCG levels. HCG determinations are, therefore, useful in detection of retained placental tissue. They are also used in following the clinical response to treatment of both malignant and nonmalignant trophoblastic tumours and in the detection of tumour recurrences or metastases.

HUMAN CHORIONIC SOMATOMAMMOTROPIN

Physiology

Prolactin-like activity was found in extracts from human placenta as early as 1936[57] and was called human placental lactogen. Growth hormone-like activity was also found in the same kind of preparation[58]. An active component containing both kinds of activity in a single molecule has subsequently been characterised as a polypeptide currently known as human chorionic somatomammotropin (HCS)[59]. A similar substance could be extracted from the placentas of 2 monkeys: macaques and baboons. Macaque chorionic somatomammotropin (MCS)[60] has partial immunological cross-reactivity with HCS and, to a greater extent, with human growth hormone (HGH). The mammotropic properties of HCS are reflected in its promotion of crop sac growth in the pigeon and of milk production in the pseudo-pregnant rabbit. HGH-like effects have been best demonstrated in patients with hypopituitarism, in whom there is little or no interference from pituitary hormones. These studies have shown reduced urinary excretion of nitrogen, potassium, and phosphorus, while urinary loss of calcium increased. However, HCS is relatively low in growth-promoting activity, having less than 1/100 of the biological activity of HGH.

Two opposing effects on carbohydrate metabolism have been found[61]; HCS is diabetogenic, probably producing insulin antagonism as does HGH. It also promotes the secretion of insulin, simulating an effect observed in HGH-deficient children given HGH. Plasma-free fatty acids are also increased by HCS. Many of these effects observed on administration of HCS are changes which occur physiologically during human pregnancy. It is difficult to attribute any one of them specifically to HCS independently of con-currently-acting hormones, particularly HGH, estrogens and cortico-steroids. Those which have been observed, and which are consistent with the action of HCS, have been interpreted as favouring the growth of the fetus largely through decreasing maternal utilisation of carbohydrate and making increased supplies available in the fetus and thereby providing an energy source for fetal protein anabolism. HCS, like HCG, has been shown to suppress the *in vitro* phytohaemagglutinin-induced lymphocyte response; as with HCG, the significance of this phenomenon is not clear at present.

In spite of the numerous effects of HCS on a variety of systems, it is difficult to assess its role in pregnancy. As with the chorionic gonadotropins, the restriction of chorionic somatomammotropins to primates indicates that mammalian reproduction has no general requirement for this protein hormone, in contrast to the generally essential nature of estrogen and progesterone.

Quantitative aspects

HCS is synthesised in the syncitial trophoblast, and, like HCG, is secreted predominantly into the maternal circulation. It becomes detectable in maternal plasma after the first month of pregnancy and subsequently rises to values of about 8 μg/ml at term[62] (Figure 7.1), when its production rate has been estimated at about 1 gram per day[63]. These values at term for both concentration and production rate are far higher than those for any other human polypeptide hormone. Unlike HCG, very little HCS appears in maternal urine.

HCS shows no circadian rhythm; its circulating half-life has been estimated at 29 minutes[63].

Biochemistry

The single polypeptide chain of HCS shows close similarities to that of HGH in its molecular weight (both are about 20 000)[64], in both its NH_2-terminal[65] and COOH-terminal[66] amino acid sequence and in its primary structure[67].

Clinical aspects

Earlier reports published before 1970 revealed no correlation between maternal urinary HCS excretion and various feto-placental disorders[40], but more recent data indicate that HCS radioimmunoassay in maternal blood affords an index of placental function in the presence of many pathological conditions during pregnancy[62]. Pregnancies ending in abortion show low or decreasing HCS levels. Values are lower than normal in pre-eclampsia, feto-placental dystrophy, multiple placental infarcts, prolonged pregnancy with chronic fetal distress, and preceding intrauterine fetal death in diabetic pregnancies. High levels are found in rhesus-isoimmunisation with hydrops fetalis, in twin pregnancies and in non-diabetic pregnancies with excessively large babies. There is a significant correlation between fetal weight and plasma HCS values up to the time of normally declining HCS values a few days before parturition.

Conclusion

In recent years, considerable progress has been made in accumulating detailed knowledge of the biochemistry and physiology of the human placental hormones. The mode of action of estrogens during reproduction is fairly well understood. For the protein hormones, detailed knowledge of the structure of HCG and HCS is available and some knowledge about their binding sites has been gained. For progesterone, progress has been less spectacular; we are still largely ignorant of its mode of action, particularly regarding its influence on uterine motility. Perhaps least satisfactory is our understanding of the need for the contribution of the human placenta to the endocrinology of pregnancy. The trophoblast has extraordinary capabilities; in addition to its manifold transfer and transport functions, it is perhaps the most versatile of endocrine organs. But, with the possible exception of HCG, it is still unclear whether the development of the placenta's endocrine roles is either essential or even beneficial. The search for significant influences of the placental hormones on the reproductive process provides ample challenge for further investigation.

References

1. Saxena, B. N. (1971). Protein-polypeptide hormones of the human placenta. *Vitam. Horm.*, **29**, 95

2. Abdul-Karim, R. W., Nesbitt, R. E. L., Jr., Drucker, M. and Rizk, P. T. (1971). The regulatory effect of estrogens on fetal growth. I. Placental and fetal body weights. *Am. J. Obstet. Gynecol.*, **109**, 656

3. Liggins, G. C., Fairclough, R. J., Grieves, S. A., Kendall, J. Z. and Knox, B. S. (1973). The mechanism of initiation of parturition in the ewe. *Recent Progr. Hormone Res.*, **29**, 111

4. Segal, S. J. and Scher, W. (1967). In: *Cellular Biology of the Uterus*. (R. M. Wynn, editor) (New York: Appleton-Century-Croft)

5. Diczfalusy, E. and Lauriken, C. (1961). *Oestrogene beim Menschen*. (Berlin: Springer Verlag)

6. Hopper, B. R. and Tullner, W. W. (1967). Urinary estrogen excretion patterns in pregnant Rhesus monkeys. *Steroids*, **9**, 517

7. Mellin, T. N. and Erb, R. E. (1965). Estrogens in the bovine—a review. *J. Dairy Sci.*, **48**, 687

8. Savard, K. (1961). The estrogens of the pregnant mare. *Endocrinology*, **68**, 411

9. Raeside, J. I. (1963). Urinary oestrogen excretion in the pig during pregnancy and parturition. *J. Reprod. Fertil.*, **6**, 427

10. Oakey, R. E. (1970). The progressive increase in estrogen production in human pregnancy: An appraisal of the factors responsible. *Vitam. Horm.*, **28**, 1

11. Bedford, C. A., Challis, J. R., Harrison, F. A. and Heap, R. B. (1972). The role of oestrogens and progesterone in the onset of parturition in various species. *J. Reprod. Fertil.*, Suppl. 16, 1

12. Hobkirk, R. and Nilsen, M. (1962). Observations on the occurrence of six estrogen fractions in human pregnancy urine. I: Normal pregnancy. *J. Clin. Endocrinol. Metab.*, **22**, 134

13. Canivenc, R. (1951). L'activité endocrine du placenta de la rate. *Arch. d'anatomie, d'histologie et d'embryologie*, **34**, 105

14. Yoshimi, T., Strott, C. A., Marshall, J. R. and Lipsett, M. B. (1969). Corpus luteum function in early pregnancy. *J. Clin. Endocrinol. Metab.*, **29**, 225

15. Telegdy, G., Weeks, J. W., Archer, D. F., Wiqvist, N. and Diczfalusy, E. (1970). Acetate and cholesterol metabolism in the human foeto-placental unit at mid-gestation. 3. Steroids synthesized and secreted by the foetus. *Acta Endocrinol. (Kbh)*, **63**, 119

16. MacDonald, P. C. and Siiteri, P. K. (1965). Origin of estrogen in women pregnant with an anencephalic fetus. *J. Clin. Invest.*, **44**, 465.

17. France, J. T. and Liggins, G. C. (1969). Placental sulfatase deficiency. *J. Clin. Endocrinol. Metab.*, **29**, 138

18. Rosenthal, H. E., Slaunwhite, W. R. and Sandberg, A. A. (1969). Transcortin: A

corticosteroid–binding protein of plasma X. Cortisol and progesterone interplay and unbound levels of these steroids in pregnancy. *J. Clin. Endocrinol. Metab.*, **29,** 352

19. Murphy, B. E. P. (1967). Some studies of the protein–binding of steroids and their application to the routine micro and ultromicro measurements of various steroids in body fluids by competitive protein–binding radioassay. *J. Clin. Endocrinol. Metab.*, **27,** 973

20. Greig, M., Coyle, M. G., Cooper, W. and Walker, J. (1962). Plasma progesterone in mother and foetus in the second half of human pregnancy. *J. Obstet. Gynaecol. Br. Commonw.*, **69,** 772

21. Wray, P. M. and Russell, C. S. (1964). Maternal urinary oestriol levels before and after death of the foetus. *J. Obstet. Gynaecol. Br. Commonw.*, **71,** 97

22. Frandsen, V. A. and Stokemann, G. (1961). The site of production of oestrogenic hormones in human pregnancy. Hormone excretion in pregnancy with anencephalic foetus. *Acta Endocrinol. (Kbh)*, **38,** 383

23. Csapo, A. (1969). In: *Progesterone: Its regulatory effect on the myometrium.* Ciba Foundation Study Group No. 34

24. Kao, C. Y. (1967). In: *Cellular Biology of the Uterus.* (R. M. Wynn, editor) (New York: Appleton–Century–Croft)

25. Kumar, D., Ward, E. F. and Barnes, A. C. (1964). Serial plasma progesterone levels and the onset of labor. *Am. J. Obstet. Gynecol.*, **90,** 1360

26. Kumar, D., Goodno, J. A. and Barnes, A. C. (1963). *In vivo* effects of intravenous progesterone infusion on human gravid uterine contractility. *Bull. Johns Hopkins Hosp.*, **113,** 53

27. Koller, G. (1952). Der Nestbau der weissen Maus und seine honmonale Auslösung. *Verh. Dtsch. Zool. Ges. Freiburg 1952,* 160

28. Zarrow, M. X., Sawin, P. B., Ross, S. and Dennenberg, V. H. (1962). Maternal behavior in the rabbit and a consideration of its endocrine basis. In: *The Roots of Behavior.* (E. L. Bliss, editor)

29. Diczfalusy, E. and Troen, P. (1961). Endocrine functions of the human placenta. *Vitam. Horm.*, **19,** 229

30. LeMaire, W. J., Conly, P. W., Moffett, A. and Cleveland, W. W. (1970). Plasma progesterone secretion by the corpus luteum of term pregnancy. *Am. J. Obstet. Gynecol.*, **108,** 132

31. Johansson, E. D. B. (1969). Progesterone levels in peripheral plasma during the luteal phase of the normal human menstrual cycle measured by a rapid competitive protein binding technique. *Acta Endocrinol.*, **61,** 592

32. Zander, J., Holzmann, K., von Münstermann, A. M., Runnenbaum, B. and Silber, W. (1969). In: *The Foeto-placental Unit.* (A. Pecile and C. Finzi, editors) (Amsterdam: Excerpta Medica Foundation)

33 Wiest, W. G. (1970). Progesterone and 20 α-hydroxypregn-4-en-3-one in plasma, ovaries and uteri during pregnancy in the rat. *Endocrinology*, **87,** 43

34. Ryan, K. J., Meigs, R. and Petro, Z. (1966). The formation of progesterone by the human placenta. *Am. J. Obstet. Gynecol.*, **96,** 676

35. Hellig, H., Lefebvre, Y., Gattereau, D. and Bolté, E. (1969). In: *The Foeto-placental Unit.* (A. Pecile and C. Finzi, editors) (Amsterdam: Excerpta Medica Foundation)

36. Appleby, T. T. and Norymberski, J. K. (1957). The urinary excretion of 17-hydroxy-corticosteroids in human pregnancy. *J. Endocrinol.*, **15,** 310

37. Allen, W. M. (1953). In discussion of Hunt, A. B., McConakey, W. M. Pregnancy associated with diseases of the adrenal glands. *Am. J. Obstet. Gynecol.*, **66,** 970

38. Telegdy, G., Weeks, J. W., Wiqvist, N. and Diczfalusy, E. (1970). Acetate and cholesterol metabolism in the human foeto-placental unit at mid-gestation. 2: Steroids synthesized and secreted by the placenta. *Acta Endocrinol.*, **63**, 105

39. Kitchin, J. D. III, Pion, R. J. and Conrad, S. H. (1967). Metabolism of progesterone by term human placenta perfused *in situ*. *Steroids*, **9**, 263

40. Klopper, A. (1970). Assessment of feto-placental function by hormone assay. *Am. J. Obstet. Gynecol.*, **107**, 807.

41. Hodgen, G. D., Dufau, M. L., Catt, K. J. and Tullner, W. W. (1972). Estrogens, progesterone and chorionic gonadotropin in pregnant Rhesus monkeys. *Endocrinology*, **91**, 896

42. Aschheim, S. and Zondek, B. (1927). Hypophysenvorderlappenhormon und Ovarialhormon im Harn von Schwangeren. *Klin. Wochenschr.*, **6**, 1322

43. Hobson, B. M. (1966). Review Pregnancy diagnosis. *J. Reprod. Fertil.*, **12**, 33

44. Geiger, W. and Post, W. (1972). The distribution of HCG, HCS, STH and TSH to various phsyiological fluids of mother and·fetus in the last trimester of pregnancy. *Acta Endocrinol.*, *(Kbh)*, Suppl. 159, 81

45. Vaitukaitis, J. L. and Ross, G. T. (1973). Recent advances in evaluation of gonadotropic hormones. *Ann. Rev. Med.*, **24**, 295

46. Hilliard, J., Saldarini, R. J., Spies, H. G. and Sawyer, C. H. (1971). Luteotrophic and luteolytic actions of LH in hypophysectomized, pseudopregnant rabbits. *Endocrinology*, **89**, 513

47. Treolar, O. L., Wolf, R. C. and Meyer, R. K. (1972). Corpus luteum of the Rhesus monkey during late pregnancy. *Endocrinology*, **91**, 665

48. Adcock, E. W. III, Teasdale, F., August, C. S., Cox, S., Meschia, G., Battaglia, F. C. and Naughton, M. A. (1973). Human chorionic gonadotropin: Its possible role in maternal lymphocyte suppression. *Science*, **181**, 845

49. Cushman, P., Jr. (1970). Effects of perfusion of chorionic and human postmenopausal gonadotropins on the secretion of cortisol and 17-ketosteroids in the dog. *Am. J. Obstet. Gynceol.*, **107**, 519

50. Canfield, R. E., Morgan, F. J., Kammerman, S., Bell, J. J. and Agesto, G. M. (1971). Studies on human chorionic gonadotropin. *Recent Prog. Horm. Res.*, **27**, 121

51. Van Hall, E., Vaitukaitis, J. L., Ross, G. T., Hickman, J. W. and Ashwell, G. (1971). Immunological and biological activity of HCG following progressive desialyzation. *Endocrinology*, **88**, 456

52. Bahl, O. P., Carlsen, R. B., Bellisario, R. and Swaminathan, N. (1972). Human chorionic gonadotropin: Amino acid sequence of the α and β subunits. *Biochem. Biophys. Res. Commun.*, **48**, 416

53. Van Hell, H., Goverde, B. C., Schuurs, A. H. W. M., DeJager, E., Matthijsen, R. and Homan, J. D. H. (1966). Purification, characterization and immunochemical properties of human chorionic gonadotropin. *Nature*, **212**, 261

54. Swaminathan, N. and Bahl, O. P. (1970). Dissociation and recombination of the subunits of human chorionic gonadotropin. *Biochem. Biophys. Res. Commun.*, **40**, 422

55. Pierce, J. G., Bahl, O. P., Cornell, J. S. and Swaminathan, N. (1971). Biologically active hormones prepared by recombination of the α chain of human chorionic gonadotropin and the hormone specific chain of bovine thyrotropin or of bovine luteinizing hormone. *J. Biol. Chem.*, **246**, 2321

56. Braunstein, G. D., Vaitukaitis, J. L. and Ross, G. T. (1972). The *in vivo* behavior of human chorionic gonadotropin after dissociation into subunits. *Endocrinology*, **91**, 1030

57. Ehrhart, K. (1936). Forschung und Klinik. Ueber das Laktationshormon des Hypophysenvorderlappens. *Munch. Med. Wochenschr.*, **83**, 1163

58. Grumbach, M. M., Kaplan, S. L., Sciarra, J. J. and Burr, I. M. (1968). Chorionic growth hormone-prolactin (CGP): Secretion, disposition, biologic activity in man, and postulated function as the 'Growth Hormone' of the second half of pregnancy. *Ann. N.Y. Acad. Sci.*, **148**, 501

59. Li, C. H., Grumbach, M. M., Kaplan, S. L., Josimovich, J. B., Friesen, H. and Catt, K. J. (1968). Human chorionic somatomammotropin (HCS): Proposed terminology for designation of a placental hormone. *Experientia*, **24**, 1288

60. Vinik, A. I., Kaplan, S. L. and Grumbach, M. M. (1973). Purification, characterization and comparison of immunological properties of monkey chorionic somatomammotropin with human and monkey growth hormone, human chorionic somatomammotropin and ovine prolactin. *Endocrinology*, **92**, 1051

61. Samann, N., Yen, S. C. C., Gonzalez, D. and Pearson, O. H. (1968). Metabolic effects of placental lactogen (HPL) in man. *J. Clin. Endocrinol. Metab.*, **28**, 485

62. Genazzani, A. R., Pocola, F., Neri, P. and Fioretti, P. (1972). Human chorionic somatomammotropin (HCS): Plasma levels in normal and pathological pregnancies and their correlation with placental function. *Acta Endocrinol.* Suppl. 167, 1

63. Kaplan, S. L., Gurpide, E., Sciarra, J. J. and Grumbach, M. M. (1968). Metabolic clearance rate and production rate of chorionic growth hormone—prolactin in late pregnancy. *J. Clin. Endocrinol. Metab.*, **28**, 1450

64. Andrews, P. (1969). Molecular weight of human placental lactogen investigated by gel filtration. *Biochem. J.*, **III**, 799

65. Catt, K., Moffat, J. B. and Niall, H. D. (1967). Human growth hormone and placental lactogen: structural similarity. *Science*, **157**, 321

66. Grumbach, M. M., Kaplan, S. L. and Vinik, A. I. (1972). In: *Peptide Hormones. Methods in Investigative and Diagnostic Endocrinology*. (S. A. Berson, editor) (Amsterdam: North Holland Publishing Co.)

67. Li, C. H., Dixon, J. S. and Chang, D. (1971). Primary structure of the human chorionic somatomammotropin (HCS) molecule. *Science*, **173**, 56

CHAPTER 8

Immunological Functions of the Placenta

J. T. Lanman

The human placenta normally serves two immunological functions: (1) it provides the fetus with immunological defences, passively transferred from the mother as a selection of her immunoglobulins, which will transiently protect the newborn infant against invading micro-organisms and (2) it protects the fetus, which is normally histoincompatible with the mother, against a maternal immunological attack that could destroy it in the same manner in which a graft of foreign tissue is destroyed. It would appear unlikely that both these functions could be carried out without conflict. However, not only is this accomplished, but also, it is becoming increasingly evident that the two processes are in some ways interrelated and complementary.

The basis for feto-maternal histoincompatibility lies with the paternal component of the fetus' genetic constitution. In all but highly inbred strains of animals, it is foreign to the mother, as reflected in the rejection of fetal tissues directly grafted to the mother. The implanted placenta has been likened to a graft, particularly in the case of the haemochorial placenta found in man, rabbits, and rodents, but despite the intimacy of the maternal-placental association, the similarity to a graft is limited. The two circulations are kept separate, and throughout pregnancy a continuous layer of tissue of fetal origin, the placental trophoblast, and later-on perhaps a sheet of fibrinoid, marks the boundary between fetal and maternal tissue. The physical separation of mother and fetus by a continuous and selective barrier is undoubtedly critical to fetal survival. However, the trophoblastic barrier, though limiting materno-fetal exchange, is imperfect, permitting passage to varying degrees of both macromolecules and the cellular elements contained in blood. In addition, the presence of fetal trophoblast in direct contact with the mother raises the question as to how trophoblast itself is protected against maternal immunological attack. Present evidence suggests that fetal protection lies not in abrogation of the maternal immune response but in its control. In particular, the relation and timing of cellular to humoral immunity which the mother develops in response to fetal antigens appears critical.

Antigenic Stimulation of the Mother by the Conceptus

The stimulus for development of homograft immunity is usually afforded by nucleated cells. Even with the human haemochorial placenta, only a very few kinds of fetal cells can reach the mother: trophoblast and the red and white cells of fetal blood. There is evidence, however, that all of these cells normally do reach the mother, some in considerable numbers. In the human, trophoblast is in extensive and direct contact with the mother in the intervillous space, decidua basalis, and myometrium and, for short distances, lining the uterine arteries. In addition, clusters of trophoblast cells are normally shed into the maternal circulation in numbers estimated at 10^5 cells per day[1]; some of these lodge in the maternal lung, where they may persist without proliferation and without visible host tissue response for months or years. Such lack of tissue response to foreign tissue is unusual, but maternal tissue unresponsiveness to trophoblast has been observed in various other normal and experimental[2] situations. The lack of visible tissue response does not negate the possibility of a maternal humoral response, and, as will be discussed later, the production of maternal circulating antibody in response to maternal exposure to fetal cells may be an essential element in the protection of the fetus against maternal cellular immunity[3].

The apparent immunological inertness of trophoblast, when regarded as a graft, may reflect either a paucity of antigenic sites or their masking by a barrier layer or both. Simmons[4] reviewed the development of antigenicity in fetal cells; antigenicity developed during fetal life, but was weak throughout gestation when compared with the antigenicity of adult cells. Such evidence does not differentiate a paucity of antigenic sites from their masking, as by a barrier layer. An amorphorous layer covering the surface of the trophoblast has been observed by some investigators and variously described as fibrinoid[5], mucopolysaccharide[6], or sialomucin[7]; its demonstration by electron microscopy has not been uniformly successful[8]. Currie and co-workers[9] found that removal of a postulated sialomucin layer from mouse ectoplacental cones by the enzyme neuranimidase rendered an otherwise immunologically inert trophoblast antigenic when transplanted to adult hosts. However, the high toxicity of the enzyme leaves the nature of the revealed antigen open to question. Recently, Adcock et al.[10] suggested that human chorionic gonadotropin (HCG) might interfere with a maternal lymphocyte-mediated attack on the trophoblast. They showed that HCG reversibly blocked the in vitro response of lymphocytes to phytohaemagglutinin; human chorionic somatomammotropin has a similar effect[10a]. The effect of these hormones, if any, on the immune response of lymphocytes to either antigens or incompatible cells is not known. Despite the various observations, the presence or absence of a barrier layer remains unsettled. A number of other studies indicate that trophoblast does carry several antigenic determinants. Histocompatibility[11] and tissue specific[14] antigens have been identified in mouse trophoblast and so-called organ-specific antigens have been found in the trophoblast of various animals including man[12, 13]; these latter antigens appear, however, always to cross-react with kidney.

Fetal red and white cells also normally cross the placenta and reach the mother. Non-nucleated human red cells are incapable of inciting homograft immunity, but antigens on the cell membrane may induce production of a variety of circulating antibodies. During the course of pregnancy, demonstrable transfer of red cells from fetus to mother occurs in about one-third of cases[15], and considerably greater transfer occurs during normal labour, again in about one-third of cases[16]. The antigenic stimulus afforded by these cells depends on their fate. If they are confronted in the maternal circulation by appropriate isoagglutinins and rapidly removed, the likelihood of a maternal immune response is sharply reduced. If not, they may remain for the remainder of their life span in the maternal circulation, and on removal with ageing exit via the spleen, where their foreign antigens may cause an immune response[15]. These contrasting results explain the reduced incidence of erythroblastosis attributable to Rh-incompatibility in those cases with a concomitant maternal–fetal major blood group incompatibility leading to rapid removal of fetal red cells from the maternal circulation. By contrast, prevention of maternal sensitisation in Rh-incompatibility with anti-Rh γ-globulin reflects the blocking or removal of antigenic sites by appropriate antibody given therapeutically. The success of such treatment given shortly after delivery suggests that the effective sensitising dose of fetal cells is that transmitted abruptly during parturition, and not the smaller but measurable dose reaching the mother more gradually before birth.

White cells move across the placenta in smaller numbers than do red cells, but passage in both directions[17, 18] has been demonstrated under normal conditions.

Fetal cells reaching the mother should afford an antigenic stimulus, but the effects of repeated or continuous transfer in low dosage are not well understood. Tolerance can be induced in adults by low[19] as well as by very high doses of antigen. While usually maternal immunological responses to pregnancy are difficult to detect, such responses as have been observed are often in the direction suggestive of tolerance or enhancement[3]. Prolonged survival of paternal-strain grafts (skin or tumour) on the mother after one or particularly after several pregnancies has been observed in humans[20], rats[21] and mice[3, 22]. Interpretation of this observation in man is rendered difficult by similarly prolonged survival in a number of other relationships, but various experiments in rodents appear beyond question. These altered maternal immunological responses cannot be attributed specifically or solely to leukocyte transfer; rather, they represent an effect of any one or more of the tissues involved in exposure of the mother to paternal-strain antigens, whether from fetal leukocytes, trophoblast, or possibly sperm.

Altered receptivity of the uterus to grafts of genetically alien tissue has been observed in rats and appears to reflect a block in the transfer of immuno-genic material to the host. Beer and co-workers[23] observed significant prolonged survival of homografts placed in the uterus specifically at the preimplantation stage of pregnancy when the decidual response was promi-nent; grafts placed elsewhere at the same stage were rejected in the usual way. It was suggested that the decidua may have blocked the antigenic stimulus to the mother; the uterine grafts were not protected against sensitivity either pre-existing or induced by other grafts or by adoptive transfer of appropri-ately sensitised lymphocytes. The situation appears to be analogous to the protection afforded grafts by the 'slime layer' of the hamster cheek pouch, which similarly prevents host sensitisation but will not protect the graft against immunological attack. These barrier layers appear to lack those afferent lymphatic channels which afford the most effective route by which antigenic material is carried to the regional lymph nodes, where their stimulus is translated into cellular immunity. By contrast, the vascular system offers a poor route by which to administer antigens to incite cellular immunity, though the ability to excite a humoral response persists.

Transfer of Immune Substances from Mother to Fetus

All birds, mammals, and at least one amphibian for which information is available provide for transfer of maternal antibodies to the offspring[24], affording transient passive protection postnatally against various bacterial, viral, and parasitic infections. Transfer in birds is to the egg yolk; in mammals it is made by a variety of routes; prenatally via the yolk sac or chorioallantoic placenta; postnatally via the gut for antibodies contained in colostrum or milk. Different species of animals use one or more of these routes. In most animals, materno-fetal transfer of protein is selective, though the kind of selectivity varies widely between species; selectivity is usually effected by the epithelium of the placenta or neonatal gut across which antibody reaches the offspring. In birds, however, it is the follicle cells of the ovary which are concerned. In ungulates, prenatal transfer does not occur; there is a brief period, usually 36 hours or less, in which massive transfer of colostral anti-bodies across the neonatal gut occurs, affording the newborn animal in that short time antibody levels approaching those in the mother. Transfer across the gut in ungulates is non-selective, but selectivity occurs in the mammary gland during secretion of colostrum. Man and primates use the chorioal-lantoic route to provide the newborn infant with plasma levels of IgG approximating or exceeding those in the mother. The human placenta does not appear to transmit other gamma globulins (IgM, IgA, IgD, IgE).

The mechanism of selective antibody transfer has been studied in both placental and gut epithelium. On both of these tissues Gitlin and Gitlin[25] have demonstrated receptors that selectively bind those proteins which have been observed to be most effectively transferred. Electron microscope studies in gut tissue suggest that initial uptake of antibody is by nonselective pino-cytosis[26], creating intracellular bodies known as phagosomes. These then appear to fuse with lysosomes, creating 'phagolysosomes'. Brambell[27] has suggested that proteolytic enzymes contributed by the lysosomes destroy part or all of the contained proteins, including antibody protein, except for those antibody proteins for which selection is operative and which are protected against lysis by binding with specific receptors in the cell. The concept of indiscriminate uptake and selective destruction does not, however, explain certain observations on antibody transfer to mammary secretion in cows[28], where selective uptake appears to be operative. In either case, competition for selective transfer may occur between two related antibodies. Such competition has been demonstrated, for example, between homologous and heterologous immunoglobulins of the same class. The resultant transfer appears to reflect the relative effectiveness of the competing gamma globulins for binding with the receptor sites[24].

In man, only IgG is transferred across the placenta from mother to fetus. The presence of IgM in the plasma of the fetus or very early neonatal infant is indicative of intrauterine antigenic stimulation of fetal immunoglobulin synthesis, a system competent for the last months of gestation but normally latent for lack of antigenic stimulus[29]. The initial immune response to a new antigen is by IgM production, affording a means of distinguishing passively transferred maternal from actively produced fetal or neonatal immuno-globulins. The placental barrier to IgM transfer usually protects the infant against maternal isohaemagglutinin, which are usually wholly or predominantly IgM antibodies. Erythroblastosis arising from Rh, ABO or other feto-maternal red cell incompatibilities can occur only when corresponding haemagglutinins of the IgG type are made by the mother. Maternal circulating antibodies against pathogenic E. Coli are also usually of the IgM type; the infant is normally denied these except for those cases in which maternal IgG antibody of this type is produced[30]. Normally, protection of the newborn infant against these organisms comes from factors in colostrum or breast milk, either as secretory IgA antibodies or, probably more important, as a poorly characterised nutritional factor promoting growth of Lactobacillus bifidus to the virtual exclusion of other flora in the breast-fed infant's intestine[31]. Maternal antibodies appearing in colostrum or milk and swallowed by the infant or in amniotic fluid and swallowed by the fetus have been shown to be locally effective in the gut against various infectious agents, but do not appear to reach the plasma.

Circulating antibodies are a significant factor in materno-fetal histoincompatibility. Tissue incompatibility stimulates not only cellular immunity but also the production of circulating antibodies variously described as cytotoxic, agglutinating, protective, or tumour neutralising[32]. The most potent cytotoxic antibodies are usually of the IgM type, and in most animals are not transferred to the offspring (though they are in the rabbit and in cattle). The weaker cytotoxic IgG antibodies, however, are usually transmitted. Despite their name, the capacity of such circulating antibodies to destroy appropriate target cells is limited. It is usually restricted to destruction of types of cells carried in the circulation, notably lymphocytes and leukaemic cells, although damage to cells in solid tissues has on occasion been demonstrated[33]. The non-lethal binding of circulating antibody to an antigenic site on cells may, however, block the ability of similarly sensitised lymphocytes to seek out and destroy the same target cells. Similarly, if another antibody without destructive potential is bound, it may interfere with the binding of cytotoxic antibody. In mice, IgG has been divided into 3 subgroups, one of which, IgG3, does not fix complement and does not lyse cells[34]. IgG3 is preferentially transferred from mother to fetus at rates 20–50 times those for IgG1 and IgG2. In the presence of maternal sensitisation against her fetuses, non-destructive IgG3 antibodies may protect against potentially damaging maternal antibodies of other types as well as against cell-mediated immunity. In man, 4 subclasses of IgG have been identified. Two (IgG2 and IgG4) bind complement less avidly than the other two; three (IgG1, 3, and 4) pass the placenta to attain levels at or somewhat above maternal serum levels; IgG2, however, is found in cord serum at about 40% of maternal levels[35]. The system in man appears to afford no means of fetal protection similar to that described for the mouse.

The protective effect of circulating antibody against cell-mediated immunity is the basis for enhancement, a phenomenon first recognised in work with transplantable tumours and in which growth of a tumour, instead of being inhibited by a tumour-specific circulating antibody, is paradoxically increased. The varying balance between cellular and humoral immunity is probably critical in explaining the wide variety of feto-maternal immune interactions which have been described. One such interaction has been described which is particularly suggestive of enhancement; Kaliss and Dagg[36] found that female mice pregnant repeatedly by males of another strain differing at the H-2 locus developed both humoral antibodies and *reduced* reactivity to paternal-strain skin and sarcoma homografts, but reactivity against leukaemic grafts was *heightened*. Protection of solid tissues against possible cellular immunity and destruction of leukocytes are contrasting responses characteristic of humoral cytotoxic antibody. A similar effect indicating the appearance of both cellular and humoral immunity in mice bearing genetically foreign fetuses has been shown *in vitro*[37]: lymph node cells from BALB/c females bearing BALB/c × C3H F_1 fetuses inhibited growth of C3H cells *in vitro*, but sera from the pregnant animals abrogated this effect.

Effects similar to those described above, when attributable to circulating antibody, should be producible by passive transfer. Such attempts have not been uniformly successful, but failures may have been attributable to inadequate dosage, and on the whole, increased acceptance of paternal-strain grafts by mothers after repeated pregnancies appears best explainable by the competition between the relatively harmless humoral and the more lethal cellular immunity.

Maternal–fetal Homograft Immunity and Graft–versus–Host Reactions

Many experiments have attempted to demonstrate an effect of homograft sensitisation of the mother against her fetuses, usually by appropriate skin grafts preceding or during pregnancy. In a study by Lanman and co-workers[38] in rabbits, fetuses genetically alien to the mother were obtained by using egg transplantation; the pregnant mother had been repeatedly sensitised by skin grafts from both the male and the female member of the egg-donor pair. Despite demonstrable sensitisation of the mother, no effect on the conceptuses or pregnancy were observed. Several other experiments of this type have had similarly negative results, but in all cases, observations terminated at the time of delivery. Experiments in which postnatal observations on the offspring have been made yielded different results. Stastny[39] found that offspring of

Sprague–Dawley rats could be rendered immune to Lewis-strain skin homografts if the mother had been sensitised by grafting during pregnancy, suggesting a significant transfer of maternal lymphocytes to the fetus. This and similar experiments led Beer and co-workers[40] to follow offspring of Fischer-strain matings, the mothers of which, preceding pregnancy, had been made chimaeric by injections of Lewis-strain bone marrow cells after immunosuppression with cyclophosphamide. Spontaneous abortion in these pregnancies was common. Surviving offspring appeared normal at birth, but postnatally, 50% died in the first 25 days with a wasting syndrome suggestive of runting. Those young which were healthy enough to permit testing demonstrated tolerance to Lewis skin grafts. Beer's experiment also appears to demonstrate significant passage of white cells from mother to fetus. More recently, Beer and Billingham[41] have induced runting in the offspring of mice, hamsters, guinea pigs and rabbits by either adoptive or active immunisation of the mothers against their fetuses. They believe that their success in inducing runting, as contrasted with numerous previous failures, reflects two factors: (1) the timing of immunisation was critical, perhaps providing during pregnancy a stage in the development of the immune response when cellular immunity was less effectively offset by humoral antibody affording target cells protection in the manner of enhancement and (2) offspring were observed for some time postnatally, a period during which runting became apparent. Previous investigators usually used mothers immunised before birth and sought an effect on the fetuses *in utero* or at birth, and carried their observations no further.

In some cases, lymphocytes inoculated into the mother and effective in producing runting in the offspring were also directed against maternal cells, but the mothers remained unharmed. The ability of the mother to destroy rapidly the incompatible cells did not appear to afford the answer to this apparent paradox, because in some combinations of experimental animals, a second litter was also affected despite the fact that no further inoculations were given to the mother. Beer and Billingham[42] also found in rats that immunologically activated lymphocytes crossed the placenta more readily than did unactivated lymphocytes. These various experiments of Beer and Billingham are not at present fully understood, and open new areas for investigation in maternal–fetal immune relationships. They strengthen the concept that fetal protection against immunological destruction reflects a controlled maternal immune response to fetal antigens in which both the timing and nature of the response are critical.

Naturally-occurring wasting syndromes occurring in human infants or young animals and attributed to graft-versus-host reactions have been recognised only very infrequently; even during the initial trials of third trimester treatment of Rh disease with blood transfusions to the fetus, when no precautions of removing leukocytes from the transfused blood were taken, wasting syndromes were rarely recognised[42], probably because in virtually all cases, the transfused leukocytes were destroyed by a fetus already sufficiently mature to have become immunocompetent. The human fetus usually develops a degree of immunocompetence by 20 weeks, before which intra-amniotic transfusions were not usually administered. There is also evidence[43] that the trophoblast itself may be immunocompetent, providing not only a physical but also an early immunological barrier between mother and offspring. However, the infrequency with which the effects of an uncontrolled maternal immunological attack on her offspring have been clinically recognised may also reflect the lack of reliable and readily available diagnostic methods; in the large group of human infants now placed in the category of 'failure to thrive', it seems likely that a group will be found whose disease is related to an abnormal materno-fetal graft-versus-host reaction.

Feto-maternal histoincompatibility has usually been regarded as a potential danger to the fetus, but advantages are also possible. James[44], using crosses of inbred strains of mice, demonstrated increased placental size which he showed to be related to feto-maternal immunological interaction; other effects probably secondary to increased placental size were increased body weight and slightly shorter gestation times. Increased placental and body weights are suggestive of hybrid vigour, in this case attributable to immunological factors. In other studies, also using inbred strains of mice[45] and rats[46] differing in respect to a given histocompatibility locus, appropriate matings have revealed modest but significant selective advantage for progeny differing from their mother with regard to certain H loci. A particularly striking example of selection favouring materno–fetal histoincompatibility was afforded by Michee and Anderon's[47] inbreeding experiments. They failed to develop an isohistogenic strain of Wistar rats despite 72 generations of sister-brother matings; their observations revealed strong selection against individuals homozygous for an (unfortunately) undefined histocompatibility locus. In such studies as these, the time at which selection becomes operative is unknown, but may be early in gestation, perhaps at the time of fertilisation, blastocyst implantation, or early placentation.

The relative antigenic ineffectiveness of trophoblast has been mentioned and related either to a paucity of antigenic sites of their masking by an amorphous barrier layer. Trophoblast also appears to be relatively inert as a potential immunological target, usually remaining unharmed in an immunologically hostile environment. The same factors which impair antigenicity could assist in affording this protection. A low density of surface antigenic determinants has been shown to protect cells against lysis by complement-fixing humoral antibodies[48]. If a placental amorphous barrier layer protects the trophoblast against a hostile immunological attack, special properties not found in other such protective layers would have to be involved, since usually barrier layers protect only against antigenic stimulation of the host and not against immunological attack against the graft. Trophoblast, however, is usually not detectably damaged when in an immunologically hostile environment, as was strikingly demonstrated by Simmons and Russell[49] by transplantation of mixed trophoblast and embryonic tissues from early mouse embryos to presensitised adult recipients. The embryonic elements were rapidly rejected, but trophoblast proliferated and was unaffected even when juxtaposed to embryonic cells undergoing lysis. However, trophoblast lost its apparent protection when grown *in vitro*. There, when grown in association with either homologous or maternal lymphocytes, Currie and Bagshaw[7] showed that trophoblast underwent cytolysis. The contrasting observations *in vivo* and *in vitro* may reflect a protective effect of humoral antibody *in vivo*, but the *selective* protection of trophoblast *in vivo* requires additional undefined influences. Heterologous antisera against trophoblast also appears to override its apparent protection. Antibody against rat trophoblast raised in rabbits caused abortion in rats but not in mice or hamsters[11]. It appears that trophoblast is usually adequately protected against immunological attack in normal situations, but not in special experimental situations.

Conclusions

Perhaps the most striking aspect of placental maternal–fetal immunological relationships is the variety of means by which essentially the same end results are accomplished. Placental structure is highly variable between species. Protection of the fetus against immunological attack presents little problem in the marsupial, in which prolonged implantation does not occur or, for the same reason, through most of gestation in ungulates, since implantation does not occur in these animals until well on in gestation. With progressively more intimate types of placentation, the problem becomes more apparent, until with the haemochorial placenta resemblance to a graft becomes closer. Even in this instance, the feto-placental unit never becomes a true graft, but the intimacy of the association is sufficient to excite materno–fetal exchanges leading to immune responses by the mother. Under normal conditions the nature and extent of these incompatibilities and associated responses produce no detectable damage and may even afford a selective advantage to the fetus. But, under abnormal conditions, a change in the maternal immune responses and death or damage to the fetus occurs. It now appears that at least with the more intimate types of placentation, fetal protection against immunological attack rests not in the avoidance of a maternal immune response, but rather in an appropriate timing and interplay of maternal cellular and humoral immunity.

The passive transfer of maternal humoral immunity to the fetus is also effected by a wide variety of mechanisms, and is reflected in a variety of placental types providing either different pathways for transfer of maternal antibody or, in a few species, no placental antibody transfer at all. Nevertheless, in all the higher vertebrates for which data are available, the fetus is in some way and by some route the recipient of passive immunity from the mother.

Species variability in structure and mechanisms is characteristic of many aspects of reproduction: hormonal, anatomical, behavioural, and genetic to a degree far greater this is encountered in other organ systems. These differences effectively prevent cross breeding, except in a few cases between closely related animals. The species variability in the reproductive process may be an expression of the high survival value of speciation, which is promoted by conservation and confinement of genetic variations that might otherwise be lost by more widespread and often inappropriate dissemination.

References

1. Ilké, F. A. and Gallen, S. T. (1964). Dissemination von Syncytiotrophoblastzellen im mütterlichen Blut während der Gravitität. *Schweiz. Akad. Med. Wiss.*, **20**, 62

2. Simmons, R. L. and Russell, P. S. (1962). Antigenicity of mouse trophoblast. *Ann. N.Y. Acad. Sci.*, **99**, 717

3. Prehn, R. T. (1960). Specific homograft tolerance induced by successive matings, and implications concerning choriocarcinoma. *J. Natl. Cancer Inst.*, **25**, 883

4. Simmons, R. L. (1969). Histoincompatibility and the survival of the fetus: current controversies. *Transplant Proc.*, **1**, 47

5. Bardawil, W. A. and Toy, B. L. (1959). The natural history of choriocarcinoma: problems of immunity and spontaneous regression. *Ann. N.Y. Acad. Sci.*, **80**, 197

6. Kirby, D. R. S., Billington, W. D., Bradbury, S. and Goldstein, D. (1964). Antigen barrier of the mouse placenta. *Nature (London)*, **204**, 548

7. Currie, G. A. and Bagshawe, K. D. (1967). The masking of antigens on trophoblast and cancer cells. *Lancet*, **i**, 708

8. Simmons, R. L. and Russell, P. S. (1967). Immunologic interactions between mother and the fetus. *Adv. Obstet. Gyn.*, **1**, 38

9. Currie, G. A., Van Doorninck, W. and Bagshawe, K. D. (1968). Effect of neuraminidase on the immunogenicity of early mouse trophoblast. *Nature (London)*, **219**, 191

10. Adcock, E. W., III, Teasdale, F., August, C. S., Cox, S., Meschia, G., Battaglia, F. C. and Naughton, M. A. (1973). Human chorionic gonadotropin: its possible role in maternal lymphocyte suppression. *Science*, **181**, 845

10a. Contractor, S. F. and Davies, H. (1973). Effect of human chorionic somatomam-motropin and human chorionic gonadotropin on phytohaemagglutinin-induced lymphocyte transformation. *Nature New Biol.*, **243**, 284

11. Kirby, D. R. S., Billington, W. D. and James, D. A. (1966). Transplantation of eggs to the kidney and uterus of immunized mice. *Transplantation*, **4**, 713

12. Koren, Z., Abrams, G. and Behrman, S. J. (1968). Antigenicity of mouse placental tissue. *Am. J. Obstet. Gynecol.*, **102**, 340

13. Bevans, M., Seegal, B. C. and Kaplan, R. (1955). Glomerulonephritis produced in dogs by specific antisera. *J. Exp. Med.*, **102**, 807

14. Kirby, D. R. S. (1968). The immunological consequences of extrauterine development of allogenic mouse blastocysts. *Transplantation*, **6**, 1005

15. Coehn, F. and Zuelzer, W. W. (1967). Mechanisms of isoimmunization. II. Trans-placental passage and postnatal survival of fetal erythrocytes in heterospecific pregnancies. *Blood*, **30**, 796

16. Beer, A. E. (1969). Fetal erythrocytes in maternal circulation of 155 Rh–negative women. *Obstet. Gynecol.*, **34**, 143

17. Walknowska, J., Conte, F. A. and Grumbach, M. M. (1969). Practical and theoretical implications of fetal/maternal lymphocyte transfer. *Lancet*, **i**, 1119

18. Oehme, J., Hundeshagen, H. and Eschenbach, C. (1966). Uber die Passage markierter Leukocyten vom Muttertier zum Feten—zugleich ein Beitrag zur Runt-Disease. *Klin. Wochenschr.*, **44**, 430

19. Nossal, G. J. V. (1967–68). The cellular basis of immunity. *Harvey Lect.*, **63**, 179

20. Peer, L. A., Bernhard, W. and Walker, J. C., Jr. (1958). Full-thickness skin exchanges between parents and their children. *Am. J. Surg.*, **95**, 239

21. Rogers, B. O., Raisbeck, A. P., Ballantyne, D. L., Jr. and Converse, J. M. (1960). The genetics of skin homografting in rats between brothers, sisters, parents and grandparents. *Trans. Int. Soc. Plastic Surgeons*, p. 421

22. Breyere, E. J. and Barrett, M. K. (1960). 'Tolerance' in postpartum female mice induced by strain-specific matings. *J. Natl. Cancer Inst.*, **24**, 699

23. Beer, A. E., Billingham, R. E. and Hoerr, R. A. (1971). Elicitation and expression of transplantation immunity in the uterus. *Transplant Proc.*, **3**, 609

24. Brambell, F. W. R. (1970). *The Transmission of Passive Immunity from Mother to Young.* (New York: American Elsevier)

25. Gitlin, J. D. and Gitlin, D. (1973). Cell receptors and the selective transfer of proteins from mother to young across tissue barriers. *Pediatr. Res.*, **7**, 290

26. Clark, S. L. (1959). The ingestion of proteins and colloid materials by columnar absorptive cells of the small intestine of suckling rats and mice. *J. Biophys. Biochem. Cytol.*, **5**, 41

27. Brambell, F. W. R. (1966). The transmission of immunity from mother to young and the catabolism of immunoglobulins. *Lancet*, **ii**, 1087

28. Brandon, M. R., Watson, D. L. and Lascelles, A. K. (1971). The mechanism of transfer of immunoglobulin into mammary secretion of cows. *Aust. J. Exp. Biol. Med. Sci.*, **49**, 613

29. Silverstein, A. M. and Lukes, R. J. (1962). Fetal response to antigenic stimulus. I. Plasmacellular and lymphoid reactions in the human fetus to intrauterine infection. *Lab. Invest.*, **11**, 918

30. Gitlin, D., Rosen, F. S. and Michael, J. G. (1963). Transient 19S-1-globulin defi-ciency in the newborn infant, and its significance. *Pediatrics*, **31**, 197

31. György, P. (1955). Lactobacillus acidophilus and lactobacillus bifidus in their relation to infant feeding. *Q. Rev. Pediatrics*, **10**, 17

32. Stetson, C. A. and Jensen, E. (1960). Humoral aspects of the immune response to homografts. *Ann. N.Y. Acad. Sci.*, **87**, 249

33. Boyse, E. A., Old, L. J. and Stockert, A. (1962). Some further data on cytotoxic isoantibodies in the mouse. *Ann. N.Y. Acad. Sci.*, **99**, 574

34. Ralph, P., Nakoinz, I. and Cohn, M. (1972). IgM–IgG 1,2,3, relationship during pregnancy. *Nature (London)*, **238**, 344

35. Hay, F. C., Hull, M. G. R. and Torrigiani, G. (1971). The transfer of human IgG subclasses from mother to fetus. *Clin. Exp. Immunol.*, **9**, 355

36. Kaliss, N. and Dagg, M. K. (1964). Immune response engendered by multiparity. *Transplantation*, **2**, 416

37. Hellström, K. A., Hellström, I. and Brawn, J. (1969). Abrogation of cellular immunity to antigenetically foreign mouse embryonic cells by a serum factor. *Nature (London)*, **224**, 914

38. Lanman, J. T., Herod, L. and Fikrig, S. (1964). Homograft immunity in pregnancy: survival rates in rabbits born of ova transplanted into sensitized mothers. *J. Exp. Med.*, **119**, 781

39. Stastny, P. (1965). Accelerated graft rejection in the offspring of immunized mothers. *J. Immunol.*, **95**, 929

40. Beer, A. E., Billingham, R. E. and Yang, S. L. (1972). Maternally induced transplantation immunity, tolerance, and runt disease in rats. *J. Exp. Med.*, **135**, 808

41. Beer, A. E. and Billingham, R. E. (1973). Maternally acquired runt disease. *Science*, **179**, 240

42. Naiman, J. L., Punnett, H. H., Destine, M. L. and Lischer, H. W. (1966). Y_y chromosomal chimerism. *Lancet*, **ii**, 590

43. Dancis, J., Jansen, V., Gorstein, F. and Douglas, G. W. (1968). Hematopoietic cells in mouse placenta. *Am. J. Obstet. Gynecol.*, **100**, 1110

44. James, D. A. (1967). Some effects of immunologic factors on gestation in mice. *J. Reprod. Fertil.*, **14**, 265

45. Hull, P. (1969). Maternal-foetal incompatability associated with the H–3 locus in the mouse. *Heredity*, **24**, 203

46. Palm, J. (1970). Maternal-fetal interactions and histocompatibility antigen polymorphisms. *Transplant Proc.*, **2**, 162

47. Michie, D. and Anderson, N. F. (1966). A strong selective effect associated with a histocompatability gene in the rat. *Ann. N.Y. Acad. Sci.*, **129**, 88

48. Humphrey, J. and Dourmashkin, R. (1969). The lesions in cell membranes caused by complement. *Adv. Immunol.*, **11**, 75

49. Simmons, R. L. and Russell, P. S. (1962). Antigenicity of mouse trophoblast. *Ann. N.Y. Acad. Sci.*, **99**, 717

Circulation in the Intervillous Space; Obstetrical Considerations in Fetal Deprivation

Karlis Adamsons and Ronald E. Myers

Introduction

The frequency with which biochemical evidence of asphyxia is encountered among newborn human infantst[1, 2] has led to the belief that the structure of the placenta itself unduly limits oxygen delivery to the fetus. This contention has received support from morphological considerations which point out the greater thickness of the tissue layers interposed between the maternal and fetal circulations in the placenta compared to those which separate alveolar air from pulmonary capillaries. Furthermore, the considerably lower oxygen tension of the fetal arterial blood compared to that of the mother has been cited as further evidence of the inferior design of the placenta as an organ of gaseous exchange. Little attention has been paid to the fact that due to the high diffusion constant of oxygen in tissue, the difference in thickness of the trophoblastic layer and of the alveolar lining is of little consequence. Indeed, it has been pointed out[3] that the operational conditions for placenta and lung are surprisingly similar, and that the safety factor with respect to oxygen transport to the fetus is at least as great as that of the adult under conditions of slight physical activity. Furthermore, within certain limits, the oxygen tension of the fetal arterial blood is a poor indicator of oxygen availability to the fetal tissues. Thus, in a situation where the oxygen tension of the fetal arterial blood is only 40% of that of the mother, its oxygen concentration is likely to be at least 80%

of that of the mother. The above considerations implicate deficiencies in convection of oxygen to the placenta rather than in its diffusion through it as the source of fetal asphyxia when it occurs.

The recognition that the structure of the placenta cannot be made responsible for the occurrence of inadequate fetal oxygenation during pregnancy or during labour and delivery requires a redirection of attention to the various mechanisms by which the maternal blood supply to the placenta is altered.

Two principal models have emerged. One deals with moderate reduction in uterine and placental blood flow of long duration which results primarily in growth retardation of the fetus. The mass of the fetus at a given gestational age is considered as an index of the adequacy of perfusion of the intervillous space. The basis for this assumption rests on experimental studies in which fetal growth retardation was produced by artificially reducing the maternal uterine or the fetal umbilical blood supplies[4, 5] and from epidemiologic data which point out a strong association between impaired growth of the fetus and conditions known to decrease blood flow to the uterus.

The second model examines a reduction in uterine blood flow which leads to asphyxia of the fetus of greater magnitude but shorter duration. This may lead to death of the fetus or, less commonly, brain injury. It will be the principal objective of the present review to survey our knowledge of conditions which affect uterine blood flow, with the intent to demonstrate that under normal circumstances the fetus possesses an excellent supply line and that substantial interferences in uterine circulation are needed in order to elicit fetal changes of lasting consequence.

Although a variety of methods exist for the measurement of uterine blood flow, none of them is suitable for a precise estimation of the flow rates through the intervillous space on a continuous basis. On the other hand, determinations of the oxygen pressure and content of the fetal arterial blood, although not capable of reflecting the absolute blood flow rates through the exchange system, nonetheless provide a satisfactory indication of both the direction and degree of any change in placental perfusion. Because interferences with fetal circulation are rare and when they occur under experimental circumstances are readily detectable, determination of oxygen pressure and content of the fetal arterial blood are good indicators of the functionally significant blood flow rate through the intervillous space. Conceptually, oxygen in this context can be viewed much in the same way as any other indicator used in indicator dilution methods for measuring flow rates. Its principal merit as an indicator in the present circumstance is its rapid removal from the fetal compartment. This permits the detection of even rapidly occurring transient changes in intervillous space perfusion.

Morphological and Functional Characteristics of the Maternal Supply of Blood to the Placenta

The uterus derives its blood supply from two major sources—the uterine arteries which are branches of the internal iliac arteries, and the ovarian arteries which take their origin from the abdominal aorta below the take-off of the renal arteries. Within the pregnant uterus these principal supplying arteries send branches to the myometrium, the decidua, and the placenta. Although measurements are not available for the human, it may be assumed that at least 80% of the total blood flow to it is allocated for the perfusion of the placenta.

It has been assumed that the principal resistance to flow of blood through the placenta on the maternal side lies in the intervillous space. The main fall in blood pressure in this interpretation occurs across the intervillous space and calls for a high pressure in the terminal portion of the spiral artery. Indeed, a pressure as high as 80 mmHg has been projected for this site[6].

There are several arguments that can be raised against this generally held hypothesis. In the primate, the uteroplacental circulation is highly reactive to a variety of pharmacological agents which affect its flow and lead to alterations in oxygenation of the fetus. For example, the catecholamines and the prostaglandins are capable of reducing intervillous space perfusion even to the extent of causing fetal death[7]. The concept of the major resistance to flow residing in the intervillous space cannot accommodate these observations demonstrating such reactivity to vasoconstrictive agents. A second argument against this hypothesis is that a pressure as high as 80 mmHg within the intervillous space would compress the capillaries of the fetal villi and would arrest the umbilical circulation in which the perfusion pressure at least early in gestation does not exceed 20–30 mmHg. Furthermore, the structure and physical characteristics of the dilated terminal portion of the spiral artery (the infundibulum) make it unlikely to resist distension by so high an intraluminal pressure.

Current studies by the authors in which direct pressure measurements from the infundibular portion of the spiral artery have been obtained in the rhesus monkey have demonstrated that the perfusion pressure of the intervillous space is exceedingly low. Under optimal conditions, the mean pressure in this segment of the spiral artery, which empties directly into the central portion of the cotyledon, is less than 25 mmHg[8]. This is confirmed by our own observations (unpublished). The pressures recorded at the same time in the uterine veins forming the venous outflow from the placental cotyledons range between 3 and 5 mmHg in the rhesus monkey in the supine position. Thus, the perfusion pressure across the intervillous space is about 15–20 mmHg.

One of the unique features of the intervillous space as a conduit of blood is the absence of a direct feedback mechanism from the tissues supplied (the placental villi) and the sites where regulation of flow occurs (the spiral arteries). In most other tissues of the body considerable changes in blood flow occur to meet the changing metabolic needs of the tissues. In these instances the mechanism involved in regulating the regional blood flow resides locally within the tissue. However, because of the relatively slight changes in metabolism of the placenta and fetus over shorter periods of time, little need exists for such regulation. Furthermore, fetal control over the conductance of the intervillous space might constitute a risk to the mother since the fetus would be in a position to divert progressively more of the cardiac output of the mother irrespective of her own circumstance.

The volume of the intervillous space near term in man is about 150 ml[9]. The oxygen contained in this reservoir which is equal to the oxygen consumption of the fetus for 1–1·5 minutes, serves to minimise the rates and extents of changes in oxygenation of the fetus during labour when uterine contractions may intermittently reduce blood flow to the intervillous space. In some pathologic states, however, this volume may be considerably reduced due to edema of the villi or to failure of the trophoblastic layer to undergo attenuation. This occurs in erythroblastosis and diabetes mellitus.

Assuming a volume for the intervillous space of about 150 ml and a flow rate through it of 600 ml/min, the mean transit time through the cotyledons would be 15 seconds. This calculated time for circulation through the intervillous space approximates that time required for disappearance of dye from the placenta as documented using cineradiography in man[10, 11]. No measurement is available of blood flow through the intervillous space in man. Technical difficulties prevent either the direct or the indirect measurement of the blood flow of the uterus particularly under conditions which are representative of normality. The values available from the literature derived using N_2O equilibration, range from 125 to 150 ml/min/kg of combined fetal and placental mass[12, 13]. A similar value is obtained by calculations which assume a mean oxygen consumption of the fetus and placenta of 5 ml/kg/min and a difference in oxygen concentration between the uterine artery and vein of 5 ml/100 ml.

The channel size of the intervillous space varies over a wide range. In the centre of the lobules and in the interlobular areas which empty into the uterine veins, the spaces are irregular and cavernous and may measure up to 2 mm in diameter. In the intermediate region which constitutes the major portion of the cotyledonary mass and serves as the principal site for exchange of materials between the maternal and fetal compartments, the channels become more regular and measure 4–20 μ in diameter (average $=15$ μ). This estimated channel diameter agrees closely with that derived from knowledge of the volume of the intervillous space (150 ml) and the surface area of the placental villi (10–12 m²) but is considerably below that given by other authors[11, 14]. Assuming a given low rate through any system, the flow velocity through each of its components is inversely proportional to the cross-sectional area. In the case of the spiral artery and the lobule, the mean flow velocity through the spiral artery can be calculated to be about 300 mm/sec in contrast to 0·1 mm/sec in the periphery of the lobule and 10 mm/sec in the intervillous space near the centre.

From the above considerations of morphology and function of the placenta it is apparent that highly favourable conditions exist for the exchange of respiratory gases between the mother and the fetus. This is substantiated by the fact that under normal circumstances only negligible differences exist in the concentrations of oxygen and carbon dioxide between the blood of the uterine and the umbilical veins. The special features of the placenta which ensure this efficiency of operation include the small channel size of the intervillous space, the long transit time of the maternal blood in passing through the lobule, the small distance between the maternal and fetal vascular channels, and the large area of the exchange surface. Additional factors which enhance respiratory gas exchange between the mother and the fetus are the high diffusion constants of carbon dioxide and oxygen, the higher affinity of the haemoglobin in the fetal red cell for oxygen, and the action of the rise in hydrogen ion concentration of the maternal blood during its transit through the intervillous space upon the affinity of hemoglobin for oxygen (the Bohr effect).

Conditions Altering Rates of Maternal Blood Flow through the Intervillous Space

The conditions which can cause a decrease in the blood flow through the intervillous space can be divided into four categories. The first encompasses those in which the net perfusion pressure across the intervillous space is altered. The second deals with changes in viscosity of maternal blood. The third is concerned with changes in intrauterine pressure while the final group considers the channel size of the intervillous space as affected by alterations in the structuring of the villi.

Conditions Affecting Perfusion Pressure

During pregnancy both the systolic and diastolic blood pressures are decreased often by as much as 10 mmHg. This results from the vasodilating effects of the placental steroids on the entire vasculature rather than from increases in vascular conductance due to the grafting on of the placental circulation. This physiological decrease in maternal blood pressure, however, does not threaten the oxygen supply to the fetus. Similar or even greater reductions in blood pressure can be produced by analgesic, anaesthetic or hypnotic agents without significant reduction in oxygen supply to the fetus. On the other hand, the effects of hypovolaemia, either relative or absolute, upon intervillous space perfusion remains to be elucidated. Clinical observations suggest that decreases in blood volume of the mother may impair fetal oxygenation. It is likely that the reduction in intervillous space perfusion under these circumstances is principally brought about by reflex vasoconstriction of the uterine arteries and their branches rather than by a reduction in mean arterial blood pressure in the aorta.

The complex haemodynamic effects of spinal and epidural anaesthesia deserve particular attention. It is beyond the scope of this communication to examine the details which are available in texts on obstetrical anaesthesia. It is generally agreed, however, that the principal factor which contributes to hypotension in the mother under these circumstances is increase in venous capacitance. This leads to a reduction in cardiac output and decrease in blood pressure. The pregnant individual near term receiving epidural or spinal anaesthesia is particularly vulnerable to compression of the vena cava and aorta in the supine position. Information is lacking regarding the ability of the spiral arteries to increase their conductance under conditions of systemic hypotension. Clinical observations, however, indicate that such a response does not occur under the circumstances described above. Such an outcome might be anticipated inasmuch as the expected response of the visceral circulation to hypovolaemia is vasoconstriction.

The autonomic innervation of uterine vessels including the spiral arteries is similar to that of other abdominal viscera which contain numerous terminals of sympathetic nerves located predominantly in the media. The relative distribution of alpha- and beta-adrenergic receptors for this vascular bed has not been determined. Preliminary information suggests that there is a paucity or perhaps a total absence of beta-receptors. The presence of the alpha-receptors accounts for the reactivity of these vessels to the electrical stimulation of sympathetic nerves[15] or to the administration of ganglionic stimulants or adrenergic drugs[7, 16, 17].

Lowering of blood pressure at the terminal portion of the spiral artery can

result from a decrease in systemic arterial blood pressure due to hypovolaemia, to certain types of myocardial disease, or to myocardial depression
due to exogenous agents. However, considerable changes in arterial blood
pressure can occur without accompanying changes in intervillous space perfusion sufficient to be detectable as changes in oxygenation of the fetus.
This has been demonstrated in the rhesus monkey in which fetal oxygenation was assessed before and after partial occlusion of the descending aorta[18].
Reduction of the systemic blood pressure of the mother by as much as 50%
by administration of flourothane also may cause no detectable changes in
fetal oxygenation[19].

A second category of abnormal states of the circulatory system associated
with diminished intervillous space perfusion includes excessive adrenergic
stimulation (either endogenous or exogenous), stimulation of the vascular
musculature by substances such as prostaglandin F_{2a}, and disease conditions
such as pre-eclampsia, essential hypertension, or kidney disease. It is presumed that all these conditions lead to a constriction of the arteries which
supply the placenta. Experimental evidence to substantiate the validity of
this contention has been obtained in the case of norepinephrine-induced
hypertension. Intravenous injection of norepinephrine in the rhesus monkey
elicits a fall in the blood pressure recorded from the infundibular portion of
the spiral artery while causing a rise of as much as 100% in the aorta. (Authors' unpublished observation.)

From a clinical point of view the group of disorders characterised by vasoconstriction within the uterine arteries and their branches account for the
majority of instances in which the welfare of the fetus is jeopardised because
of inadequate delivery of blood of normal composition to the intervillous
space. Under these circumstances, the blood pressure at the site of inflow
into the intervillous space is inadequate despite the fact that the pressure in the
major supplying vessels may be elevated.

The deranged state of the vessels may be structural in nature as occurs in
atherosclerosis or the collagen vascular diseases or the impaired flow may be
secondary to a tonic constriction of the normal vascular smooth muscle in
the uterine vessels as in essential hypertension or pre-eclampsia. These two
categories are not always mutually exclusive in that longstanding hypertension or toxaemia may be associated with structural changes in the vessels
along with the vasospastic component.

Atherosclerosis is an infrequent cause of reduced uterine perfusion during
pregnancy because this disorder is chiefly encountered, with the exception of
juvenile diabetics, among older individuals. However, it is the occasional
cause of fetal hypotrophy in juvenile diabetics with far-reaching vascular
involvement. Angiographic studies in patients with atherosclerosis have

revealed focal narrowing of the arterial lumina[20]. Involvement of the uterine vasculature in the collagen-vascular diseases is rare. The implications for the fetus are dependent on the extent to which the supplying blood vessels are affected. In extreme cases, the outcome is fetal growth retardation, premature labour and intrauterine death; in milder cases, the effect upon the fetus may be negligible[21].

As alluded to above, the uterine vasculature responds to a variety of stimuli in a manner analogous to that of other abdominal viscera. It is highly probable that the uterine blood flow is maximal when the mother is in a non-stressed state. Studies with non-human primates have demonstrated that activation of either the alpha- or the beta-receptors or their blockade lead to impairments in oxygenation of the fetus. Administration of epinephrine or nonepinephrine to the pregnant rhesus monkey has documented the potency of these agents in reducing intervillous space perfusion and, hence, fetal oxygenation[7]. It was possible to produce death of the fetus when the adrenergic agonists were administered in sufficient doses to the mother. These findings were not unexpected since stimulation of alpha-adrenergic receptors has been known to decrease visceral blood flow. It was unexpected, however, that a beta-adrenergic stimulant (isoproterenol) had a similar effect on the oxygenation of the fetus when administered to the mother. The mechanism by which such an agent can lead to decreases in intervillous space perfusion is not immediately apparent. Because of the slightness of the decrease in mean perfusion pressure one cannot satisfactorily entertain the argument that it is this reduction that decreases the blood flow through the intervillous space. Rather, it may be assumed that beta-stimulation leads to vasoconstriction in the spiral arterial system to account for the decrease in po_2 in the blood of the umbilical artery.

Clinically, activation of the sympathetic nervous system of the mother occurs in two ways: from endogenous release of catecholamines secondary to emotional and other stress states and from ingestion, injection or inhalation of exogenous materials capable of stimulating either the sympathetic ganglia or the adrenergic receptors of the effector cells.

Satisfactory studies have not been carried out in which the effects of stress in the human free from other associated variables have been related to altered fetal growth and neonatal outcome. Evidence has been presented which favours the contention that exaggerated sympathetic activity can occur throughout gestation among 'would be' smokers[22]. The birth weight of the offspring of 'would be' smokers was significantly less than that of women who never took up smoking. It is also possible that the poor fetal outcome among chronic alcoholics[23] and heroin addicts is not solely due to the pharmacological and toxic effects of these agents but may also relate to aspects of the mothers' life style and specific autonomic reactivity. That aspects of the personality of life styles of the mother may affect the fetal environment has received support from studies which show that anxious mothers give birth to babies of smaller weight than non-anxious mothers[24]. Studies carried out with rhesus monkeys have also provided both epidemiological[25] and direct physiological evidence[26] of the adverse effects of maternal psychological stress upon the fetus.

Perhaps the most dramatic example of endogenous catecholamine release is observed in patients with pheochromocytoma. These patients may present an appearance similar to that of essential hypertension or pre-eclampsia of pregnancy characterised by periodic episodes of marked exacerbation of symptoms. Because of the rarity of this condition it is difficult to assess with precision the risk to the fetus under these circumstances. Often the correct diagnosis has not been established prior to autopsy. From data available in the published literature, however, one can estimate that the incidence of fetal loss during the 2nd and 3rd trimesters in this disease approaches 50%[27]. A marked increase is also seen in the frequency with which premature separation of the placenta occurs among this group of patients.

Among the exogenous agents capable of reducing uterine vascular conductance nicotine has been presented as of the greatest epidemiological importance[28]. Through its properties as a stimulant to the sympathetic ganglia, it releases both norepinephrine and epinephrine from the adrenal medulla and the terminals of sympathetic nerves throughout the body resulting in a generalised vasoconstriction. Thus, it is expected that the chronic inhalation of nicotine during pregnancy would result in decreased growth of the fetus due to a subnormal perfusion of the intervillous space. This has been found to be the case by a variety of investigators[28, 29]. On average, the birth weight of a fetus of a heavy smoker is about 300 g less than that of a matched control while the duration of gestation is not significantly shortened. Although it is generally accepted that it is the exposure of the mother to nicotine that reduces growth of the fetus, it remains possible that the sympathetic reactivity of the smoker *per se* may play the more important role in reducing fetal growth.

The use of adrenergic agonists in clinical practice is limited to treatment of hypotensive states, such allergic reactions as bronchial asthma, and as decongestants of mucosal surfaces. Although there is no question that adrenergic agonists can diminish uterine circulation as alluded to above, this is rarely of clinical significance because of their relatively short durations of action. More significant fetal asphyxia may result when alpha-receptor agonists are administered for longer periods or when compounds of longer duration of action such as ephedrine are used. It cannot be overemphasised that in the presence of systemic hypotension, visceral vasoconstriction is already considerable. In such circumstances, it is advantageous to restore perfusion pressure by an increase in cardiac output rather than by a further decrease in vascular conductance. Needless to say, the first effort should be directed towards the restoration of blood volume and the normalisation of venous return.

There is another group of diseases in which the mechanisms leading to decreased intervillous space perfusion reside within small arteries and arterioles. In the initial stages of these disorders the decrease in vascular conductance is largely due to an increased tonus of the vascular musculature. In later stages morphological abnormalities may supervene and ultimately dominate. These diseases include essential hypertension, toxaemia, unilateral kidney disease, and a variety of other disorders including Kimmelstiel–Wilson disease of diabetics and nephrosclerosis. The outcome for the fetus varies according to the degree of decrease in vascular conductance to the intervillous space and its duration. In the early stages of these diseases the impact upon the fetus may not be demonstrable which would permit the inference that the degree of reduction of blood flow was well within the tolerance limits for normal growth. In more advanced stages of these diseases, there is impairment of fetal growth, and an increased incidence of premature onset of labour and intrauterine death. Because of reduced uterine circulation and the resulting decrease in oxygen stores in the blood of the intervillous space, these fetuses are particularly susceptible to the adverse effects of labour and agents known to alter the cardiovascular performance of the mother.

The time in gestation at which a decreased conductance to the intervillous space emerges as a limiting variable is of clinical significance. Deprivation from early in the second half of gestation appears to be less hazardous to the fetus than that occurring later. In the former instance, the fetus responds to the reduced availability of nutrients and oxygen by decreased growth. Thus, the discrepancy between requirements and supply may often be maintained within the limits of tolerance. Such a fetus is in many ways comparable to a fetus of a multiple gestation. Any reduction in the uterine circulation which emerges late during gestation and affects a fetus which had hitherto exhibited a normal growth rate, will elicit a greater discrepancy between the impaired supply and the demand. In support of this interpretation, one can cite the markedly higher perinatal mortality and morbidity among patients with toxaemia and those with essential hypertension or twin gestations.

Altered conductance through the intervillous space

From theoretical considerations it is evident that flow through the intervillous space is affected by changes in the viscosity of blood. Thus, it is anticipated that in circumstances which increase blood viscosity such as active sickling, the conductance through the intervillous space is greatly reduced. Hypergammaglobulinaemias also lead to a decrease in perfusion rate for any given perfusion pressure.

There are two categories of morphological conditions in which the conductance of the intervillous space is below normal. The first comprises conditions in which the gross and fine structure of the villi and the intervillous space are normal and where the decrease is solely due to a reduced placental mass. Examples in this category are the individual placentas in cases of multiple gestation. This results in reduced growth rates of the fetuses in the last trimester of pregnancy and some reduction in duration of gestation. There is no evidence in the human that fetal oxygenation is adversely affected.

The second category of conditions is characterised by an altered structure of the placental villi with a resultant decrease in channel size and, hence, in conductance of the intervillous space. Such changes in architecture of the villi are most conspicuous in the presence of high umbilical venous pressure as occurs in cases of erythroblastosis, fetal syphilis, or neoplasia of the fetal liver. The presence of the high venous pressure leads to an edema of the villi and a diminished cross-sectional area of the intervillous space. As has already been described, a small volume of the intervillous space decreases the tolerance of the fetus to interruptions in circulation through it.

The situation in patients whose mothers suffer from diabetes mellitus and anaemia has been only partially clarified. It is currently assumed that in the presence of hyperinsulinaemia, all fetal organs with the probable exception of the central nervous system undergo accelerated cell division and increase in cell size. In the case of the placenta, this leads to a prolonged proliferation of the cyto- and syncytiotrophoblast and to a failure of their attenuation during the second half of gestation. It is not known whether the increase in placental mass as observed in these two conditions can entirely compensate for the decrease in the conductance of the intervillous space.

The deposition of fibrin within the channels of the intervillous space or the development of placental infarcts may have less influence on the total blood flow through the intervillous space than on fetal oxygenation. The oxygenation of the fetus is diminished in such instances largely because of the exclusion of still perfused fetal villous capillaries from the maternal circulation through the intervillous space.

Alterations in outflow conductance and intervillous space flow

In view of the low pressures which exist in the infundibulum of the spiral artery (15–20 mmHg), it might appear at first that the blood flow through the intervillous space would be greatly affected by alterations in the pressures in the veins draining the cotyledon. Closer examination of the system, however, disqualifies such a contention. The principal determinant of the low blood pressure in the infundibular portion is the high conductance through the intervillous space in relation to the volume of blood delivered to it per unit time from the high resistance part of the afferent circuit, the spiral artery. When the pressure in the uterine veins rises, as occurs with compression of the vena cava, a proportionate increase in the intraluminal pressure is transmitted throughout the entire conduction system proximal to the occlusion site. Since the proportion of the pressure required for the perfusion of the intervillous space is small in relation to the total pressure gradient across the system as a whole (less than 20%) it is apparent that only extraordinary increases in venous pressure will significantly reduce the flow rates through the intervillous space. There is, however, an additional aspect to consider regarding changes in venous pressure and fetal oxygenation. Assuming that it were possible to elevate the venous pressure in the inferior vena cava to as high as 30 mmHg, this pressure would be transmitted through the intervillous space and a proportionately higher pressure would develop in the terminal portion of the spiral artery. Because the net pressure gradient across the intervillous space would remain largely unchanged, it can be assumed that its perfusion would be maintained. The abnormally high pressure within the intervillous space, however, would compress the villous capillaries leading to a decrease in perfusion of villi and hence to fetal asphyxia. The relative immunity of the flow rate through the intervillous space to changes in venous pressure, as projected above would seem to run contrary to clinical observations. It is well documented that compression of the vena cava by the gravid uterus with the patient in a supine position frequently causes asphyxia of the fetus. Although there is unquestioned radiological evidence that the vena cava is compressed effectively, there is no evidence that fetal asphyxia develops under such circumstances unless there is evidence of maternal hypotension secondary to decreased venous return. In this context it is noteworthy that ligation of the inferior vena cava even during advanced gestation in the human, does not significantly affect fetal oxygenation. Reflex vasoconstriction in the visceral circulation of the mother in response to functional hypovolaemia may also contribute substantially to decreased perfusion of the intervillous space.

Effects of Uterine Contractions on Intervillous Space Perfusion

It can be considered as an established fact that uterine contractions decrease the rate of perfusion of maternal blood through the intervillous space. For the primate, the strongest and most direct evidence of this effect comes from angiographic studies. These studies show an impaired filling of the lobules with the contrast medium when the material is injected into the aorta during uterine contractions. Additional evidence comes from the demonstration that the oxygen tension in the fetal arterial blood shows a phasic decrease which follows the onset of any uterine contraction by a 30–45 second interval. In the asphyxiated fetus, this is accompanied by commensurate decreases in the fetal heart rate known as late decelerations. In the sheep, decrease in uterine blood flow during contractions has been demonstrated by electro-magnetic flow meter studies[15].

Controversy still prevails regarding the mechanism by which uterine contractions cause reductions in intervillous space perfusion. One hypothesis proposes that the contracting myometrium reduces intervillous space perfusion by impeding the venous outflow from the uterus and thus reducing the pressure gradient across the intervillous space. The other hypothesis emphasises the occlusion of the afferent artery by the myometrium by a pseudo-sphincter action. A third hypothesis identifies the intraluminal pressure of the uterus as a modulator of the pressure gradient which exists between the uterine and ovarian arteries on the one hand and the venous outflow from the intervillous space on the other.

When one considers the structure of the uterus and its contents it becomes apparent that the decidual portion of the spiral artery is always exposed to the same pressure as is the fetus and the placenta. This follows from the fact that the contractile elements, mainly the myometrium, are located entirely external to these vessels. Because the uterine contents are essentially non-compressible, contractions of the uterus lead to increases in the tensions in the uterine wall but to no gross shortening of the wall until cervical dilatation begins. This speaks against venous compression as a major mechanism in reducing arterial inflow into the intervillous space during uterine contractions and emphasises the changes in the pressure gradient between the uterine and spiral arteries as the responsible modulator of flow rate through the inter-villous space. Because the mean blood pressure in the uterine arteries is sub-stantially greater than that normally reached during a uterine contraction, it can be inferred that uterine blood flow continues, though attenuated, through-out the contraction phase.

Clinical Conditions Associated with Abnormal Composition of Maternal Blood

The impact of low arterial P_{O_2} secondary to living at high altitude has been most extensively studied in regard to perinatal morbidity, mortality and neonatal birth weight. Perhaps the best data are found from studies which have compared pregnancy outcome in Denver, U.S.A. (5000 feet above sea level) with that of Baltimore, U.S.A. (at above sea level). The mean birth weight for the Denver population was only one per cent less than that for Baltimore. It is difficult to interpret the data gathered on human populations living at elevations above 15 000 feet such as in the Peruvian Andes or in the Himalayan Region because of the influence of social, economic, and ethnic factors. It should be noted, however, that the mean birth weight in Lake County, Colorado (10 000 feet above sea level), is nearly 300 g less than that for the population of Denver.

Studies in various laboratory animals such as rats and sheep do not support the view that altitude has a significant impact on the ability of the mother to supply the fetus with the required quantity of oxygen. This is not unexpected in view of the compensatory mechanisms such as increased concentration of red cells in the maternal circulation, and increase in alveolar ventilation which reduces the P_{O_2} difference between inspired air and gas mixture in the alveoli.

Interference with oxygen transport from the lung to the intervillous space in the presence of normal blood viscosity and normal vascular conductance is seen in carbon monoxide poisoning and following the exposure of the mother to oxidizing agents leading to methemoglobinemia (e.g. Mepivicaine). The net effect in this circumstance is a decrease in the quantity of oxygen delivered to the intervillous space per unit time and a concomitant fall in fetal P_{O_2}. Because of the very high affinity of carbon monoxide for haemoglobin only minimal amounts of carbon monoxide are transferred to the fetus in cases of carbon monoxide poisoning of the mother. Hence, the fetus in this situation is subjected to a normocarbic hypoxia.

The most common abnormal composition of maternal blood in pregnancy is anaemia. Although reduction in red cell concentration is inevitably linked to a decrease in oxygen carrying capacity or oxygen content in the blood perfusing the intervillous space, the impact upon the fetus of such a condition appears to be minimal unless the anaemia has reached extreme degrees. There are two explanations for this phenomenon. In the presence of low haemoglobin concentrations the partial pressure of oxygen in the blood of the intervillous space is higher than when the same quantity of oxygen is carried by a larger quantity of haemoglobin. Since not only the quantity of oxygen but also the oxygen tension determines the amount of oxygen transferred from mother to the fetus, it is evident that maternal anaemia is less hazardous to the fetus than maternal hypoxaemia. Maternal anaemia is usually associated with a decrease in viscosity of the blood which leads to an increase flow rate through the intervillous space for a given perfusion pressure. The circumstances in sickle cell anaemia are grossly different. The oxygen supply of the fetus in this instance is not so much affected by the reduced concentration of haemoglobin in the maternal blood as it is by the large increase in blood viscosity during the phases of active sickling.

Polycythaemia either primary or secondary due to low arterial P_{O_2} seem to have little effect on fetal oxygen supply unless complicated by other factors.

Fetal Circulation to the Placenta

Because of the protected position of the fetus within the uterus adverse environmental influences are far less likely to affect the circulation to the placenta from the fetal side in comparison to that occurring on the material. Indeed, even gross malformations of the fetal heart and great vessels which are incompatible with survival after birth—such as interventricular septal defects, atresia of the pulmonary arteries—may not affect the perfusion of the placenta and somatic tissues of the fetus. There is circumstantial evidence that pharmacological agents such as certain local anaesthetics may have a specific propensity to suppress the fetal myocardium leading to bradycardia and perhaps a decrease in fetal cardiac output.

The disturbances which are brought about by the mechanical compression of the fetal vessels leading to the placenta are rare and are limited to the compression of the umbilical cord which may follow the rupture of membranes and the torsion or compression of it due to rotation of the fetus or the wrapping of the umbilical cord around the fetal neck or extremity. True knots in the cord are also known and are the likely cause of stillbirth in such cases. An additional form of abnormality that predisposes the fetus to impaired villus circulation is abnormal insertions of the umbilical cord.

The umbilical arteries which originate as major branches of the internal iliac arteries are supplied with blood from the combined output of the right and left ventricles, with the right ventricle contributing the major portion. Accurate measurements of the part of the total cardiac output allocated to the placenta are not available in the human. Data from rhesus monkey and sheep indicate that at least 50% of the total cardiac output is assigned to the umbilical circulation. However, this fraction is variable and affected by the conductance through the ductus arteriosus and of the pulmonary arteries. The umbilical vessels and their chorionic and villous branches are unique in their relationship to vasoactive agents. Neither increases nor decreases in hydrogen ion concentration, carbon dioxide or catecholamines appear to affect the villous vascular conductance *in vivo*. According to present knowledge, prostaglandins are the only biological materials which can decrease the vascular conduction of the umbilical circulation upon administration directly to the fetus[30]. It is also generally agreed that the umbilical vessels lack autonomic nerves and hence are not sensitive to activation of the sympathetic nervous system.

The villous capillaries when examined in a fresh state under the phase contrast microscope exhibit a diameter of 7–8 μ, just large enough to allow a rouleau formation of fetal red blood cells to be circulated. Controversy still exists regarding the distance that separates a fetal capillary from the maternal blood in the intervillous space. This appears at least partly to be due to the fact that the wall of the villus varies considerably in its thickness from location to location in addition to the variations induced by fetal age. In the mature human placenta unfixed specimens provide unequivocal evidence that at least in some villi the capillaries are separated from the intervillous space by not more than 2 or 3 μ. In other portions the separation involves a greater thickness of connective tissue core and includes multiple layers of synthiotrophoblast nuclei and a greater mass of cytoplasmic material giving a total diffusion distance as much as 20–30 μ.

Therapeutic Considerations

In the foregoing paragraphs a number of conditions were examined under which the transport of vital materials from the mother to the fetus is impaired. Most of them evolve as an inevitable consequence of some medical disorder in the mother or in the fetus, leaving little opportunity for the physician to apply prophylactic or therapeutic measures. Among the few exceptions were diabetes melitus of the mother and the presence of anti-D antibody in maternal circulation secondary to her previous exposure to Rh positive red cells. In the former situation, prevention of maternal hyperglycaemia could prevent fetal hyperinsulinemia and its sequelae upon the fetus and placenta. In the latter, appropriately timed administration of donor blood to the fetus is effective not only to correct fetal anaemia but also to circumvent changes in the placenta which are known to reduce its transport capacity.

There are conditions in which treatment of the mother may actually threaten the supply line of the fetus. Among examples are hypertensive cardiovascular disorders including some forms of toxaemia of pregnancy. According to presently available data antihypertensive therapy either by antiadrenergic agents, ganglionic blocking agents or non-specific relaxant of the smooth muscle are likely to reduce rather than enhance perfusion of the intervillous space. This may be explained on the basis that the spiral arteries of the uterus are less responsive to the vasodilatory actions of these agents than the arterioles of other vascular beds. Often the decisive factor in planning therapy is whether or not the hypertension *per se* constitutes a risk to the mother. In the absence of such a risk the obstetrician might elect to postpone the initiation of therapy in order not to jeopardise further the already impaired uterine blood flow. This might be particularly so in patients with essential hypertension.

The minimisation of physical activities during the second half of gestation appears to maximise uterine and, hence intervillous space perfusion. Although no specific measurements regarding this aspect are available, support in favour of this contention is rendered by the observation that bed rest often decreases uterine irritability if such occurs prior to term. It also appears to account for delaying onset of labor in patients with multiple gestation.

Reducing the level of maternal anxiety without altering her circulatory state is likely to be beneficial to the fetus. Hence, in some patients hypnotics or tranquillisers may actually be required during the antipartum course if optimal conditions for uterine perfusion are to be maintained. Because the mildly sedated patient is more likely to rest than the untreated counterpart, the above therapy often exerts an additional favourable influence on uterine circulation. Prevention of severe maternal and, hence fetal hyperthermia in the febrile patient is essential for fetal safety. It has been documented at least in the monkey that the fetus is seriously at risk when maternal temperature exceeds $41 \cdot 5°C$. It remains to be elucidated to what extent the tolerance limits are lowered in patients with already impaired fetal oxygenation.

Controversy still prevails regarding the mode of delivery of the fetus 'at risk'. There appears to be, however, a concensus that fetuses with partial premature separation of the placenta should not be exposed to labour unless analyses of fetal blood negate the required assumption that fetal P_{O_2} is already abnormally low in the absence of uterine contractions. The protagonists of hysterotomy as a method of choice in delivering patients with impaired placental function stress the elimination of further reduction of fetal oxygenation brought about by uterine contractions. They assume that anaesthesia and preparation of the patient for Caesarean section such as positioning, have rarely an adverse effect on uterine circulation and fetal oxygenation. The antagonists point out that a well conducted labour seldom affects fetal oxygen supply even in the 'high risk' population to the extent which might lead to a neurological injury to the fetus. In addition, they emphasise the advantages of the vaginally born infant regarding the establishment of ventilation vis-à-vis that delivered by Caesarean section.

The introduction of more precise surveillance techniques of the fetus during labour has made the difference between the two schools of thought more apparent than real. Electronic monitoring of fetal heart rate by means of ultrasound has enabled the obstetrician to ascertain fetal tolerance to uterine contractions long before the fetus is accessible for sampling of blood and the precise determination of the state of oxygenation. The availability of agents capable of suppressing virtually instantaneously spontaneous or oxytocin induced uterine contractions (e.g. diazoxide) has further increased the safety of the so-called trial of labour in patients with borderline placental function. The contemporary obstetrician is also cognisant of the relative hazards of the supine position whether during labour or during the preparation phase for Caesarean section. He also bears in mind the importance of normovolemia and he is taught to resort to prophylactic measures when administering agents which increase the capacitance of the circulatory system of the mother. Although he has not yet found the cure—and perhaps he is unlikely ever to find it—for many of the conditions which impair the supply of the fetus with substances needed for optimal growth and development, he has made a substantive progress in assessing the impairment of fetal environment, in determining its impact upon the rate of fetal maturation, in elucidating the mechanism by which extraneous factors either spontaneous or iotrogenic aggravate the existing liability. This has placed him in a favourable position to determine when the extrauterine environment constitutes less risk to the fetus than that prevailing *in utero*.

References

1. Kubli, F., Ruttgers, H. and Henner, H.-D. (1972). Clinical aspects of fetal acid-base balance during labor. In: Longo, L. D. and Bartels, H., *Respiratory Gas Exchange and Blood Flow in the Placenta*. DHEW publ. No (NIH) 73-361, p. 487
2. Apgar, V., Holaday, D. A., James, L. S. and Weisbrot, I. M. (1958). Evaluation of the newborn infant. Second report. *J. Amer. Med. Ass.*, **168,** 1985
3. Adamsons, K. (1965). Transport of organic substances and oxygen across the placenta. Proceedings of a Symposium on the Placenta. Birth Defects Original Article Series, The National Foundation—March of Dimes. **1,** 27
4. Wigglesworth, J. S. (1964). Experimental growth retardation in the fetal rat. *J. Path. Bact.*, **88,** 1
5. Myers, R. E., Hill, D. E., Holt, A. B., Scott, R. E., Mellits, E. D. and Cheek, D. B. (1971). Fetal growth retardation produced by experimental placental insufficiency in the rhesus monkey. I. Body weight, organ size. *Biol. Neonate.*, **18,** 379
6. Ramsey, E. M. (1954). Circulation in the maternal placenta of primates. *Amer. J. Obstet. Gynecol.*, **67,** 1

7. Adamsons, K., Mueller-Heubach, E. and Myers, R. E. (1971). Production of fetal asphyxia in the rhesus monkey by administration of catecholamines to the mother. *Amer. J. Obstet. Gynecol.*, **109**, 248

8. Moll, W., Künzel, W., Stolte, L. A. M., Kleinhout, J., DeJong, P. A., and Veth, A. F. L. (1974). The blood pressure of the decidual part of the uteroplacental arteries (spiral arteries) of the rhesus monkey. *Pflügers Arch.*, **346**, 291

9. Aherne, W. and Dunnill, M. S. (1966). Quantitative aspects of placental structure. *J. Path. Bact.*, **91**, 123

10. Freese, U. E., Ranniger, K. and Kaplan, H. (1966). The fetal-maternal circulation of the placenta. II. An x-ray cineradiographic study of pregnant rhesus monkeys. *Amer. J. Obstet. Gynecol.*, **94**, 361

11. Freese, U. E. (1972). Vascular relations of placental exchange areas in primates and man. In: Longo, L. D. and Bartels, H., *Respiratory Gas Exchange and Blood Flow in the Placenta.* DHEW Publ. No. (NIH) 73-361, p. 31

12. Metcalfe, J., Romney, S. L., Ramsey, L. H., Reid, D. E. and Buswell, C. S. (1955). Estimation of uterine blood flow in normal human pregnancies at term. *J. Clin. Invest.*, **34**, 1632

13. Assali, N. S., Douglas, R. A., Baird, W. W., Nicholson, D. B. and Sugemoto, R. (1953). Measurement of uterine blood flow and uterine metabolism. *Amer. J. Obstet. Gynecol.*, **66**, 248

14. Bartels, H. and Moll, W. (1964). Passage of inert substances and oxygen in the human placenta. *Pflugers Arch. Ges. Physiol.*, **280**, 165

15. Greiss, F. C. and Gobble, F. L. (1967). Effect of sympathetic nerve stimulation on the uterine vascular bed. *Amer. J. Obstet. Gynecol.*, **97**, 962

16. Misenhimer, H. R., Margulies, S. I., Panigel, M., Ramsey, E. M. and Donner, M. W. (1972). Effects of vasoconstrictive drugs on the placental circulation of the rhesus monkey. *Invest. Radiol.*, **7**, 496.

17. Ladner, C. N., Brinkman, C. R., Weston, P. and Assali, N. S. (1970). Dynamics of uterine circulation in pregnant and nonpregnant sheep. *Amer. J. Physiol.*, **218**, 257

18. Myers, R. E. (1972). Two patterns of perinatal brain damage and their conditions of occurrence. *Amer. J. Obstet. Gynecol.*, **112**, 246

19. Morishima, H. O., Allen, I. H., Adamsons, K., James, K. L. (1971). Anesthetic management for fetal surgery in the subhuman primate. *Amer. J. Obst. Gynec.*, **110**, 926

20. Borell, U., Fernstrom, I., Lindblom, K., and Westman, A. (1952). Diagnostic value of arteriography of iliac artery in gynecology and obstetrics. *Acta Radiol.*, **38**, 247

21. Mund, A., Simson, J. and Rothfield, N. (1963). Effect of pregnancy on course of systemic lupus erythematosis. *J. Amer. Med. Ass.*, **183**, 917

22. Yerushalmy, J. (1971). The relationship of parent's cigarette smoking to outcome of pregnancy—implications as to the problem of inferring causation from observed associations. *Amer. J. Epidemiol.*, **93**, 443

23. Jones, K. L. (1974). Outcome in offspring of chronic alcoholic women. *Lancet*, **i**, 1076

24. Shaw, J. A., Wheeler, P. and Morgan, D. W. (1970). Mother-infant relationship and weight gain in the first month of life. *J. Amer. Acad. Child Psychiat.*, **9**, 428

25. Myers, R. E. (1972). The pathology of the rhesus monkey placenta. *Acta Endocrinol.*, Suppl. **166**, 221

26. Myers, R. E. (1975). Maternal psychologic stress and fetal asphyxia: A study in monkey. *Amer. J. Obstet. Gynecol.* (In press)

27. Dean, R. E. (1958). Pheochromocytoma and pregnancy. *Obstet. Gynecol.* **11**, 35

28. MacMahon, B., Alpert, M. and Salber, E. J. (1965). Infant weight and parental smoking habits. *Amer. J. Epidemiol.*, **82,** 247

29. Rush, D., Kass, E. H. (1972). Maternal smoking: a reassessment of the association with perinatal mortality. *Amer. J. Epidemiol.*, **96,** 183

30. Myers, R. E., Comas-Urrutia, A., Lazotte, L. A. and Adamsons, K. (1974). Cardio-vascular effects of prostaglandins on fetal and uterine circulations of rhesus monkey. *Gynecol. Invest.*, **5,** 61

CHAPTER 10

Abnormalities of Composition of Maternal Blood

Henning Schneider and Joseph Dancis

Maternal homeostatic mechanisms provide the major protection to the mammalian fetus. In the absence of illness or severe environmental stress, pathogens are excluded from the maternal blood stream and the composition of the blood is maintained within narrow limits. Under these circumstances, the fetus easily derives its nutrients and eliminates its excretory products through the placenta, remaining sheltered from the external world.

The fetus exists as a parasite in the sense that it derives its sustenance from the mother without making any notable contributions to maternal welfare. In fact, it appears that the fetus may modify maternal metabolism for its own benefit. It has been suggested that the role of the large amounts of chorionic somatomammotropin liberated from the placenta into the maternal blood stream is to alter metabolism so that glucose is partially replaced by fatty acids as maternal fuel, conserving carbohydrate for the fetus[1].

The term, 'fetal parasitism', has developed the additional subtle connotation that the fetus will thrive in spite of severe maternal deprivation or other disturbances. The concept has been fostered by clinical observations of normal infants issuing from abnormal pregnancies. We shall review some of the limited available information concerning the welfare of the baby in pregnancies in which maternal homeostasis is disturbed. We shall avoid the extensive literature accumulated by experimental teratologists even though the subject is interesting and to some extent pertinent.

Starvation

Nutrients are generally distributed according to metabolic needs, the more metabolically active organs receiving a greater proportion of materials.

During pregnancy, the fetus participates in this partition[2]. Consistent with its rapid growth rate, it receives more nutrition per unit weight than does the mother (Figure 10.1).

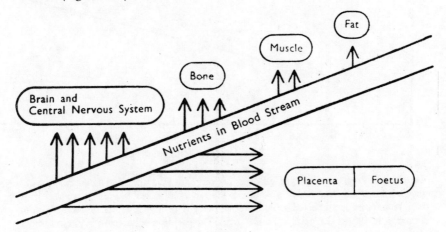

Figure 10.1 Schematic representation of partition of nutrients according to metabolic activity. (From Hammond, J. (1960). *Farm Animals*. (London: Edward Arnold) with permission from the author)

Limiting the food intake of pregnant experimental animals reduces the size of the young[3]. As the limitation becomes more severe, there is some indication that the fetus derives more than its appropriate share of protein and calories (Figure 10.2). However, the drain upon maternal nutrients is greater in most animals than in primates, because of the relatively extended gestation period and slow rate of fetal growth in the latter[4].

It is not possible to gather such well-controlled information in the human. Generalised malnutrition in the human as seen today in a large part of the world is usually accompanied by infection and specific deficiencies. An exceptional situation occurred during World War II when Holland was subjected to starvation conditions which lasted less than a year. The diet remained well-balanced but severely restricted, and there were no major epidemics. Comparison of reproductive records before and after this acute episode revealed the the major impact was on fertility. Over half the women became amenorrhoeic. Successful pregnancies yielded infants with birth weights averaging 9% less than those born in non-starvation periods, a relatively small but significant difference. The major impact was on pregnancies in which starvation occurred during the last trimester, when the fetus gains weight most rapidly[5].

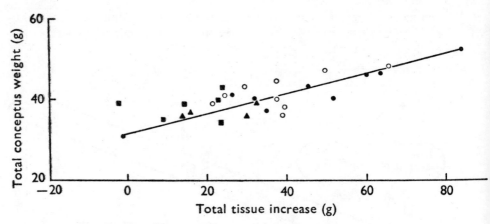

Figure 10.2 Pregnant rats were fed *ad lib* and on reduced intakes. Total maternal weight increase from day 10 to 21 of gestation is plotted against total conceptus weight. Fetal weight appears less affected than maternal weight at lowest levels of intake. (From Frazer, J. F. D. and Huggett, A. St. G. (1970). The partition of nutrients between mother and conceptuses in the pregnant rat. *J. Physiol.*, **207**, 783 with permission from the authors)

It is not apparent from such observations what the mechanism of fetal growth impairment is. It is possible that nutrients circulating in maternal blood are reduced so that the fetus is starved much as the mother is. There may be endocrinological complications or other secondary factors.

Water and Electrolyte Disturbances

Biological membranes, including the placenta, are readily permeable to *water*. Any change in osmolarity in maternal plasma, results in a rapid water shift across the placenta with establishment of a new equilibrium[6]. Electrolyte transfer also occurs, but at a slower rate.

Acid-base balance of blood is maintained by a series of buffer mechanisms. Upsetting the equilibrium in the mother by an infusion of ammonium chloride induces a metabolic acidosis which is not reflected in the infant twenty minutes later[7], probably because of the slow transfer of chloride ions. Chronic acidosis, lasting for days in the mother, will produce fetal acidosis[8]. Animal experiments suggest that the disturbances of ammonium chloride acidosis are reflected in the fetus within a period of hours[9]. It may be suspected that, during equilibration, the differential rates of transfer of such ions as chloride, bicarbonate and phosphate may cause fetal disturbances that differ significantly from those in the mother.

Sodium, Potassium, Magnesium

These 3 ions will be discussed together because experimental studies have clearly demonstrated the variability of the effect of the fetus of specific maternal nutritional deprivations[10, 11].

Rats were placed on a low *sodium* diet throughout pregnancy, a period of 3 weeks. At term, the maternal plasma sodium was reduced, and a similar reduction was evident in the fetus (Figure 10.3).

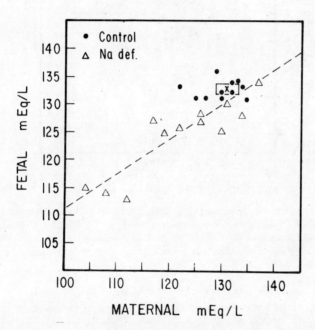

Figure 10.3 Sodium deprivation in rat. Small box indicates mean ± twice standard error of mean. Maternal and fetal plasma sodium level are both reduced as a result of sodium deprivation. (From Dancis, J. and Springer, D. (1970). Fetal homeostasis in maternal malnutrition: Potassium and sodium deficiency. *Pediat. Res.*, **4**, 345 with permission from author and journal)

A low *potassium* diet also caused a rapid fall in maternal plasma level. At term, maternal muscle was severely depleted of potassium, and the animals were clearly sick. However, the newborn pups, although a little small, were vigorous and healthy. Fetal plasma levels were normal and there was relatively little reduction in tissue potassium concentration (Figure 10.4).

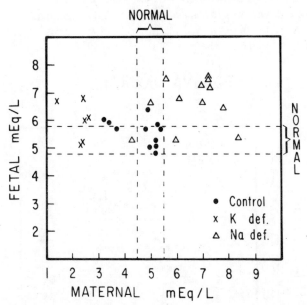

Figure 10.4 Potassium deprivation in rat. Interrupted lines indicate normal range. Fetal plasma levels are not depressed when maternal levels are considerably reduced. (From Dancis, J. and Springer, D. (1970). Fetal homeostasis in maternal malnutrition: Potassium and sodium deficiency. *Pediat. Res.*, **4,** 345 with permission from the journal)

A low *magnesium* diet produced a rapid drop in the level in maternal plasma. If the diet was instituted early in pregnancy, the mothers failed to carry to term. When the low magnesium diet was delayed until 10 days gestation, pregnancy was completed but the pups were runted, weak and suffered from a severe haemolytic anaemia.

Maternal plasma levels were sharply reduced but the changes in tissue concentration did not achieve statistical significance. The plasma level in cord blood, which is normally higher than the maternal, was as low as and often lower than the maternal. Fetal tissue concentrations were also reduced (Table 10.1).

In all 3 instances, the fetus behaved as a parasite, drawing upon a deficient mother for its nutrition. With sodium, the burden of the deficiency was

Table 10.1 Magnesium deprivation

| | Maternal tissue | | | Fetal tissue | | |
	Plasma	Bone	Muscle	Plasma	Fetus	Placenta
Control	1·6±0·04	213±13·7	23±0·8	2·4±0·07	14·2±0·39	8·8±0·15
Deficient	0·33±0·03*	176±12·1	24±0·5	0·31±0·02*	8·9±0·22*	7·8±0·50

* $p < 0.01$

Pregnant rats were placed on low magnesium diets at 10 days gestation. Analyses were done at term. Results presented in milliequivalents per litre or per kilogram.

distributed relatively equally between mother and conceptus. In potassium deprivation, the fetus fared much better than the mother, maintaining potassium levels that were close to normal in spite of serious maternal deficiencies. In contrast, the mother resisted magnesium deprivation far more successfully than the fetus. Most maternal magnesium is 'bound' to maternal tissue and is unavailable to the young.

Calcium offers an interesting contrast to magnesium. A pregnant rat placed on an essentially calcium-free diet throughout pregnancy is capable of producing a healthy litter with tissues containing normal amounts of calcium[12]. The mother evidently has a large easily mobilised reserve of calcium. However, clinical experience in old China indicates that these reserves are not inexhaustible. Mothers suffering from osteomalacia as a result of a chronic calcium deficiency often bore children suffering from congenital rickets. In a very few cases, blood analyses were done and the maternal serum calcium and phosphorus were shown to be very low and fetal levels were similarly depressed. For example, in one case report the determinations were: mother, calcium 4·0, phosphorus 2·6 mg%; newborn infant, calcium 6·4, phosphorus 4·2 mg%[13].

Such florid cases of dietary insufficiency have not been reported in the West. However, infants with severe hypocalcaemia have been born to mothers deprived of calcium because of intestinal malabsorption[14]. The clinical manifestations of maternal disease have at times been so subtle as to be detected only after the diagnosis of congenital rickets in the child.

Amino Acids

The concentration of amino acids is normally higher in the fetal than in the maternal blood (see Chapter 6). It is not known whether this gradient serves to protect the fetus against maternal amino acid deficiencies associated with a reduction of maternal blood levels. However, the gradient is maintained when the maternal level is raised[15,16] and the elevated fetal levels can be toxic to the rapidly growing organism. This observation has become clinically important now that phenylketonurics are reaching adulthood in larger numbers because of dietary regimens. Phenylketonuric mothers with elevated phenylalanine blood levels have given birth to severely retarded children who do not have the enzyme defect[17]. The damage is presumed to result from the hyperphenylalaninaemia. A low phenylalanine diet administered to the mother should prevent this tragic complication.

Summary

There is relatively little information on the effect of maternal stresses on fetal homeostasis. However, a few general principles can be identified.

Under normal circumstances, the fetus derives adequate nutrients from the mother, which the mother then replaces from environmental supplies. When environmental sources are insufficient, maternal tissues may be drawn upon to maintain a normal composition of her blood. Maternal blood represents the major 'environmental' exposure of the fetus so that, as long as normal blood composition is maintained it is reasonable to assume that the fetus will have no problem with nutrition. The success with which maternal blood composition can be maintained depends on the amount of mobilisable supplies in the mother relative to demand. Continuing deprivation will deplete even large reserves and maternal blood levels will fall. Under these circumstances, one must expect the fetus to share in the malnutrition. The effect on the fetus depends on how essential the particular nutrient is to the rapidly growing organism.

Potassium deprivation is the sole exception identified so far to the above generalisations in that the placenta appears to protect the fetus against maternal hypokalaemia. There are no examples of the placenta protecting the fetus against elevations of maternal blood constituents.

Acute disturbances, such as abrupt changes in acid–base balance, may not be immediately reflected in the fetus. After a latent period, there is a period of readjustment between maternal and fetal circulations in which different rates of transfer of the individual ions may induce fetal changes that differ from the mother's. In time, a new equilibrium is established.

It is clear that, although the fetus exists as a parasite within the mother, it is not independent of maternal welfare. Considerably more information is needed to fill in these broad outlines.

References

1. Burt, R. L., Leake, N. H. and Busdon, J. P., Jr. (1970). Whither placental lactogenic hormone? *Obstet. Gynec.*, **36,** 306

2. Hammond, J. (1960). Farm Animals, 3rd edition (London: Edward Arnold Publishers)

3. Frazer, J. F. D. and Huggett, A. St. G. (1970). The partition of nutrients between mother and conceptuses in the pregnant rat. *J. Physiol.*, **207,** 783

4. Payne, P. R. and Wheeler, E. F. (1967). Comparative nutrition in pregnancy. *Nature (London)*, **215,** 1134

5. Smith, C. A. (1947). Effects of maternal undernutrition upon the newborn infant in Holland (1944–1945). *J. Pediat.*, **30,** 229

6. Battaglia, F., Prystowsky, H., Smisson, C., Hellegers, A. and Bruns, P. (1960). Fetal blood studies. XIII. The effect of administration of fluids intravenously to mothers upon the concentrations of water and electrolytes in plasma of human fetuses. *Pediat*, **25,** 2

7. Blechner, J. N., Stenger, V. G., Eitzman, D. V., *et al.* (1967). Effects of maternal metabolic acidosis on human fetus and newborn infant. *Amer. J. Obstet. Gynec.*, **99,** 46

8. Kaiser, I. H. and Goodlin, R. C. (1958). The effect of ammonium chloride induced maternal acidosis on the human fetus at term: II. Electrolytes. *Amer. J. Med. Sci.*, **235,** 549

9. Dancis, J., Worth, M., Jr. and Schneidau, P. B. (1957). Effect of electrolyte disturbances in the pregnant rabbit on the fetus. *Amer. J. Physiol.*, **188,** 535

10. Dancis, J. and Springer, D. (1970). Fetal homeostasis in maternal malnutrition. I. Potassium and sodium deficiency. *Pediat. Res.*, **4,** 345

11. Dancis, J., Springer, D. and Cohlan, S. Q. (1971). Fetal homeostasis in maternal malnutrition. II. Magnesium deprivation. *Pediat Res.*, **5,** 131

12. Bodansky, M. and Duff, V. B. (1941). Dependence of fetal growth and storage of calcium and phosphorus on the parathyroid function and diet of the pregnant rat. *J. Nutr.*, **22,** 25

13. Maxwell, J. P., Pi, H. T., Lin, H. A. C. and Kuo, C. C. (1939). Further studies in adult rickets (osteomalacia) and foetal rickets. *Proc. Royal Soc. Med.*, **32,** 287

14. Begun, R., Coutinko, Mde. L., Dormandy, T. L. and Yudkin, S. (1968). Maternal malabsorption presenting as congenital rickets. *Lancet*, **i,** 1048

15. Cockburn, F., Farquhar, J. W., Forfar, J. O., Giles, M. and Robins, S. P. (1972). Maternal hyperphenylalaninaemia in the normal and phenylketonuric mother and its influence on maternal plasma and fetal fluid amino acid concentrations. *J. Obstet. Gynaec. Brit. Comm.*, **79,** 698

16. Kerr, G. R., Chamove, A. S., Harlow, H. F., *et al.* (1968). Fetal phenylketonuria: The effect of maternal hyperphenylalaninemia during pregnancy in the rhesus monkey. *Pediat.*, **42,** 27

17. Fisch, R. D., Doeden, D., Lansky, L. L. and Anderson, J. A. (1969). Maternal phenylketonuria. Detrimental effects on embryogenesis and fetal development. *Amer. J. Dis. Child.*, **118,** 847

CHAPTER 11

Ill-defined Maternal Causes of Deprivation

Peter Gruenwald

Various empirically recognised clinical conditions lead to retarded fetal growth. In some of these but not in others, we have some clue regarding the mechanism. In none has this mechanism been fully elucidated. Detailed accounts of the subject have been given by Brent and Jensch[1] and by Ounsted and Ounsted[2].

Multiple Birth

McKeown and Record[3] showed more than 20 years ago that growth of multiple births in man begins to be retarded when litter weight exceeds 3000 g—as it is in singletons. This has been confirmed in my own observations on twins[4]. The somewhat smaller size of monochorionic as compared with dichorionic twins, as well as other peculiarities of the former group, may be explained by the fact that monochorionic twinning represents a malformation arising within one single ovum[4]. This has been vividly expressed by naming these twins choriopagus in analogy with thoracopagus, etc. In spite of the earlier onset of growth retardation, twins usually have a much higher combined weight than even a large singleton of the same gestational age. McKeown and Record[3] ascribed the earlier onset of growth deceleration in multiple births to properties of the 'maternal organism' which is what we have here called the maternal supply line. They also discussed the effect of crowding in the uterus, particularly in mammals; this should not necessarily be considered as mechanical constraint of growth, but may well be a limitation of maternal blood supply. The placenta proper is apparently not a source of growth limitation: it is proportionately larger in twins than in singletons[4].

Litter size and position effects have been studied particularly in the mouse[5], rat[6], and guinea pig[7]. The relationship to maternal vessels supplying the uterus, and with it the explanation of the effect is different in the mouse and the rat[6]. What is important to us in the present context, is the fact that multiple pregnancy imposes increased and peculiar strains on the maternal supply line, and should therefore help elucidate some of the mechanisms, in experimental animals as well as in man.

Prolonged Pregnancy

This is another instance in which human fetal growth is adversely affected, though not as regularly as in multiple pregnancy. If, as we have seen, the fetal supply line declines late in pregnancy to the extent that in most populations growth decelerates before term, then it should be expected that this deprivation makes itself felt more strongly if pregnancy continues past term. This is, in fact, true and it is common knowledge that the 'postmaturity' syndrome as described by Runge[8], Clifford[9] and others includes not only wasting and other skin changes, but more significantly a high stillbirth rate. The gradual decline in adequacy of the supply line interacts with other factors having a similar effect. Primiparity ordinarily is associated with a slightly lower birth weight for gestational age when compared with infants of multiparae; in prolonged pregnancy the severe sequelae are almost limited to first pregnancies. Twin pregnancy is another example: Dunn[10] holds that if trends of fetal growth and well-being are applied to twins as they are to singletons in delineating post-term pregnancy, then the limit should be set two weeks earlier, at 40 weeks of gestation.

The striking effects of a supply line declining past term are but one end of a spectrum which is otherwise covered up by the use of empirical birth weight standards. Post-term infants with a birth weight within one standard deviation from the mean by these standards, show at post-mortem examination trends of organ growth which are similar to those in obvious growth retardation, though less severe: the brain is little affected, and the thymus very severely[11] (Figure 11.1). If one therefore accepts that the *average* post-term infant has suffered the effects of deprivation, then extrapolated standards (Table 11.1) are in order to indicate how adequately supplied fetuses would grow, and sometimes do. When this is done, the number of small-for-dates infants increases sharply (Figure 11.2).

Deprived post-term fetuses are the best examples of subacute fetal distress, unless their growth was modified in addition by chronic fetal distress (Figure 11.3). Skin changes such as greenish-brown staining and wrinkling ('washerwoman's hands') are characteristic of the condition occurring past

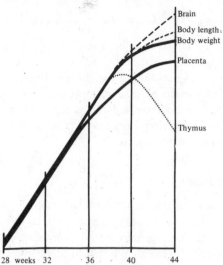

Figure 11.1 Increments in weights and length after 38 weeks of gestation. Growth between 30 and 38 weeks is assumed to be linear, and all values are adjusted so that the values from 30 to 38 weeks coincide (except for the placenta). The trends are the same as in obvious fetal growth retardation, only to a lesser extent

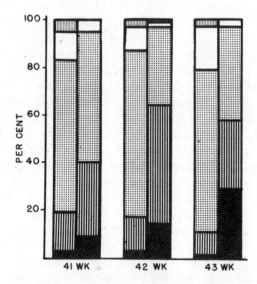

Figure 11.2 Body weight scores of all births during the forty-first, forty-second and forty-third week, by empirical (left) and extrapolated (right) standards. Score − 2 (below mean minus 2 standard deviations) is at the bottom. By extrapolated standards the proportion of low scores increases as pregnancy proceeds past term. (From Gruenwald, P.: The fetus in prolonged pregnancy, *Am. J. Obst. Gynecol.*, **89**, 503–509 (1964), by permission of C. V. Mosby, St. Louis)

term; subacute fetal distress with a low weight/length index terminating at or before term is not usually associated with these skin changes.

We can only speculate about the role of placental and maternal factors in post-term deprivation. Morphological and physiological data suggest that there may be an absolute (not just relative) decline in placental function past term (Chapters 6, 12). On the other hand, we know that the relative adequacy of the supply line, probably maternal, begins to decline before term, and this effect must be expected to increase past term, producing a relative insufficiency with regard to the increasing demands of the fetus. The fact that the fetus actually loses weight as indicated by wasting, is consistent with this possibility since the fetus may have to cover its needs at the expense of its

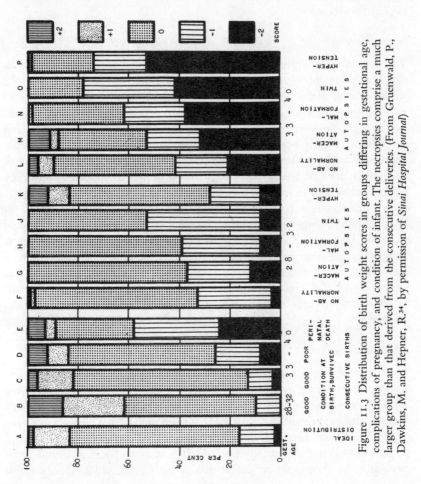

Figure 11.3 Distribution of birth weight scores in groups differing in gestational age, complications of pregnancy, and condition of infant. The necropsies comprise a much larger group than that derived from the consecutive deliveries. (From Gruenwald, P., Dawkins, M. and Hepner, R.[34], by permission of Sinai Hospital Journal)

stores of energy such as subcutaneous fat. Here again, as in multiple pregnancy, is a condition that may be used in the future to pinpoint specific
factors in the supply line in experiments and in man, because it tends to
exaggerate sensitivity to deprivation.

Maternal Conditions

It is impossible to separate clearly maternal from environmental effects on
the fetal supply line since the mother is affected by the environment. Environmental factors are influenced, and probably cushioned by the maternal
organism before affecting the fetus. Thus, the following distinction is
necessarily arbitrary.

Maternal stature

This is known to correlate positively with fetal size. Interpretation of this
observation is, however, very difficult. This pertains not only to the
determination of the genetic component[1], but also to environmental factors
which interact with length and weight of the mother in various ways[12]. Thus,
nutrition and socio-economic factors not only influence maternal stature, but
are related to each other, and to fetal growth beyond the effect possibly
accounted for by maternal size. The environmental portion of the effect of
maternal stature on fetal growth is mediated in part by influences upon her
own development in early life, including her fetal growth. Socio-economic
status and its change have, in addition to the striking, short-term effects on
fetal growth[13], long-term influences through effects on the mother. It must
therefore be expected that improvement of socio-economic status which is
now occurring in several parts of the world, will take several generations of
slow change for its full effect on fetal size by way of maternal condition. The
entire subject of the relation of maternal to fetal size, including the study of
proband infants' parents, has been investigated and reviewed by Ounsted and
Ounsted[2].

Maternal diseases

A number of maternal diseases affect fetal growth. Foremost among them is
hypertensive disease, pre-pregnant as well as pre-eclamptic. The increased
number of growth-retarded fetuses associated with these diseases is well
known, and has been linked with the reduction in maternal blood flow to the
intervillous space. Less well known is the fact that there is also an excess of
larger-than-normal infants, particularly late in pregnancy, as found independently in three studies and reviewed by Gruenwald[14]. One possible

explanation lies in the observation of Bieniarz et al.[15] that the usual inter-ference of the pregnant uterus with circulation in the lower aorta is lessened in hypertension. Thus, the changes at both ends of the spectrum are probably explained by a circulatory abnormality of the maternal supply line.

There are other circumstances in which the maternal circulation is thought to be involved in fetal deprivation. According to a group of Finnish investi-gators[16,17] failure of the maternal heartsize (as determined radiographically) to increase with progressing pregnancy, is associated with subnormal fetal growth, though not necessarily to the extent that would qualify as small-for-dates. This matter is undecided since some of those who undertook similar studies, failed to confirm the relationship. Also, correction for maternal height has been said to eliminate the effect[18]. Women with severe, congenital or acquired heart disease have growth-retarded infants whom Barnes[19] called classical examples of intrauterine growth retardation. It is not known whether the effect is mediated by poor circulation or poor oxygenation, or both. Furthermore, morphometry showed that in women with decompensated heart disease the villous surface area is enlarged as if attempting to compensate for poor oxygenation or circulation[20]. Maternal anaemia also results in smaller fetuses[21, 22] with a relatively large placenta[23].

Some women without any demonstrable disease have, either sporadically or repeatedly small-for-dates infants: Radio-angiography shows in these cases that the uterine vessels are small and fill slowly[24]. Among other maternal characteristics, parity or at least the difference between the first and any subsequent pregnancy has the most pronounced and best known effect. The cause is unknown; it has been suggested that the uterine vasculature does not adapt adequately at the first pregnancy. Maternal age, the spacing of preg-nancies, antigenic relationships and other factors affect fetal growth; these have been reviewed in detail by Ounsted and Ounsted[2].

Environmental Factors

As has been said, these factors cannot be separated completely from maternal ones. An example of interaction of these two is the condition to be discussed first, *pregnancy at high altitude*. In high locations in the Andes, a long period of adaptation is required before women who had lived at lower altitudes will have a successful pregnancy at all, but even after adaptation, or in women who grew up at high altitude, fetal growth is retarded. Data from the United States (Lake County, Colorado, 3000 m) and the South American Andes (higher than 4000 m) are reviewed by Ounsted and Ounsted[2]. In addition, McClung[25] compared Peruvian births in Lima (200 m) and Cuzco (3400 m) and also found a reduction of birth weights in the latter. All those who examined placenta weights at high altitude, found an increase relative to birth weight as compared with values near sea level. This, along with the above mentioned maternal adaptations, buffers the ill effects that low oxygen tension at high altitude would have on the fetus.

Maternal nutrition

This is obviously a significant factor in the maintenance of an adequate supply line to the fetus. Specific information is reviewed in Chapter 10. Correlation of the outcome of human pregnancy with the level and quality of maternal nutrition is inconclusive beyond the fact that gross undernutrition interferes with normal fetal growth. In his *Foetal and Neonatal Physiology* Dawes[26] questions in a brief but thoughtful section that under *usual* circumstances maternal nutrition limits fetal growth. He questions in particular the early work in sheep because the pregnant ewe is so sensitive to experimentation that maternal changes not directly reflecting nutrition may affect the fetus. Yet there are experiments and human data as summarised in a report of the National Academy of Sciences[30] which strongly suggest an effect of the mother's nutrition, not only during the pregnancy in question but also during her early life.

Relevant information comes from studies during and after the two world wars. It will become clear, however, that in none of these studies is nutrition the only means by which fetal growth could have been affected. Peller's[28] observations during and after the first world war relate to the custom of the woman's clinics in Vienna to admit indigent, unmarried pregnant women several weeks before term to give them a period of rest and adequate nutrition. This offset the unfavourable environment and, in fact, yielded infants with a birth weight equal to that of well-to-do families. Since this effect was achieved late in pregnancy, it obviously offset subacute fetal distress. In addition to improved nutrition, these women also had rest, away from work at home or on a job, and this surely contributed to an unknown extent. Similar results were achieved in women of a low economic group in India[29]. The serum albumin levels of women hospitalised for 4 weeks were slightly higher, and those of the infants significantly higher than those of controls, and the birth weight difference was about 300 g. The hunger winter in Holland (1944–45)[30] and the siege of Leningrad (1942)[31] accounted for birth weight reductions of about 200 and 500 g, respectively. The severity of deprivation was not comparable and, in addition, the past experience of the women in the two areas may have predisposed them as good providers for their fetuses to different degrees. In a study of fetal growth in Japan in 1945–1964, following the war[13], the contribution of factors other than nutrition was probably greater than in the other instances just reviewed.

Socio-economic status

Socio-economic status has been extensively studied as a determinant of fetal growth. Nutrition is one of many factors entering into this ill-defined conglomerate, along with, to mention just a few, health care, sanitation, and psychic factors influencing people's attitudes and priorities with regard to attaining their status in life. Racial differences are ass·iated in most if not all societies with socio-economic one: nd it has therei re been impossible to separate their effects on the fetal supply line, as was mentioned above. The identification of social classes is particularly difficult in the United States both, because of the basic heterogeneity of the population and because of its social mobility. Data coming from that country must therefore be viewed with caution. In those instances in which differences between groups or changes within one population have been investigated by means of birth weight in relation to gestational age, it has invariably been found that none of the observed differences were due to length of gestation. One may therefore use mean birth weights of entire populations as presumptive evidence of fetal growth characteristics, although data relating to gestational age are, of course, preferable. This lends significance to compilations from many parts of the world, such as a table put together by McClung[25]; some of these figures strongly suggest genetic differences.

It is inescapable to conclude from all information on nutritional and other socio-economic effects, that the mother's own past experience including her prenatal growth (as suggested by her birth weight) influences her ability to provide for her fetus *in utero*, even while living under adequate conditions during her pregnancy. Chow's work (quoted in the report of the National Academy of Sciences[27]) showed that when rats were given a restricted diet for several generations, more than one generation was needed for the off-spring to attain normal size again. Chow also found metabolic changes in the offspring of rats on a restricted diet which reduced efficiency of utilisation of nutrients and thus increased the need for nutrition. It has been suggested that the same changes occur in humans[32]. It is not known to what extent these two observations are related. As has already been suggested, rapid changes of fetal growth in response to socio-economic change will be followed by a much slower change as the mothers of subsequent generations adjust to the change. It is not known whether this phenomenon is mediated by chemical mechanisms such as changing utilisation of nutrients, or circulatory differences between well-grown and deprived mothers.

There is ample evidence that *maternal smoking* inhibits fetal growth. After a period during which pharmacological effects of nicotine on the circulation were suspected, it now appears likely that a high concentration of carboxyhaemoglobin in maternal and fetal blood (up to 10% in the latter) is responsible[33]. As in most instances of fetal deprivation, the length of pregnancy is within 2 days of that in controls. Reports of the extent of weight deficit at birth range up to 300 g[33]. It is now also accepted that perinatal mortality is adversely affected.

Summary

Among specific conditions which have an adverse effect on fetal growth, twin pregnancy and that associated with hypertension furnish the largest numbers of small-for-dates infants (below mean minus 2 standard deviations). However, in a series of consecutive births, and necropsies from a larger group of births[34] some additional trends appear (Figure 11.3): low birth weight scores as defined in Chapter 1 are infrequent up to 32 weeks. Between 33 and 40 weeks, survivors in poor condition at birth have about twice the incidence of low scores as do those in good condition, and cases of perinatal deaths have even higher incidences of low birth weight scores. Among these, hypertension and twin pregnancy yield the highest numbers with score − 2; malformed and macerated infants do not concern us here; a sizable number of cases are unassociated with any detectable maternal or fetal causative factor. Looked at from a different angle, study populations in Great Britain, the United States and Japan have, at or above 37 completed weeks of gestation, 44–70% infants weighing 1001–2500 g.

Various conditions mentioned here produce in a variety of time, duration and intensity lesser degrees of birth weight deficit by subacute or mild chronic fetal distress. This is usually insufficient to transfer a fetus who has the potential to attain an average birth weight, to the small-for-dates category. There is, however, a shift of the entire birth weight distribution and thus more fetuses will be in the small-for-dates group as has been shown by Papaevangelou et al.[35] for social class, maternal age and parity. It will be the task of future research to relate all these ill-defined conditions under which a fetal supply line becomes relatively insufficient earlier than usual, with known factors described in the two preceding chapters, and others yet to be recognised and understood.

Animal Models

Work on experimental animals was referred to at many points throughout this chapter. There is, in addition, some unpublished evidence which was discussed informally at a conference[35], to the effect that rhesus monkeys and probably other species of primates react strongly to what one might regard as counterparts of socio-economic differences by variations in fetal growth. It was, for instance, well known at the Perinatal Physiology Laboratory in Puetro Rico that the offspring of rhesus monkeys imported from India were considerably smaller than those from nearby Cayo Santiago where living conditions in the well-kept colony were near-ideal. Also, the former group lived in small cages which may have affected their circulatory system. While primates are, of course, very expensive experimental animals, the fact that they react to environmental differences at least as strongly as humans, should be kept in mind for crucial experiments.

References

1. Brent, R. L. and Jensch, R. P. (1967). Intra-uterine growth retardation. *Adv. Teratol.*, **2,** 140
2. Ounsted, M. and Ounsted, C. (1973). On fetal growth rate (its variations and their consequences). *Clinics Develop. Med.*, **46,** 1
3. McKeown, T. and Record, R. G. (1952). Observations on foetal growth in multiple pregnancy in man. *J. Endocrin.*, **8,** 386
4. Gruenwald, P. (1970). Environmental influences on twins apparent at birth. *Biol. Neonat.*, **15,** 79
5. McLaren, A. (1965). Genetic and environmental effects on foetal and placental growth in mice. *J. Reprod. Fertil.*, **9,** 79
6. Barr, Jr., M. and Brent, R. L. (1970). The retation of uterine vasculature to fetal growth and the intrauterine position effect in rats. *Teratol.*, **3,** 251.
7. Eckstein, P. and McKeown, T. (1955). Effect of transection of one horn of the guinea pig's uterus on foetal growth in the other horn. *J. Endocrin.*, **12,** 97
8. Runge, H. (1939). Die lange dauernde Schwangerschaft. *Deutsche med. Wochenschr.*, **65,** 541
9. Clifford, S. H. (1954). Postmaturity—with placental dysfunction. *J. Ped.*, **44,** 1
10. Dunn, P. M. (1965). Some perinatal observations on twins. *Develop. Med. Child Neurol.*, **7,** 121
11. Gruenwald, P. (1964). The fetus in prolonged pregnancy. *Am. J. Obstet. Gynec.*, **89,** 503
12. Thomson, A. M. (1960). Maternal stature and reproductive efficiency. *Eugenics Rev.*, **51,** 157
13. Gruenwald, P., Funakawa, H., Mitani, S., Nishimura, T. and Takeuchi, S. (1967). Influence of environmental factors on foetal growth in man. *Lancet*, **i,** 1026
14. Gruenwald, P. (1966). Growth of the human fetus. II. Abnormal growth in twins and infants of mothers with diabetes, hypertension, or isoimmunisation. *Am. J. Obst. Gynec.*, **94,** 1120
15. Bieniarz, J., Maqueda, E. and Caldeyro-Barcia, R. (1966). Compression of aorta by the uterus in late human pregnancy. I. Variations between femoral and brachial artery pressure with changes from hypertension to hypotension. *Am. J. Obst. Gynec.*, **95,** 795
16. Kauppinen, M. A. (1967). The correlation of maternal heart volume with the birth weight of the infant and prematurity. *Acta Obst. Gynaec. Scand.*, **46,** suppl. 6: 1
17. Räihä, C. E., Johansson, C. E., Lind, J. and Vara, P. (1957). Heart volume during pregnancy, with special consideration of its reduction. *Ann. Paed. Fenniae*, **3,** 65

18. Hytten, F. E., Paintin, D. B., Stewart, A. M. and Palmer, J. H. (1963). The relation of maternal heart size, blood volume and stature to the birth weight of the baby. *J. Obst. Gynaec. Brit. Cwlth.*, **70**, 817

19. Barnes, A. C. (1963). In discussion of: Cannell, D. E. and Vernon, C. P. Congenital heart disease and pregnancy. *Am. J. Obst. Gynec.*, **85**, 749

20. Clavero, J. A. and Botella Llusia, J. (1963). Measurement of the villus surface in normal and pathologic placentas. *Am. J. Obst. Gynec.*, **86**, 234

21. MacGregor, M. W. (1963). Maternal anaemia as a factor in prematurity and perinatal mortality. *Scot. Med. J.*, **8**, 134

22. World Health Organization (1970). The prevention of perinatal mortality and morbidity. *Wld. Hlth. Org. Tech. Rep. Series*, **457**, 1

23. Beischer, N. A., Sivasamboo, R., Vohra, S., Silpisornkosal, S. and Reid, S. (1970). Placental hypertrophy in severe pregnancy anaemia. *J. Obst. Gynaec. Brit. Cwlth.*, **77**, 398

24. Caldeyro-Barcia, R. (1970). Fetal malnutrition: the role of maternal blood flow. *Hosp. Pract. June 1970*, 33

25. McClung, J. (1969). *Effects of high altitude on human birth: observations on mothers, placentas, and the newborn in two Peruvian populations.* (Cambridge: Harvard Univ. Press)

26. Dawes, G. S. (1968). *Foetal and Neonatal Physiology.* (Chicago: Year Book Med. Publ.)

27. National Academy of Sciences (1970). *Maternal nutrition and the course of pregnancy.* (Washington: National Academy of Sciences)

28. Peller, S. (1919). Rückgang der Geburtsmasze als Folge der Kriegsernährung. *Wien. klin. Wochenschr.*, **32**, 758

29. Iyenger, L. (1967). Effects of dietary supplements late in pregnancy on the expectant mother and her newborn. *Ind. J. Med. Res.*, **55**, 85

30. Smith, C. A. (1947). The effect of wartime starvation in Holland upon pregnancy and its product. *Am. J. Obst. Gynec.*, **53**, 599

31. Antonov, A. N. (1947). Children born during the siege of Leningrad in 1942. *J. Ped.*, **30**, 250

32. Chow, B. F., Blackwell, R. Q., Blackwell, B. N., Hou, T. Y., Anilane, J. K. and Sherwin, R. W. (1968). Maternal nutrition and metabolism of the offspring: studies in rats and man. *Am. J. Pub. Hlth.*, **58**, 668

33. Haddon, Jr., W., Nesbitt, R. E. L. and Garcia, R. (1961). Smoking and pregnancy: carbon monoxide in blood during gestation and at term. *Obst. Gynec.*, **18**, 262

34. Gruenwald, P., Dawkins, M. and Hepner, R. (1963). Panel discussion: Chronic deprivation of the fetus. *Sinai Hosp. J. (Baltimore)*, **11**, 51

35. Papaevangelou, G., Papadatos, C. and Alexiou, D. (1973). The effect of maternal age, parity and social class on the incidence of small-for-dates newborns. *Acta Paediat. Scand.*, **62**, 527

36. Gruenwald, P. (1969). Comparative aspects of the supply line of primate fetuses. *Ann. New York Ac. Sci.*, **162**, 242

CHAPTER 12

Morphological Pathology of the Placenta

H. Fox

The student of placental pathology is faced with several unique problems. Firstly, the terminology used to describe placental lesions has been, until quite recently, quaintly archaic; one may cite, for instance, the application of the terms 'white infarct' and 'red infarct' to a wide variety of unrelated lesions and the usage of 'fibrin' and 'fibrinoid' as synonyms. Most of this outdated nomenclature has now sunk into oblivion but traces of it still remain to pollute the obstetric literature. Secondly, many placental lesions have a vascular origin and the pathologist is therefore often forced to study abnormalities the cause of which lies in vessels that are outside the placenta and not regularly available for examination. Thirdly, the placenta differs from most other organs in that its pathology is largely quantitative rather than qualitative; for example infarcts are common in placentas from normal pregnancies and hence their mere presence cannot strictly be considered as pathological, a significance which they only assume if they are unduly large or numerous. It is therefore insufficient simply to enumerate placental abnormalities; all must be quantified and their significance assessed in relation to the nature and outcome of the pregnancy, and any lesion, no matter how impressive pathologically, must be considered unimportant if it does not interfere with fetal growth and maturation. Fourthly, it would at first sight appear that pathological examination of placentas from cases of intrauterine fetal death would be of considerable value. This is not, however, necessarily the case for following fetal death the placenta both survives and undergoes extensive histological changes[1]. These changes are so marked that histological examination of placentas from all except very fresh stillbirths is of very little value and hence one of the most promising avenues for relating placental changes to fetal death is closed to the pathologist. Finally, the placenta is not histologically uniform and the villi normally vary considerably in appearances from one area to another; fortunately this variability is not totally random and can be overcome by taking standard blocks and invariably using the appearances in these as a point of reference. Villous appearances should be studied in a block taken from the central area of the placenta and it is preferable to limit examination to those villi lying near to the basal plate, this being the area in which the villi are most numerous and best adapted for gas transfer[2].

In this chapter stress is placed on the functional significance of morphological placental abnormalities and those which lack such significance are only considered at length if they are of some importance for the understanding of placental pathophysiology. Certain subjects, such as twin placentation, hydatidiform mole and chorionepithelioma, are not discussed, partly because they fall outside the general pattern of placental pathology and partly because they have been fully considered in recent publications[3, 4].

Macroscopic Abnormalities of the Placenta

These can be usefully, though somewhat arbitrarily and artificially, divided into four groups, between which there is, of course, some overlap:—
   (i) Developmental abnormalities.
  (ii) Lesions that reduce the population of functional villi.
 (iii) Lesions that obstruct or alter the blood flow through the placenta.
 (iv) Lesions that do not influence placental function.

DEVELOPMENTAL ABNORMALITIES

Some of these, e.g. the fenestrate placenta and the tripartite placenta, are so rare that their clinical significance cannot be estimated whilst others, such as bipartite placenta, accessory lobe, velamentous insertion of the cord and placenta accreta are primarily of obstetric interest and do not apparently influence either placental function or fetal development; both velamentous insertion of the cord and accessory lobe may, however, cause fetal bleeding during labour and it is of interest that velamentous insertion is associated unduly frequently with abortion and fetal malformation[5].

The commonest developmental anomaly of the placenta is placenta extrachorialis. This is found to some degree in about a quarter of all placentas and is characterised by the chorionic plate being smaller than the basal plate. The transition from villous to membranous chorion therefore takes place at some distance within the fetal margin of the placenta and if this transition is marked by an elevated ridge-like fold the placenta is classed as 'circumvallate'; if the chorionic margin is flat the placenta is 'circummarginate'. Either of these two anomalies may be complete or partial whilst a placenta may be circumvallate in one area and circummarginate in another (Figure 12.1). The

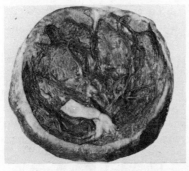
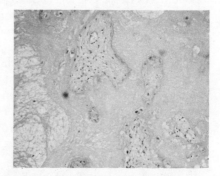

12.1

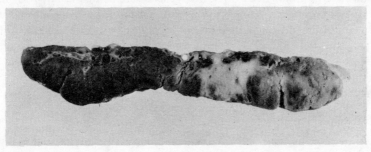

12.3

Figure 12.1 A partial form of placenta extrachorialis. This is normal above and circumvallate below

Figure 12.2 Histological appearances of perivillous fibrin deposition. The intervillous space is filled in with fibrin which envelops fibrotic villi. The villous trophoblast is degenerate and lost but cytotrophoblastic cells are seen in the fibrin. (Van Gieson × 80)

Figure 12.3 An irregular white plaque of perivillous fibrin

debate as to the clinical significance of this abnormality has been confused by the consideration of the extrachorial placenta as a single entity and by a failure to distinguish between the complete and the partial forms; studies[6, 7] which have avoided this pitfall have shown that the circummarginate placenta is of no clinical significance but that all forms of the circumvallate placenta are associated with an unduly high incidence of fetal growth retardation. The totally, but not the partially, circumvallate placenta is also linked with a relatively high incidence of fetal hypoxia and premature labour; nevertheless, circumvallate placentation is not accompanied by any increase in perinatal mortality and whether this type of placenta is relatively inadequate in its functioning or whether there is a common factor causing both the abnormal development of the placenta and the poor fetal growth is unknown. Indeed, the pathogenesis of placenta extrachorialis is far from clear; though of the various suggested theories that attributing it to unusually deep implantation of the ovum[8] is the least implausible.

A rare anomaly is placenta membranacea in which all of the maternal surface of the membranes is covered by villi. This is not only often complicated by antepartum bleeding and premature labour but is also associated with deficient fetal growth. The aetiology of this condition is obscure but the fact that this form of placenta is also often of the accreta type lends credence to the view that an endometrial hypoplasia or deficiency may play a role in its development.

A single artery is found in about 1% of umbilical cords from mature liveborn singletons, though the incidence is considerably higher in twins and in aborted or premature fetuses[5, 9]. This abnormality has a definite association with fetal malformations and trisomic syndromes but, in the absence of these factors, the lack of one umbilical artery does not appear to affect fetal growth[10].

LESIONS REDUCING POPULATION OF FUNCTIONAL VILLI

Perivillous fibrin deposition

Deposition of fibrin around villi occurs in almost all placentas and in a proportion is sufficiently extensive to be macroscopically visible either as a firm white plaque or as an area of irregular whitish mottling (Figure 12.3). Such lesions are found most commonly in the lateral area of the placenta and consist histologically of widely separated villi embedded in fibrin which fills in the intervillous space (Figure 12.2). The syncytiotrophoblast of the entrapped villi degenerates and disappears but their cytotrophoblast is frequently retained and may proliferate not only to form a cellular mantle around individual villi but to infiltrate into the surrounding fibrin. The stroma of the villi becomes markedly fibrotic and their fetal vessels undergo complete sclerosis.

This lesion is found in about a quarter of placentas from uncomplicated mature pregnancies but is relatively uncommon in those from prematurely terminating pregnancies; its incidence is not increased in prolonged pregnancy or in pre-eclamptic toxaemia.

The villi embedded in fibrin are not infarcted but nevertheless are of no functional value to the fetus as they are obviously incapable of participating in any transfer activity. However, macroscopically visible perivillous fibrin deposition, whilst clearly decreasing the total population of functional villi, not only lacks any clinical significance but tends to be associated with an unduly low incidence of fetal hypoxia[11]; this applies not only to small lesions but also to those in which as many as 20% of the villi are entrapped in fibrin. The clinical triviality of this lesion is, however, explicable in terms of its pathogenesis. There is no doubt that the fibrin is formed by thrombosis of maternal blood in the intervillous space; as the villous syncytiotrophoblast is in direct contact with this blood and can thus be considered as playing an endothelial-like role it was in the past thought that thrombosis occurred as a consequence of syncytial 'degeneration'. Electron microscopy has, however, shown that the initial stage in the development of this lesion is deposition of platelets on healthy syncytiotrophoblast[12] and it is almost certain that this occurs as a result of eddy currents and stasis of maternal blood in the intervillous space; the entrapped villi are thus only accidently included within the thrombus and the syncytial damage is a secondary phenomenon. The low incidence of perivillous fibrin deposition in placentas from toxaemic women and the inverse relationship between this lesion and fetal hypoxia suggests that it tends to develop particularily in placentas with a good maternal blood supply; clearly, the greater the blood flow through the closed irregular intervillous space the greater is the possibility of turbulence, stasis and fibrin deposition.

The banality of this lesion indicates that the placenta is, in the presence of a good maternal blood supply, unaffected by the functional loss of a considerable proportion of its villous population and thus bears eloquent witness to the considerable reserve capacity of this organ.

Infarction

Placental infarcts are usually wedge shaped and always have a point of contact with the basal plate. When fresh they are well demarcated, dark red and moderately firm (Figure 12.4), as they age they become converted into hard white structureless plaques. Histologically, the villi in a fresh infarct are closely packed and the intervillous space is narrowed or obliterated; the villous capillaries are widely dilated and markedly congested whilst the trophoblast shows early necrotic changes. As the infarct ages the red cells in the fetal vessels lyse and the villi undergo a progressive coagulative necrobiosis so that the well established lesion is formed solely of crowded 'ghost' villi. The necrotic area is often infiltrated by polymorphonuclear leukotyces and not infrequently the basal plate immediately underlying the infarct is also necrotic.

Small areas of infarction, involving less than 5% of the parenchyma, are found in almost a quarter of placentas from normal pregnancies and are of no

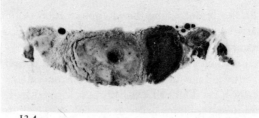

12.4

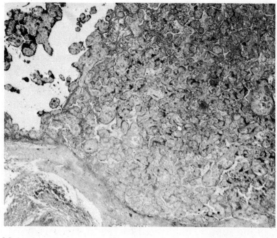

12.5

Figure 12.4 A well demarcated fresh infarct: it is darker and firmer than the surrounding tissue

Figure 12.5 Histological appearances of an infarct. The villi are aggregated together and the intervillous space is almost obliterated. The villi show early necrobiosis and the infarct is in contact below with the basal plate. (Haematoxylin and eosin × 42)

clinical significance. Extensive infarction, that is involving more than 10% of the villous substance, is associated with a high incidence of fetal hypoxia, low birth weight and fetal death and is virtually confined to placentas from patients suffering either from the hypertensive complications of pregnancy or from large retroplacental haematomas[13-15]. It is tempting to attribute the fetal complications simply to the loss of viable villous tissue but, as discussed above, a similar loss of villi due to entrapment in fibrin is of no consequence to the fetus. This is an apparent paradox unless it is borne in mind that the villi are oxygenated by the maternal blood and that although many maternal vessels open into the intervillous space there is little or no mixing of the streams from individual arterioles; these vessels can therefore be considered as end arteries and an infarct is due to a localised obstruction to the utero-placental circulation either by a retroplacental haematoma or by occlusion of a maternal arteriole. If one excludes those infarcts which are a consequence of retroplacental bleeding it follows that extensive infarction is due to occlusion of multiple maternal arterioles; the usual occluding lesion is a thrombus, which can often be demonstrated in a spiral arteriole supplying an infarcted area (Figure 12.6)[16, 17]. It would not be expected that multiple

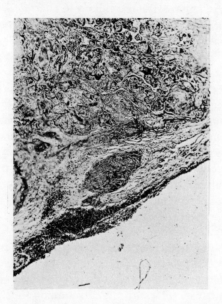

Figure 12.6 A thrombosed maternal vessel is seen in the basal plate immediately under-lying an infarct. (Haematoxylin and eosin × 56)

thrombi would occur in a healthy vascular tree and, indeed, it has been clearly shown that the hypertensive complications of pregnancy, i.e. those conditions specifically associated with a significant degree of placental infarction, are regularly accompanied by marked abnormalities of the utero-placental vessels[18]. Thus extensive infarction only occurs against a background of an inadequate maternal circulation through the placenta and it is this, rather than the simple loss of placental villi, that is the cause of the fetal complications. Although the loss of the infarcted villi will clearly further deplete the functional capacity of the placenta the principal significance of placental infarcts is that they are, when extensive, a visible indication of a severely compromised utero-placental circulation.

Small placenta

Not uncommonly a low fetal birth weight is attributed to an unduly small placenta, the assumption being in such cases that the placenta has an abnormally small villous population and is therefore unable to fulfil adequately the nutritional demands of the fetus. It has already been pointed out that the placenta has a considerable functional reserve and that a simple reduction in villous population is, unless extreme, unlikely to interfere with fetal nutrition or growth. It is therefore not surprising that the authors of a very extensive survey[19] were unable to correlate changes in placental weight with fetal hypoxia and were forced to the conclusion that weight is a poor indicator of placental adequacy. That a rough correlation between placental weight and fetal birth weight exists, however, is almost certainly true, especially if the true blood-free weight of the placenta is measured rather than the extremely inaccurate (and uninformative) gross weight[20]. This does not, however, necessarily mean that the fetus is small because the placenta is small; indeed, the reverse is more probably the case and the placenta, being a fetal organ, is small because the fetus is, for unrelated reasons, small. In this respect it may be noted that the placenta/fetal weight ratio is often normal or even slightly increased, in infants of low birth weight[21].

Fetal artery thrombosis

Thrombosis of a fetal stem artery produces a roughly triangular area of pallor in the placental substance, the apex of the triangle being near the chorionic plate. Histologically there is a sharply localised group of avascular villi which contrast markedly with the surrounding fully vascularised villi (Figure 12.7). The fetal vessels in these villi show an obliterative sclerosis and the villous stroma is markedly fibrotic; the trophoblast is intact and usually shows an excessive formation of syncytial 'knots'. An organising thrombus in a fetal stem artery can always be found at the apex of the lesion.

Single lesions of this type are found in 3–4% of placentas from live births but are rather more common in placentas from diabetic women; these, though reducing the population of functional villi, are of no clinical significance. Occasionally, however, there may be thrombosis of multiple stem arteries and this may cause fetal death, though this does not occur until about 40% of the villi have been rendered avascular.

The thrombosis usually occurs in otherwise morphologically normal arteries and its aetiology is unknown.

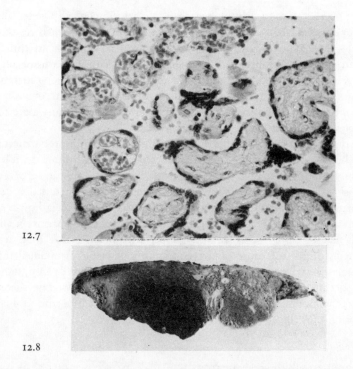

12.7

12.8

Figure 12.7 Avascular villi (below and right) resulting from a thrombosis of a fetal stem artery. These contrast markedly with the adjacent fully vascularised villi (above and left). (Haematoxylin and eosin × 280)

Figure 12.8 A retroplacental haematoma which is compressing the overlying placental substance

LESIONS THAT OBSTRUCT OR ALTER BLOOD FLOW THROUGH THE PLACENTA

Retroplacental haematoma

This is apparent on the maternal aspect of the placenta and bulges up towards the fetal surface thus compressing the overlying placental substance which is often, though not invariably, infarcted (Figure 12.8). An old haematoma is firmly adherent to the placenta and although a fresh one may become dislodged during delivery it leaves a characteristic crateriform depression in the maternal surface. It should be noted that simple adherent clot is always easily detached from the placenta and does not indent the surface.

Retroplacental haematomas are evidence of premature placental detachment but they are found in between 4 and 5% of all placentas[22] and their incidence is therefore much higher than is that of clinically detectable abruptio placentae. A high proportion of those haematomas which are only detectable pathologically are, however, small and of little or no clinical significance. Large retroplacental haematomas are associated with a high incidence of fetal hypoxia and death, largely because a very considerable proportion of the villi are acutely separated from the maternal uteroplacental circulation; despite its reserve capacity the placenta cannot compensate for an abrupt loss of 40–50% of its functioning villi.

The retroplacental haemorrhage probably comes from a ruptured maternal arteriole but the pathogenesis of this vascular accident is far from clear. It has been widely thought that it occurs particularly as a complication of the hypertensive diseases of pregnancy, it being argued that the maternal vessels are abnormal in such diseases and thus more likely to rupture. It has, however, been denied that any true association between antecedent hypertension and retroplacental bleeding exists and it has been maintained that folic acid deficiency is the prime cause of this condition[23], it being maintained that faulty nucleic acid metabolism during placentation could lead to an unstable placento-decidual attachment. This is not a particularly convincing theory and indeed has not been supported by subsequent studies[24]. The true etiology of this lesion thus remains obscure.

Chorangioma

Haemangiomas, which are hamartomatous malformations rather than true neoplasms, are present in about 1% of placentas; although usually solitary they may be multiple and occasionally there is a diffuse haemangiomatosis of the placenta. The vast majority of haemangiomas are small firm, apparently encapsulated, intraplacental nodules which are brown, tan or plum coloured a minority are large (more than 5 cm in diameter) and form obvious tumours on the fetal or maternal surface of the placenta. Most have the usual histo-logical appearances of a haemangioma but a few are of the 'cellular' variety and are formed largely of loose connective tissue in which there are only a few ill-formed vessels: hyaline or myxoid change is common.

Small haemangiomas are of no clinical importance but the larger ones are sometimes associated with polyhydramnios or antepartum bleeding; even more importantly they are accompanied by a relatively high incidence of fetal hypoxia and low birth weight, this being particularly the case when there are multiple or diffuse lesions[25]. These fetal complications have been attributed to fetal blood being shunted through the haemangioma rather than through the placenta and thus being returned to the fetus in an un-oxygenated state. A large haemangioma can also be considered as a peripheral arterio-venous shunt and this may be the cause of the transitory cardiomegaly that is sometimes seen in neonates whose placentas have contained such a lesion.

Subamniotic haematoma

These are readily visible as effusions of blood onto the maternal surface of the placenta and whilst some are due to tearing of surface chorionic veins by excessive cord traction others result from spontaneous rupture of a surface tributary of the umbilical vein; in this latter group the chorionic veins usually show degenerative changes and contain organising mural thrombi[26]. Vascular abnormalities of this type are often found to be associated with a low fetal birth weight though the nature of this association is far from clear.

LESIONS OF NO CLINICAL SIGNIFICANCE

These include septal cysts, subchorionic fibrin plaques, marginal haematomata and intervillous thrombi; the latter often contain nucleated red blood cells[27] and mark the site of fetal bleeding, presumably from a ruptured villous capillary, into the intervillous space but are otherwise of no importance. Macroscopically visible calcification, often in the past thought to be a feature of either placental degeneration or senescence, is of no clinical or pathological significance; it is no more common or extreme in placentas from prolonged pregnancies or from pregnancies complicated by pre-eclamptic toxaemia than in those from normal term pregnancies and is not associated with any fetal complications. The cause of the calcification is unknown but it occurs most commonly in first pregnancies and its incidence is related directly to low maternal age, high maternal socio-economic status and delivery during the summer months[28,29]; local factors within the placenta must, however, also play some role for the placentas of bichorionic twins may show significantly different degrees of calcification[30].

Histological abnormalities of the placenta

VILLOUS LESIONS

When examining the villi histologically attention has to be paid to the syncytiotrophoblast, the cytotrophoblast, the subtrophoblastic basement membrane, the villous stroma and the fetal capillaries. It is, however, preferable to classify villous abnormalities on a functional rather than a purely morphological basis. Thus they may be grouped into:—

(i) Changes secondary to a reduced maternal uteroplacental blood flow.
(ii) Changes secondary to a reduced fetal blood flow through the villi.
(iii) Abnormalities of maturation and differentiation.
(iv) Abnormalities of unknown, but possibly immunologic, origin.

Changes secondary to a reduced maternal utero-placental blood flow

The villi depend on the maternal blood for their oxygen supply and the villous response to a utero-placental blood flow which though reduced is sufficient to maintain viability is characterised by cytotrophoblastic hyperplasia and thickening of the trophoblastic basement membrane.

Cytotrophoblastic hyperplasia is seen most strikingly in placentas from women suffering from pre-eclamptic toxaemia or essential hypertension (Figure 12.9) and its presence can be correlated with a high incidence of fetal hypoxia and intrauterine death. These findings led to the suggestion[31] that cytotrophoblastic hyperplasia is a response to villous ischaemia and this concept has been reinforced by studies[32] which have shown that this change can be specifically induced under *in vitro* conditions by subjecting cultured villi to a low oxygen tension (Figure 12.10).

There is now no doubt that the cytotrophoblastic cells are the stem cells of the villous trophoblast and thus function as a germinative zone from which the syncytiotrophoblast is formed by a process of cell fusion and dissolution of cell membranes. Although the villous cytotrophoblastic cells, so prominent in the first trimester placenta, become progressively smaller and fewer as pregnancy proceeds they are nevertheless still present in many of the villi of the normal mature placenta, though admittedly rather inconspicuous and easily overlooked. If the syncytiotrophoblast suffers ischaemic damage (and there is no convincing evidence that any other factor does produce syncytial damage) the cytotrophoblast will proliferate in an attempt to replace the damaged tissue. Cytotrophoblastic hyperplasia is thus a repair phenomenon and under ischaemic conditions these cells are both numerous and prominent; mitotic figures can often be seen. Hyperplasia of the cytotrophoblast must be distinguished from a failure of the normal cytotrophoblastic regression. This latter phenomenon is seen in villi which have failed to mature and, indeed, is one of the defining features of villous immaturity; mitotic figures are not seen. By contrast, cytotrophoblastic hyperplasia is usually seen in otherwise normally mature villi and its proliferative nature is indicated by the presence of mitotic activity.

It will be clear that the degree of cytotrophoblastic hyperplasia is related to the extent of the syncytial damage and thus serves, by inference, as a rough quantitative index of the severity of the ischaemia to which the villi have been subjected.

Thickening of the villous trophoblastic basement membrane, beyond its normal width of 1000–3000 Å, is also commonly seen in placentas from women suffering from the hypertensive complications of pregnancy and this change can also be reproduced *in vitro* by subjecting cultured villi to

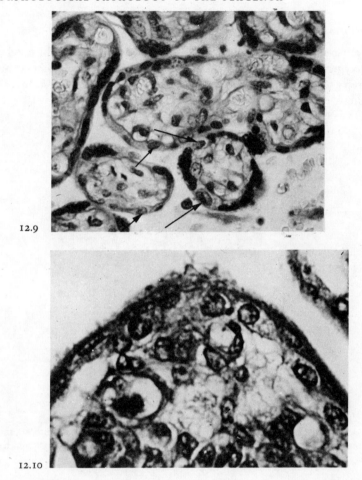

12.9

12.10

Figure 12.9 Villi in a placenta from a woman suffering from moderately severe pre-eclamptic toxaemia. Prominent cytotrophoblastic cells (arrowed) are easily visible in many of the villi. (P.A.S. × 476)

Figure 12.10 Villus cultured under conditions of low oxygen tension. Numerous large cytotroblastic cells are seen in the trophoblast. This change was not present in villi cultured under fully oxygenated conditions. (P.A.S. × 1170)

hypoxia[32]. It thus seems certain that thickening of the basement membrane can be a consequence of utero-placental ischaemia but this change is seen also in other conditions in which there is no suggestion of a reduced maternal blood flow through the placenta and is therefore, unlike cytotrophoblastic hyperplasia, a non-specific change.

Changes secondary to a reduced fetal blood flow through the villi

These are seen in their purest form in the localised group of villi which, whilst fully oxygenated by the maternal blood, have been rendered avascular by a fetal artery thrombosis. Such villi show a marked fibrosis of their stroma and a strikingly excessive number of syncytial knots (Figure 12.11); the latter are

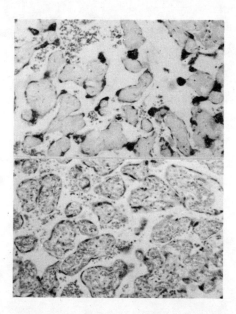

Figure 12.11 Avascular villi (above) resulting from a fetal artery thrombosis show numerous syncytial knots. Fully vascularised villi (below) from the same placenta have relatively few syncytial knots. (Haematoxylin and eosin × 280)

formed of syncytial nuclei which are focally clumped to form a multi-nucleated protrusion from the villous surface and it is by no means clear whether they are formed by a simple aggregation of pre-existent syncytial nuclei or by a true proliferation of the trophoblast. The avascular villi do not show cytotrophoblastic hyperplasia or thickening of the trophoblastic basement membrane. It is of interest to note that this lesion has been reproduced experimentally in the monkey placenta by ligation of a single fetal artery[33]; this produces exactly the same villous changes as are seen in avascular villi in the human placenta.

These characteristic changes of stromal fibrosis and excess syncytial knot formation occur in generalised form whenever the fetal circulation through the villi appears to be reduced. Thus they are seen most strikingly in placentas from prolonged pregnancies in some of which, but by no means all, there is a marked hypovascularity of the villi, the fetal villous capillaries being small and inconspicuous instead of sinusoidally dilated, as is the norm[34]. As the fetal stem arteries are usually normal in prolonged pregnancy the cause of this reduction in villous perfusion is unclear though it could be due to the accumulation of a vasoconstrictor substance, possibly a prostaglandin. Villous hypovascularity can also be secondary to an elevated pressure in the intervillous space; this results in a decreased blood flow through the fetal vasculature of the placenta, possibly by a simple squeezing mechanism which collapses the fetal capillaries[10]. A reduced fetal perfusion also occurs when the fetal stem arteries are partially occluded by an 'obliterative endarteritis' (see p. 216) as is the case of some placentas from patients with pre-eclamptic toxaemia, maternal diabetes mellitus or materno-fetal rhesus incompatibility.

Irrespective of the mechanism which is responsible for reducing fetal blood flow through the villi the inevitable result is stromal fibrosis and excess syncytial knot formation both of which are good indices of the degree of reduction in villous perfusion; thus, for instance in placentas with an obliterative endarteritis of the fetal stem arteries there is a direct relationship between the severity of the arterial lesion and the intensity of villous fibrosis[35]. Why these particular changes of fibrosis and syncytial knot formation should result from an impairment of fetal blood flow through the villi is unknown. Some collagen is normally present in the villous stroma from a quite early stage in gestation and does not, in the presence of an adequate fetal circulation, increase appreciably as gestation proceeds; syncytial knots are a normal feature of the mature placenta, being found on up to 30% of the villi, and their presence in normal, as opposed to excessive, numbers is clearly not related to villous underperfusion.

It is of interest that a reduction of fetal blood flow though the placenta does not in itself appear to be of any great consequence as far as fetal well-being is concerned for neither stromal fibrosis nor excess syncytial knot formation are associated with any excess incidence of fetal hypoxia, death or growth retardation.

Abnormalities of maturation and differentiation

Abnormal villous maturation is of very considerable importance and is considered more fully in a subsequent chapter. Suffice it to say here that placental and fetal maturation are not always synonchronous, that a proportion of prematurely delivered babies, normally developed for their gestational age, have placentas in which the villi are morphologically fully mature and that a persistent morphological immaturity of the villi may have serious consequence for the continued growth of the fetus[36].

The factors controlling placental maturation are unknown but although both fetal and maternal influence undoubtedly play a role, probably a dominant one, those cases in which placental and fetal maturation are disassociated indicate that there must also be some intrinsic mechanism within the placenta itself. Perhaps it would not be too far fetched to suggest that villous maturation may be dependent upon the fetal circulatory system through the placenta. Unduly immature villi contain, as one of their defining morphological features, small non-dilated fetal capillaries which are often at some distance from the trophoblast; it is usually thought that this failure to attain full vascularisation of the villi is due to villous immaturity but the reverse may be the case and the failure to reach full villous maturity be due to a relative failure of villous vascularisation. It must be stressed, however, that this is a purely speculative hypothesis.

It is not always fully appreciated that villous maturation appears to be accompanied by a progressive differentiation of the trophoblast, the two processes being intertwined though probably independent of each other. The villous syncytiotrophoblast has both a synthetic and a transfer function and it would be reasonable to assume that this tissue shows topographic functional differentiation so that different areas become adapted for one or other of these two roles. Recently, this assumption has received support from electronoptical studies of the first trimester villous syncytiotrophoblast which have shown that despite the apparent morphological homogeneity of this tissue at light microscopic level there is considerable ultrastructural evidence of functional regional differentiation[37]. In the mature placenta the villous syncytiotrophoblast is clearly not morphologically homogeneous for there are, in many villi, thinned anuclear areas of trophoblast which directly overlie and, on light microscopy, appear to fuse with the wall of a dilated fetal capillary. These attenuated areas have been called 'vasculo-syncytial membranes'[38] and although electron microscopy shows that there is no real fusion between trophoblast and vessel wall it is clear that they differ markedly from the non-thinned nucleated areas of the trophoblast (Figure 12.12).

The membranous areas tend to bulge into the intervillous space and they are not simply due to mechanical stretching of the trophoblast by dilated fetal vessels for scanning electron microscopy shows that they are randomly sited and very localised[39], often occurring along the course of a vessel as a dome-shaped swelling protruding from the lateral wall of a villus (Figure 12.13); this pattern of distribution argues strongly against a mechanical explanation for their formation and it has been suggested that they are specialised areas of trophoblast for the facilitation of gas transfer across the placenta. This suggestion has been principally based on the fact that where

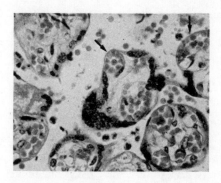
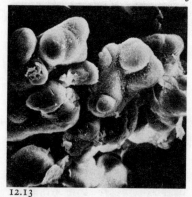

12.12

12.13

Figure 12.12 Villi from a mature normal placenta. Several vasculo-syncytial membranes (arrowed) are seen. (Haematoxylin and eosin × 340)

Figure 12.13 Scanning electron micrograph of a mature normal placenta. The vasculo-syncytial membranes are seen as dome-shaped protrusions from the villous surface. (S.E.M. × 230)

the trophoblast is focally thinned the fetal and maternal circulations come into their closest approximation to each other; this would, however, only facilitate gas transfer across the placenta if membrane resistance was an important limiting factor in this process and recent work suggests that this is not the case[10]. The trophoblastic thinning is, however, only one indication of the specialised nature of the membranous areas for not only do they differ both histochemically[40] and ultrastructurally[41] from the non-membranous areas of the trophoblast but scanning electron microscopy shows that there is a sharply localised loss of microvilli over their surface[39]. It thus appears that the functional segregation which is present in the trophoblast during the first trimester becomes accentuated in the mature placenta and the view that trophoblastic transfer function is largely confined to the membranous areas and synthetic activity to the non-membranous areas[41] would appear to be a reasonable one.

This concept is supported by the finding that a deficiency of vasculo-syncytial membranes in the mature placenta, i.e. present on less than 5% of the villi, is associated with a high incidence of fetal hypoxia[42]; this paucity of membranous areas can be considered as a failure of trophoblastic differentia-tion—a failure that appears to subject the fetus to considerable risk. A lack of trophoblastic differentiation may be simply one facet of villous immaturity and it is possibly this associated failure of differentiation that lends to villous immaturity its serious import. In some placentas which lack vasculo-syncytial membranes the villi are, however, fully mature and here there appears to be solely a defect in trophoblastic differentiation. If the fetal vessels within the villi become small and inconspicuous, as is the case in some placentas from prolonged pregnancies, the vasculo-syncytial membranes will no longer be clearly apparent; whether this morphological regression is also accompanied by a functional decline in the transfer activity of the membranous areas is as yet unknown.

Abnormalities of unknown but possibly immunological origin

Amongst these the most interesting is fibrinoid necrosis of placental villi. The first stage in the evolution of this villous abnormality is the appearance of a small nodule of homogeneous, strongly PAS-positive material at one point in the deep part of the trophoblastic layer; this lies external to the tropho-blastic basement membrane but is covered on its outer aspect by syncytio-trophoblast. This nodule progressively enlarges as fresh fibrinoid material is laid down on its deep aspect (Figure 12.14) so as to form a mass which

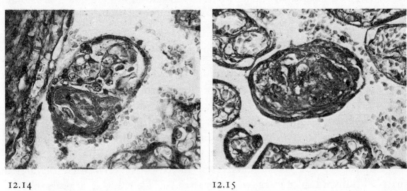

12.14   12.15

Figure 12.14 A villus showing partial fibrinoid necrosis. (P.A.S. × 340)

Figure 12.15 A villus showing complete fibrinoid necrosis. (P.A.S. × 340)

gradually bulges into and compresses the villous stroma; the underlying trophoblastic basement membrane remains intact but is pushed inwards before the expanding mass. The syncytiotrophoblast of the affected villus is normal in the early stages of the development of this lesion but later under-goes a progressive atrophy and degeneration, though even in the final stages a few remnants of this tissue remain. The eventual appearance is, therefore, that of a villus which has been totally replaced by fibrinoid material but which still retains a few degenerate syncytial nuclei around its perimeter (Figure 12.15).

It has been thought that this lesion is due to deposition in the villus of fibrin derived either from the maternal blood in the intervillous space or from the fetal blood in the villous capillaries. This concept is, however, incompatible with the observation that the fibrinoid change appears initially in the trophoblast and electronoptical studies[43] have confirmed that the fibrinoid material, which at the ultrastructural level has a fibrillar structure, accumulates first in villous cytotrophoblastic cells and only later appears extracellularly. Recently, it has been suggested that the fibrinoid material has many of the characteristics of amyloid[44] but this remains to be proven.

Villi that have undergone fibrinoid necrosis are seen in many placentas from uncomplicated pregnancies but usually the proportion of such villi does not exceed 3% and an incidence in excess of this is abnormal[45]; an unduly high incidence is found in placentas from diabetic women, from cases of materno-fetal rhesus incompatibility, from cases of pre-eclamptic toxaemia and in some placentas from cases of idiopathic premature onset of labour. The aetiology of villous fibrinoid necrosis is obscure but the possibility that it is due to an immunological reaction within the villous cytotrophoblast is worthy of consideration. Thus, fibrinoid necrosis is well recognised as one of the hallmarks of immune damage, the fibrinoid material in the affected villi contains a considerable quantity of immunoglobulins[46] and anti-D antibodies localise to villi showing fibrinoid change in placentas from cases of materno-fetal rhesus incompatibility[47]; those who consider the fibrinoid material to be amyloid postulate that this substance is comparable to senile amyloid and due to immune attack on trophoblastic cells with mis-specified proteins. All these observations are, of course, open to varying interpretations and are, in themselves, inconclusive whilst it is recognised that the whole question of immune-mediated placental damage is highly controversial. Nevertheless, villous fibrinoid necrosis merits further study as a possible index of an immunological attack on cytotrophoblast.

It has already been pointed out that undue thickening of the villous trophoblastic basement membrane may be due to villous ischaemia but that it also occurs in conditions such as maternal diabetes mellitus or materno-fetal rhesus incompatibility in which normally the maternal blood flow through the placenta is not reduced. The pathogenesis of this lesion under these circumstances is obscure but it has been suggested that it is due to the deposition of antigen-antibody complexes on the basement membrane[47]; this is an attractive but completely unproven hypothesis.

Another lesion of unknown aetiology is villous edema which may occur in a wide range of conditions but is seen most strikingly in placentas from diabetic women and from cases of materno-fetal rhesus incompatibility. Whether or not the accumulation of fluid is due to a functional insufficiency of the fetal circulation is not known but it has been suggested that the increased size of the edematous villi may decrease the capacity of the inter-villous space and thus limit the maternal blood flow through the placenta[48]; haemodynamic studies to confirm this suggestion are lacking and there is as yet no clear evidence that villous edema has, in itself, any effect on fetal growth or nutrition.

LESIONS OF THE FETAL STEM ARTERIES

Fibromuscular sclerosis

This is characterised by fibromuscular thickening of the arterial wall and an ingrowth of subintimal fibrous tissue into the vascular lumen (Figure 12.16).

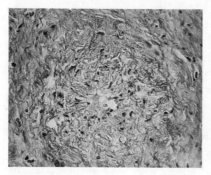 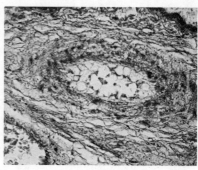

12.16   12.17

Figure 12.16 Fibromuscular sclerosis of a fetal stem artery. The lumen is being obliterated by an ingrowth of subintimal fibrous tissue. From the placenta of a macerated stillbirth. (Van Gieson × 280)

Figure 12.17 Obliterative endarteritis of a fetal stem artery. There is swelling and pro-liferation of the intimal cells from a placenta. From a woman with pre-eclamptic toxaemia. (P.A.S. × 280)

Fibromuscular sclerosis is seen in localised form distal to an occluding throm-bus and in generalised form in the stem arteries of placentas from stillbirths; it is important to emphasise, however, that this vascular lesion is not present in placentas from fresh stillbirths and that its severity and extent is directly proportional to the length of time elapsing between fetal death and delivery. The abnormality is therefore almost certainly one which is secondary to cessation of fetal blood flow through the artery, whether this is due to fetal death or thrombotic occlusion.

Obliterative endarteritis

This rather inapt term is applied to a vascular lesion characterised by swelling and proliferation of the intimal cells of the fetal stem arteries together with thickening and reduplication of the endothelial basement membrane; the intimal changes may be sufficiently marked as to diminish, and sometimes almost to occlude, the vascular lumen (Figure 12.17).

This lesion is seen most strikingly in placentas from women suffering from the hypertensive complications of pregnancy but also occurs in placentas from diabetic women[49-51]. Its pathogenesis is obscure but in placentas from hypertensive women the vascular lesion may be secondary to the haemo-dynamic changes that occur in the fetal circulatory system as a response to placental ischaemia. Thus, there is experimental evidence that a reduction of maternal utero-placental blood flow, or fetal hypoxia, is followed by a rise in fetal blood pressure[52] and it is possible that this may stimulate the changes in the fetal stem arteries. It has been suggested[47] that in placentas from diabetic women the arterial lesion may be secondary to the deposition, or formation, of antigen–antibody complexes in the vessel walls.

The obliterative endarteritis is of importance simply because it reduces fetal villous perfusion and thus produces the villous changes characteristic of this; it does not appear to be, in itself, a lesion that has any serious consequence for fetal well being.

GENERAL COMMENTS

It will be clear from the preceding account that most macroscopic abnormalities of the placenta are of little importance. In the past these have received undue attention, partly because they are easily noted and thus serve as a convenient peg upon which to hang the facile diagnosis of 'placental insufficiency' and partly because the reserve capacity of the placenta was underestimated, thus allowing for the elevation to an undeserved status of those lesions which simply reduce the total villous population. It is true that very large or multiple lesions, such as extensive infarction, thrombotic occlusion of multiple fetal arteries, large haemangiomas or large retroplacental haematomas can seriously affect fetal nutrition and oxygenation but these are found in only a small proportion of placentas from fetuses that have failed to thrive.

It is clear therefore that any serious attempt to correlate placental pathology with fetal well being must be concerned largely with villous abnormalities and it must be confessed that interpretation of these is not always easy. In this account an attempt has been made to define in isolation those changes which are due to a particular factor, e.g. placental ischaemia, and the changes seen in specific complications of pregnancy, in which several factors are operating simultaneously, have not been described. This is partly because the final picture is often very complicated and partly because no particular complication of pregnancy produces specific morphological changes within the placenta which allow one to make a specific morphological diagnosis.

Consider, for example, the placental changes in placentas from cases of moderately severe pre-eclamptic toxaemia. Here, a reduced maternal utero-placental blood flow produces villous cytotrophoblastic hyperplasia, tropho-blastic basement membrane thickening and, possibly, an obliterative endarteritis of the fetal stem arteries, the latter leading in turn to villous fibrosis and excess syncytial knot formation; in addition there is often an excess of villous fibrinoid necrosis whilst in some cases there is also a failure of trophoblastic differentiation and villous maturation. None of these changes are specific to pre-eclamptic toxaemia and, indeed, little purpose is served by attempting to define a specific pattern of changes. It is of far more importance, in any particular case, to assess the degree of ischaemia to which the placenta has been subjected and to estimate the role played by decreased fetal perfusion or failure of villous maturation. This type of analysis allows for the placental changes to be defined in functional and meaningful terms.

Finally, it will be apparent that most of the important changes seen in the placenta are secondary to an extraplacental cause, usually an alteration in either the maternal or the fetal circulation through the placenta. If the placenta fails in its nutritive function this is hardly, if ever, due to a primary fault within the placenta; hence the term 'placental insufficiency' is to be deplored, partly because it is incorrect and partly because it diverts attention away from the true basis for the failure of the fetus to survive and develop.

References

1. Fox, H. (1968). Morphological changes in the human placenta following fetal death *J. Obstet. Gynaec. Brit. Cwlth.*, **75,** 839

2. Alvarez, H., Benedetti, W. L., Morel, R. L. and Scavarelli, M. (1970). Trophoblas development gradient and its relationship to placental haemodynamics. *Amer. J Obstet. Gynec.*, **10,** 416

3. Strong, J. J. and Corney, G. (1967). The placenta in twin pregnancy. (Oxford Pergamon Press)

4. Mainwaring, A. R. (1973). Hydatidiform mole and chorion-carcinoma *in Post-graduate Obstetrical and Gynaecological Pathology*, p. 441. (H. Fox and F. A. Langley, editors) (Oxford: Pergamon Press)

5. Benirschke, K. and Driscoll, S. E. (1967). *The Pathology of the Human Placenta.* (Berlin: Springer-Verlag)

6. Benson, R. C. and Fujikura, T. (1969). Circumvallate and circummarginate placenta. *Obstet. Gynec.*, **34,** 799

7. Fox, H. and Sen, D. K. (1972). Placenta extrachorialis: a clinico-pathological study. *J. Obstet. Gynaec. Brit. Cwlth.*, **79,** 32

8. Torpin, R. (1958). Human placental anomalies: etiology, evolution and histological background. *Missouri Med.*, **55,** 353

9. Kristofferson, K. (1969). The significance of absence of one umbilical artery. *Acta Obstet. Gynec. Scand.*, **48,** 195

10. Longo, L. D. (1972). Disorders of placental transfer *in Pathophysiology of Gestation*. Vol. II, Fetal-Placental Disorders. (N. S. Assali, editor) (New York and London: Academic Press)

11. Fox, H. (1967). Pervillous fibrin deposition in the human placenta. *Amer. J. Obstet. Gynec.*, **98**, 245.

12. Moe, N. and Jorgensen, L. (1968). Fibrin deposits on the syncytium of the normal human placenta: evidence of their thrombogenic origin. *Acta Path. Microbiol. Scand.*, **72**, 519

13. Fox, H. (1967). The significance of placental infarction in perinatal morbidity and mortality. *Biol. Neonat.*, **11**, 87

14. Wallenburg, H. C. S. (1969). Uber den Zusammenhang zwischen Spatgestose und Placentarinfarkt. *Arch. Gynak.*, **208**, 80

15. Wentworth, P. (1967). Placental infarction and toxemia of pregnancy. *Amer. J. Obstet. Gynec.*, **99**, 318

16. Brosens, I. and Renaer, M. (1972). On the pathogenesis of placental infarcts in pre-eclampsia. *J. Obstet. Gynaec. Brit. Cwlth.*, **79**, 794

17. Wallenburg, H. C. S., Stolte, L. A. M. and Janssens, J. (1973). The pathogenesis of placental infarction. I. A morphologic study in the human placenta. *Amer. J. Obstet. Gynec*, **116**, 835

18. Robertson, W. B. and Dixon, H. G. (1969). Utero-placental pathology *in Foetus and Placenta*, p. 33. (A. Klopper and E. Diczfalusy, editors) (Blackwell Scientific Publications)

19. Thomson, A. M., Billewicz, W. Z. and Hytten, F. E. (1969). The weight of the placenta in relation to birthweight. *J. Obstet. Gynaec. Brit. Cwlth.*, **76**, 865

20. Garrow, J. S. and Hawes, S. F. (1971). The relationship of the size and composition of the human placenta to its functional capacity. *J. Obstet. Gynaec. Brit. Cwlth.*, **78**, 22

21. Younoszai, M. K. and Haworth, J. C. (1969). Placental dimensions and relations in preterm, term and growth-retarded infants. *Amer. J. Obstet. Gynec.*, **103**, 265

22. Wilkin, P. (1965). *Pathologie du Placenta*. (Paris: Masson et Cie)

23. Hibbard, B. M. and Hibbard, E. D. (1963). Aetiological factors in abruptio placentae. *Brit. Med. J.*, **2**, 1430

24. Whalley, P. J., Scott, D. E. and Pritchard, J. A. (1969). Maternal folate deficiency and pregnancy wastage. I. Placental abruption. *Amer. J. Obstet. Gynec.*, **105**, 670

25. Fox, H. (1967). Vascular tumors of the placenta. *Obstet. Gynec. Surv.*, **22**, 697

26. deSa, D. J. (1971). Rupture of fetal vessels on placental surface. *Arch. Dis. Childh.*, **46**, 495

27. Wentworth, P. (1964). A placental lesion to account for foetal haemorrhage into the maternal circulation. *J. Obstet. Gynaec. Brit. Cwlth.*, **71**, 379

28. Russel, J. G. B. and Fielden, P. (1969). The antenatal diagnosis of placental calcification. *J. Obstet. Gynaec. Brit. Cwlth.*, **76**, 813

29. Wentworth, P. (1965). Macroscopic placental calcification and its clinical significance. *J. Obstet. Gynaec. Brit. Cwlth.*, **72**, 215

30. Tindall, V. R. and Scott, J. S. (1965). Placental calcification: a study of 3025 singleton and multiple pregnancies. *J. Obstet. Gynaec. Brit. Cwlth.*, **72**, 356

31. Wigglesworth, J. S. (1962). The Langhans layer in late pregnancy: a histological study of normal and abnormal cases. *J. Obstet. Gynaec. Brit. Cwlth.*, **69**, 355

32. Fox, H. (1970). Effect of hypoxia on trophoblast in organ culture. *Amer. J. Obstet. Gynec.*, **107**, 1058

33. Myers, R. E. and Fujikura, T. (1968). Placental changes after experimental abruptio

placentae and fetal vessel ligation of rhesus monkey placenta. *Amer. J. Obstet. Gynec.*, **100,** 846

34. Fox, H. (1969). Histological features of placental senescence *in The Foeto-placental Unit*, p. 3. (A. Pecile and C. Finzi, editors) (Amsterdam: Excerpta Medica Foundation)

35. Fox. H. (1968). Fibrosis of placental villi. *J. Path. Bact.*, **95,** 573

36. Becker, V. (1963). Funktionelle Morpholgie der Placenta. *Arch. Gynäk.*, **198,** 3

37. Dempsey, E. W. and Luse, S. A. (1971). Regional specialisation in the syncytial trophoblast of early human placentas. *J. Anat.*, **108,** 545

38. Getzowa, S. and Sadowsky, A. (1950). On the structure of the human placenta. *J. Obstet. Gynaec. Brit. Emp.*, **57,** 388

39. Fox, H. and Agrafojo-Blanco, A. (1974). Scanning electron microscopy of the human placenta in normal and abnormal pregnancies. *Europ. J. Obstet. Gynec. Rep. Biol.* (in press)

40. Amstutz, E. (1960). Beobachtungen uber die Reifung der Chorionzotten in menschlichen Placenta mit besonderer Beruchsichtigung der Epithelplatten. *Acta Anat. (Basel)*, **42,** 12

41. Burgos, M. H. and Rodriguez, E. M. (1966). Specialised zones in the trophoblast of the human term placenta. *Amer. J. Obstet. Gynec.*, **96,** 342

42. Fox, H. (1967). The incidence and significance of vasculo-syncytial membranes in the human placenta. *J. Obstet. Gynaec. Brit. Cwlth.*, **74,** 28

43. Liehard, M. (1971). Some observations on so-called fibrinoid necrosis of placental villi. An electron-microscopic study. *Path. Europ.*, **6,** 217

44. Burstein, R., Frankel, S., Soule, S. D. and Blumenthal, H. T. (1973). Aging of the placenta: autoimmune theory of senescence. *Amer. J. Obstet. Gynec.*, **116,** 271

45. Fox, H. (1968). Fibrinoid necrosis of placental villi. *J. Obstet. Gynaec. Brit. Cwlth.*, **75,** 448

46. McCormick, J. N., Faulk, W. P., Fox, H. and Fudenberg, H. H. (1971). Immuno-histological and elution studies of the human placenta. *J. Exp. Med.*, **133,** 1

47. Burstein, R., Berns, A. W., Hirata, Y. and Blumenthal, H. T. (1963). A comparative histo- and immunopathological study of the placenta in diabetes mellitus and in erythroblastosis fetalis. *Amer. J. Obstet. Gynec.*, **86,** 66

48. Alvarcz, H., Sala, M. A. and Benedetti, W. L. (1972). Intervillous space reduction in the edematous placenta. *Amer. J. Obstet. Gynec.*, **112,** 819

49. Paine, G. G. (1957). Observations on placental histology in normal and abnormal pregnancies. *J. Obstet. Gynec. Brit. Emp.*, **64,** 668

50. Rolfini, G., Pavone, G. and deCello, L. (1963). Studio comparativo pra gli aspetti microistofluoroscopiti della placenta nel diabete e della isoimmunizzazione anti RH. *Rec. Med.*, **2,** 235

51. Fox, H. (1967). Abnormalities of the foetal stem arteries in the human placenta. *J. Obstet. Gynaec. Brit. Cwlth.*, **74,** 734

52. Dawes, G. S. (1962). The umbilical circulation. *Amer. J. Obstet. Gynec.*, **84,** 1634

CHAPTER 13

Examination of Fresh Villi

Silvio Aladjem

Following the first reports on the study of fresh placental tissue by phase contrast microscopy[1] it has become apparent that this method must be viewed as a complementary one to the classic histological and electronmicroscopic techniques[2-5]. In this chapter we propose: (1) to briefly review the technique of specimen preparation; (2) to systematise the normal and abnormal appearance of the human placental tissue as seen by phase contrast microscopy and (3) to discuss those areas of physiological and/or clinical significance that relate to the phase contrast microscopic study of the placenta.

Immediately after delivery the placenta is kept refrigerated in a plastic bag, but not frozen. If studied within 24 hours of delivery one can be sure that the findings are not influenced by the time elapsed[2,6]. However, after 36 hours certain changes appear that could mislead the diagnosis and after 72 hours a significant number of villi present changes which are different from those observed at the time of delivery.

After the placenta has been stripped of its appendages and its macroscopic characteristics recorded in the usual fashion[7] the maternal surface of the placenta is divided into four imaginary quadrants. Assuming there are no macroscopic pathological findings, (infarcts, calcifications, etc.) four specimens are obtained at random in each quadrant from the basal towards the chorionic plate. The specimens are obtained using a fine non-traumatic tissue forceps and scissors or by aspiration using a 14 gauge needle and a syringe. Each specimen is then placed on a slide with a few drops of an isotonic solution, (5% Dextrose in water or similar) covered with a cover slide (Figure 13.1), and observed with a phase contrast microscope. Microphotographs are obtained for permanent record. 200–250 terminal villi may be seen in each specimen. This random sampling of the placenta allows the study of

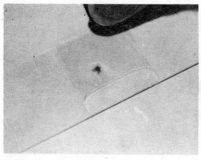 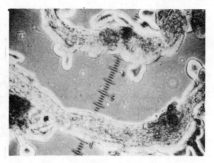

13.1   13.2

Figure 13.1 Specimen in the process of being covered with a cover slide after aspiration from the maternal aspect of the placenta. The tissue is floating in a 5% Dextrose in water solution

Figure 13.2 10 weeks placental specimen from a therapeutic abortion, normal pregnancy. Note multiple syncytial sprouts characteristic of early gestation (× 100). (From Aladjem, S. (1967). *Obstet. Gynecol.*, **30,** 408 with permission from Harper and Row)

approximately 4000 terminal villi. When a greater number of specimens were studied the evaluation based on the random sampling did not change. In those cases in which macroscopic changes are present, samples are taken centrifugally around the macroscopic finding until the samples compare with those taken at random.

The morphological appearance of the fresh placental tissue is a function of gestational age. In early pregnancy the sprouting capacity of the syncytium is its most outstanding characteristic (Figure 13.2). These sprouts become subsequently vascularised to form the terminal villi and as pregnancy progresses the number of sprouts decreases while the vascularisation becomes more prominent (Figure 13.3). Not all of these sprouts become vascularised since a great number of them loosen their attachment to the syncytial surface and freely migrate towards the maternal circulation and may be recovered in the maternal blood as syncytial globules (Figure 13.4). During the third trimester there is a rapid increase in the degree of vascularisation of the terminal villi and a marked thinning of the syncytium. The stroma all but disappears and its place is taken by either an extremely dilated or a markedly looped capillary which thus becomes the predominant villus structure (Figure 13.5).

The normal characteristics of the syncytium, stroma and capillary of the terminal villi as seen by phase contrast microscopy form the basis for the systematisation of the pathological findings. These are summarised in Table 13.1. Variation in the normal activity of the syncytium, either in the form of hypoplasia (Figure 13.6) in early pregnancy or hyperplasia (Figure

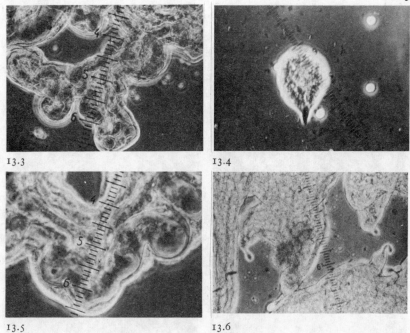

13.3

13.4

13.5   13.6

Figure 13.3 39 weeks placental specimen, normal pregnancy. (×100)

Figure 13.4 Syncytial globule recovered from the maternal circulation. Compare its size to adjacent red cells (×250)

Figure 13.5 High magnification of a villus in a normal term pregnancy (40 weeks). Observe the dilated terminal capillary approaching an extremely thin syncytium. Note the scarce stroma (×250)

Figure 13.6 Minimal sprouting in a placenta at 25 weeks gestation. Clinically abruption placenta (×62). (From Aladjem, S. (1967). *Obstet. Gynecol.*, **30,** 408 with permission from Harper and Row)

Table 13.1 Morphologic description of the normal and pathological findings of the terminal villus

Terminal Villus	Normal	Pathological
Syncytium	Syncytial sprouting in early pregnancy Thinning at term	Hypoplasia in early pregnancy Hyperplasia at term
Stroma	Abundant up to 32 weeks Decreasing thereafter Minimal at term	Edema Vacuolation
Capillary	Limited vascularisation in early pregnancy Predominant characteristic at term	Haemorrhage Avascularity

13.7) in late pregnancy are easily identified in an objective way by using the Sprout:Villus Index (Figure 13.8).

The edema of the villus stroma (Figure 13.9) may increase the diameter of the villi threefold or more. The villi acquire the characteristic club-shaped

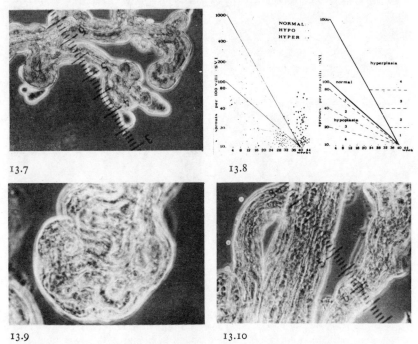

13.7

13.8

13.9   13.10

Figure 13.7 Hyperplasia of the syncytium at 42 weeks gestation. Clinically toxaemia of pregnancy. Note the characteristic appearance of the term villus, with thin syncytium, reduced stroma and with the capillary being the predominant structure. The presence of syncytial sprouting is abnormal ($\times$ 62). (From Aladjem, S. (1972). *Obstet. Gynecol.*, **39**, 591 with permission from Harper and Row)

Figure 13.8 Left side of the picture shows on semi-log paper the plotting of the number of syncytial sprouts per 100 villi (Sprout: Villus Index) against gestational weeks. Each case represents the mean value of approximately 4000 villi. At the right side the normal cone-shaped zone as determined by this plot is shown. Deviations from this normal zone are considered as hypoplasia or hyperplasia respectively. Degrees, as determined by dotted lines, are arbitrarily proposed. (From Aladjem, S. (1968). *Am. J. Obstet. Gynecol.*, **101**, 704 with permission from C. V. Mosby Company)

Figure 13.9 Edematous villus. Clinically Diabetes 37 weeks gestation. The increase in the size of the villus and its club shaped appearance is characteristic. Compare with Figure 13.2 ($\times$ 62)

Figure 13.10 Avascular degeneration of terminal villi in clinically toxaemia of pregnancy ($\times$ 62)

form and at times the edema is so severe that not more than one villus can be observed per field at × 200 magnification in which case the edema is considered to be severe[6]. The degeneration and disappearance of the terminal capillary in its entirety characterises the avascular degeneration (Figure 13.10), while the presence of extravasated blood at the terminal villus level is diagnostic of stromal haemorrhage of fetal origin (Figure 13.11). A common finding in term placentas is the subsyncytial edema, which appears as an accumulation of fluid just underneath the syncytium slightly displacing but apparently not impairing the circulation in the terminal capillary (Figure 13.12). When fixed and processed for histological sections this subsyncytial edema has a similar appearance (Figure 13.13). It is not unusual for this

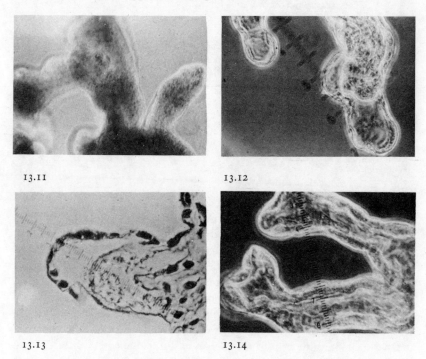

13.11

13.12

13.13

13.14

Figure 13.11 Intravillus haemorrhage of fetal origin (× 125)

Figure 13.12 Subsyncytial edema in a placenta at term. Normal pregnancy. Note the accumulation of fluid underneath the syncytium displacing, but not apparently impairing the underlying circulation (× 62)

Figure 13.13 Histological section of the same specimen as in Figure 13.12. The specimen was fixed under the microscope and only subsequently embedded and cut (× 80)

Figure 13.14 Vacuolation of the villus at term. Clinically normal pregnancy (× 62).

(From Aladjem, S. (1968). *Obstet. Gynecol.*, **32**, 28 with permission from Harper and Row)

phenomenon to involve the entire villus which then acquires the characteristic appearance of vacuolation (Figure 13.14). The significance of this
phenomenon is not clear but it may be related to normal ageing of the
placenta.

When approached in a systematic way the pathology of the terminal villi
as seen by phase contrast microscopy appears well defined both in its terminology and its description. (Table 13.1). The attempt at correlating these findings
with histological studies, however, is not a fruitful one. Table 13.2 summarises the result of such an attempt. This lack of correlation is but the result

**Table 13.2* Comparison of concurrent pathological diagnosis by phase
contrast microscopy and histology**

	No. of cases diagnosed by phase microscopy	Concurrent histological diagnosis	No. of cases diagnosed on histological sections	Concurrent phase diagnosis
Hypoplasia	15	—	5	—
Hyperplasia	11	1	5	2
Edema	43	2	1	1
Ischaemia	58	3	2	2
Avascularity	65	8	14	10
Haemorrhage	1	—	—	—

* Modified from Aladjem et al.[6]

of the different type of information provided by these two different techniques which are not to be interpreted as invalidating each other.

Two factors that relate to the technique account probably for most of
this apparent lack of correlation. One is the sampling as we devised it for our
studies which is a much more exhaustive one than the routine used for
histological sections. Gruenwald[8] has pointed out the normal and pathological
variation in the structure of terminal villi as they relate to the placental lobule.
By sampling routinely the four quadrants of the placenta, at different levels
and with a minimum of four samples in each quadrant, the phase contrast
microscopic study is more likely to faithfully represent a cross section of this
variation.

The classic concept of the placenta being a heterogenous organ 'par
excellence'[9] has thus been challenged by the fresh tissue studies[6,10]. Indeed
when macroscopic alterations have not occurred, the microscopic aspect of
the terminal villi is homogenous rather than heterogenous, to the extent that
based on the percentage of villi affected, a grading of placental findings is
possible[10]. While not all villi are affected by any one pathological change the

percentage of villi affected by the same type of pathology in any given specimen is the same[10].

The second factor is the tissue alteration secondary to the processing of histological sections. A point in case is the observation of moderate degrees of edema which cannot be observed in histological sections due to tissue shrinkage as a result of the fixation process. It has been shown that the passage through alcohol of an edematous villus may produce a shrinkage of up to 75% of the original size[11]. Another distinct advantage of the observation of the fresh placental tissue resides also in the ability to visualise 200–250 intact terminal villi in their entirety without the need for mental reconstruction of any single villus. For example the difference in appearance between the richly vascularised term villus (Figure 13.5) as opposed to the avascular degeneration where no capillary is present (Figure 13.10) is readily appreciated in fresh tissue while a histological section may tangentially miss the vessel and appear with no capillary.

The possibility of observing the terminal villus capillary in its entirety has made possible the study of the correlation between the total trophoblastic area and the functional capillary area in normal and complicated pregnancies. It has been estimated in these studies that in normal pregnancies at term approximately 75% of the total villus area corresponds to the terminal capillary while in toxaemia of pregnancy, diabetes and prematurity this is significantly reduced[12]. In planimetric studies of histological sections, however, the trophoblastic area will be measured disregarding the fact that this may be a non-functional area if the capillary is absent. On the other hand when cellular details are important, histological sections cannot be substituted for fresh specimens.

Two of the findings, as seen by phase microscopy, that have been correlated with fetal distress in labour, as determined by fetal heart rate monitoring and fetal blood-gas studies, are the edema and the avascular degeneration[13]. In both cases the common physiopathological ground is prenatal fetal hypoxia. In the presence of placental edema, a phenomenon which involves the entire placenta, the overall reduction of the intervillous space volume compromises the feto-maternal exchanges with the consequent fetal hypoxia. In the presence of avascularity the degree of hypoxia is probably a function of the percentage of villi affected, and the resulting hypoxia may therefore be less severe or indeed not occur altogether. When the functional reserve of the placenta is challenged by the stress of labour, fetal decompensation and acidosis may occur at an early stage with an edematous placenta but occurs late, if at all, in cases of avascularity (Figure 13.15).

Perhaps the most rewarding area of clinical investigation of the phase contrast microscopic study of the placenta is the correlation between certain

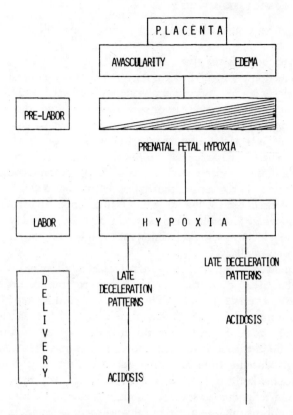

Figure 13.15 Schematic representation of the relationship between the prelabour influence of placental pathology with the consequent intrauterine fetal hypoxia and fetal behaviour during labour. Note that in the presence of prelabour fetal hypoxia, as when placental edema is present, the added hypoxia that occurs during uterine contractions will decompensate the fetus more rapidly. (From Aladjem, S. (1972). Risks in Prenatal Obstetrics, in *Risks in the Practice of Modern Obstetrics*. (Aladjem, S., editor) with permission from C. V. Mosby Company)

alterations of the terminal villus of the human placenta and the fetal outcome[2-5, 10]. In order to quantify the observed placental pathology more objectively an arbitrary scoring system was devised and this has been related to perinatal outcome[6]. The three elements considered are the syncytium, the stroma and the capillary. A score of 0 implies a normal appearance for the structure studied. Increasing scores have been given to pathological findings on a scale 0 to 10 with the intent of reflecting the severity of the observed alteration (Table 13.3). On this scale the intravillous haemorrhage (Figure 13.11) has been assigned a score of 10 based on previous observations of the

Table 13.3 Guideline for placental score*

	Pathology			Score
Syncytium	None			0
			1st degree	1
	Hypoplasia†		2nd degree	2
			3rd degree	3
			4th degree	4
			1st degree	
	Hyperplasia†		2nd degree	1
			3rd degree	
			4th degree	2
Stroma	None			0
		Partial {	Moderate	1
			Severe	2
	Edema			
		Universal {	Moderate	3
			Severe	4
Capillary	None			0
	Avascular degeneration‡ (%)	10		0
		25		2
		50		4
		51		8
	Ischaemia‡ (%)	10		0
		25		2
		50		4
		51		8
	Intravillous haemorrhage			10

* From Aladjem, *et al.*[6]
† Degrees determined using the Sprout-Villus Index
‡ Percentage of all villi

high incidence of perinatal morbidity and mortality that associated with it[2, 3, 11]. The final score is the sum of all assigned scores.

The attempt made at correlating the placental score with neonatal outcome indicates that with high placental scores a significant number of infants died or had Respiratory Distress Syndrome[6]. In fact with a score of 5 or more, 50% of all infants died and 36% had RDS. It was also apparent that the type of the observed placental pathology bears a definite influence on fetal outcome. The association of hypoplasia of the syncytium, e.g. as defined by the Sprout: Villus Index (Figures 13.6 and 13.8), was an indication of guarded neonatal prognosis, since 40% of the infants that died presented with hypoplasia of the syncytium whether associated or not with other findings.

More recent and ongoing studies suggest that the placental score is particularly useful in pre-term infants, i.e. infants with gestational age of less than 37 weeks. The risk of abnormal extrauterine adaptation and higher incidence of respiratory problems is increased with placental scores greater than 5. In term infants who suddenly develop respiratory problems or are born asphyxiated for reasons that may not necessarily reflect placental compromise, the index does not appear to be of value[14].

Conclusion

The pathological study of the human placenta has, from a clinical point of view, a longstanding history of unrewarding experiences in spite of significant advances made in the overall understanding of placental structure, ultrastructure and physiology[15,16]. If placental study is to become meaningful, it must be: (a) an accurate study of placental morphology; (b) predictive of neonatal outcome and (c) simple, reliable and readily available to the clinician[6].

None of the current methods completely fulfil these requisites. The technique of phase contrast microscopy, as reviewed here, suggests, however, that a thorough study of the fresh placental tissue may be correlated with fetal and neonatal conditions and it may provide a means of evaluating neonatal prognosis. With further experience, and with an understanding of its limitations particularly in terms of the lack of cellular details, it may prove to be a valuable tool in the evaluation of the newborn's adaptation to extra-uterine life.

References

1. Alvarez, H. (1964). Morphology and physiopathology of the human placenta. *Obstet. Gynecol.*, **23**, 813
2. Aladjem, S. (1966). Perinatal evaluation and prognosis of the premature fetus and newborn infant through phase contrast microscopy of the placenta. *Am. J. Obstet. Gynecol.*, **95**, 935
3. Aladjem, S. (1968). Phase contrast microscopic observations of the human placenta from six weeks to term. *Obstet. Gynecol.*, **32**, 28
4. Marino Iglesias, M., Gamisans, O. O., Domenech, R. G. R. (1970). Estudio de la placenta mediante el microscopio de contraste de fase. Su importancia como medio asesor del estado perinatal fetal. *Acta Ginec.* (Madrid), **21**, 355
5. Werner, C. (1971). Methodik und Wert der Phasenkontrast-mikroskopie für die Plazentadiagnostik. *Geburtsh Frauenheilk.*, **6**, 575
6. Aladjem, S., Perrin, E. and Fanaroff, A. (1972). Placental score and neonatal outcome. *Obstet. Gynecol.*, **39**, 591
7. Benirschke, K. (1961). Examination of the placenta. *Obstet. Gynecol.*, **18**, 309

8. Gruenwald, P. (1966). The lobular architecture of the human planenta. *Bull. Johns Hopkins Hosp.*, **119**, 172

9. Wilkin, P. (1965). Pathologie du Placenta, (Paris: Masson and Cie)

10. Aladjem, S. (1969). Fetal assessment through biopsy of the human placenta. In: *The Foeto-placental Unit*, p. 392 (A. Pecila and C. Finzi, editors) (Amsterdam: Excerpta Medica Foundation)

11. Alvarez, H., De Bejar, R., Aladjem, S., Alvarez Santin, C., Pemedio, M. R. and Sica Blanco, Y. (1964). La placenta humana. In: *Actas IV Congreso Uruguayo de Ginecoto-cologia*, Vol. I, p. 190

12. Aladjem, S. (1970). Studies in placental circulation. *Am. J. Obstet. Gynecol.*, **107**, 88

13. Aladjem, S., Kahn, K., Dingfelder, J. *et al.* (1971). Placental aspects of fetal heart rate patterns. *Obstet. Gynecol.*, **38**, 671

14. Aladjem, S., Fanaroff, A. and Perrin, E. (1973). (Unpublished observations)

15. Benirschke, K. and Driscoll, S. (1967). The pathology of the human placenta. *Handbuch d. spez. path. Anat. u. Histol.* p. 97 (E. Uehlinger, editor) (New York: Springer)

16. Longo, L. and Bartels, H., editors (1972). *Respiratory gas exchange and blood flow in the placenta. Proceedings of a Symposium, Hanover,* 1971—U.S. Dept. of Health, Education and Welfare. Publication No. (NIH) 73-361, Bethesda, Md.

CHAPTER 14

Abnormal Maturation of Villi

Volker Becker*

The principle of maturation of villi consists of the improvement of the structural basis of transfer mechanisms. This is done by enlargement of the areas of contact, and thinning of the distance to be traversed between maternal and fetal circulations. Maturation means improved exchange and thus reduced metabolic cost. Disturbance of maturation leads to a potentially fatal deterioration of exchange. Any elements of the placental villi which take part in the process of maturation can be the seat of a disturbance of this process.

The exchange function of the human placenta is localised in the terminal villi. Here maternal and fetal circulation are in closest contact. The terminal villi are also the site of maturation. The maternal blood within the inter-villous capillary spaces[1] is separated from the fetal blood only by a thin plate of syncytiotrophoblast and the capillary wall[2-4]. In these areas the thickness of the tissue through which exchange takes place, has been reduced in every possible way. The distance to be permeated between maternal and fetal circulations is one parameter of maturation, and the size of the area of close apposition the other. These specialised areas have been termed syncytio-capillary membranes or, according to Hörmann[1], *syncytio-sinusoidale Stoff-wechselmembranen*. The dimensions of these areas of exchange are measures of maturation and functional economy, but also of disturbances of maturation. Bender[5, 6] calculated a quotient of vascularity, consisting of the measured intravillous fetal blood volume divided by the volume of the terminal villi. This quotient is 0·47 in the normal mature placenta (range 0·44–0·50), considerably higher than in immature placentas found at term.

* Translated by the editor.

As a model of such immature placentas, Bender[5, 6] used the placenta in Rh-isoimmunisation, and calculated a quotient of vascularity of 0·12 (range 0·08–0·18). These studies of Bender showed that the critical limit of adequacy of the immature placenta is contingent on a surface area of the syncytio-vascular membranes of at least 3·6 m². Another limiting factor is an intra-villous fetal blood volume of at least 45 ml. The critical quotient of vascularity is, according to these investigations, 0·1. No fetuses in whose placentas a lower quotient was determined survived.

The terminal villus experiences a steady diminution of its diameter in the course of its maturation, from 618 μ about the 100th day to 268 μ at term[8]. The total area of contact is thereby increased and this also enters into Bender's quotient of vascularity.

The most severe disturbance of maturation of the terminal villi is char-acterised by inhibition of this process of diminution of villus size. The most impressive example of this change is the hydatidiform mole. Here the diameter of villi not only does not diminish, but is even greatly enlarged by intravillous edema and lymphorrhagias (Figure 14.1). There is no possibility of regular exchange and the embryo dies at an early stage.

Another example of generalised inhibition of maturation of the terminal villi is, as has been mentioned, blood group incompatibility. The villi in

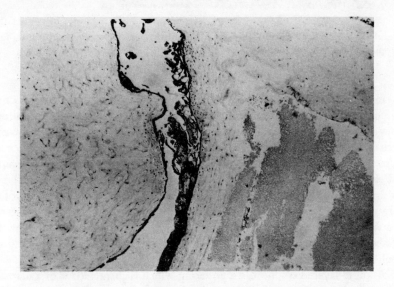

Figure 14.1 Hydatidiform mole. Large villi with edematous distension. On the right is seen lymphorrhagia with a collection of lymph. On the left, the trophoblast is stretched and low. In the villus on the right there is proliferation of trophoblast

Rh-isoimmunisation remain large (Figure 14.2); they are distended by intravillous edema. There are also other disturbances of maturation such as a double-layered trophoblastic lining, failure of formation of syncytio-capillary membranes and of the sinusoidal change of the capillaries.

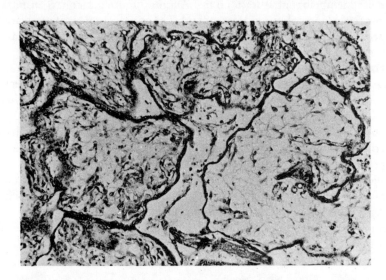

Figure 14.2 Villi in Rh-incompatibility. Large, edematous villi with few capillaries; the trophoblast is stretched. On the lower right there are nucleated erythrocytes

In the mature placenta one always finds upon careful examination varying numbers of so-called 'young villi'[9]. This is also a disturbance of maturation but only of single villi which are particularly conspicuous in comparison with other, much more mature villi[10] nearby. (Figure 14.3). Sometimes there is also a distinct double-layered trophoblastic covering. Schuhmann and Wehler[11] contend that these villi are so well supplied with oxygen that there is no functional need for vascularisation. They have found the 'young villi' always at the best supplied portions of the placental lobule. These villi are particularly numerous in diabetes mellitus[12]. The inhibition of exchange in diabetes is also marked by a number of large, paddle-shaped, undivided villi[13-16] (Figure 14.4).

A single-layered trophoblastic covering which is characteristic of a mature placenta, is one form of diminution of the distance to be permeated by transmitted materials. The dislocation of nuclei forming syncytial knots, and between them the syncytio-capillary membranes is a further mechanism of

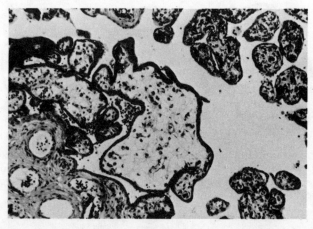

Figure 14.3 Group of villi containing immature ones. These are large, edematous, and not vascularised, among many mature villi with a small diameter

maturation which may be delayed and thereby result in a functional disturbance. This process is correlated with a diminution in diameter of the villi.

The space within the villi is greatly diminished during maturation by the reduction in size of villi (Figure 14.5). At the same time, this space is further reduced by an enlargement of fetal blood vessels. The capillaries of the villi

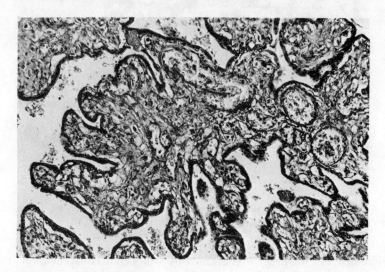

Figure 14.4 Placenta in embryopathia diabetica: a large, paddle-shaped villus (giant villus) with only minimal vascularisation

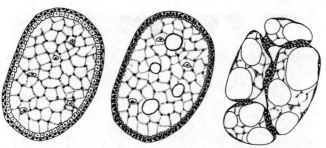

Figure 14.5 Diagram of the maturation of villi. *Left:* immature villi, double-layered trophoblast, Hofbauer cells. *Middle:* trophoblast still double-layered, some vessels present. *Right:* Diminution of villous diameter: 4 villi in the same area. Large sinusoids, synctio-vascular membranes, conglomeration of nuclei of syncytium

attach themselves to the base of the syncytium and their lumen enlarges four- to six-fold. Their wall remains that of a capillary (Figure 14.6). By this process the stroma of the villi is extensively displaced. Its central portion is

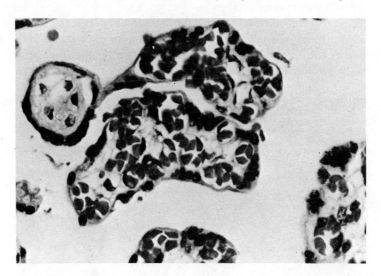

Figure 14.6 Mature villus with extensive replacement of the stroma by hyperaemic vessels, syncytio-capillary membranes next to syncytial knots

diminished, but markedly strengthened by a moderate collagenisation. The mature villus is therefore characterised by:
(1) a small circumference

(2) larger sinusoids which apply themselves to the syncytium and therefore form the

(3) syncytio-capillary membranes flanked by syncytial knots

(4) a diminished content of connective tissue stroma.

The immature villus has a large circumference, contains only small vessels, has a relatively large amount of connective tissue stroma and a uniform, often double-layered covering by trophoblast.

A delay in maturation resulting in diminution of the exchange mechanism, exists also when the villi are avascular, that is, when the stimulus for the formation of capillaries in the villi is absent. This occurs in the terminal villi particularly when the vessels in villous stems are occluded by endarteritis obliterans and the peripheral villi therefore remain avascular (Figure 14.7).

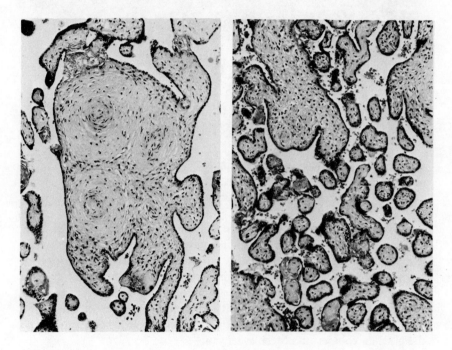

Figure 14.7 Old, now quiescent endarteritis obliterans in a villous stem (*left*) and avascularity of terminal villi supplied by this stem (*right*)

This change in the villous stems happens very early, sometimes even in the first trimester, often under the influence of maternal (virus) infections. Maternal rubella infection is a particularly good example of this intrauterine damage to blood vessels (Figure 14.8). The fetuses die as a result of inadequate exchange function of the placenta at the turn of the sixth month of pregnancy, and are expelled. The peripheral villi remain avascular because the connection

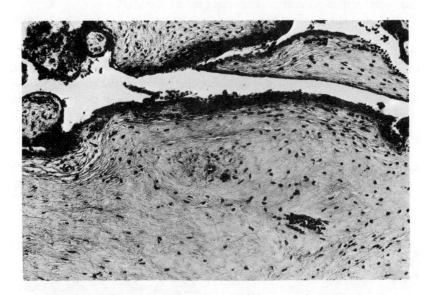

Figure 14.8 Placenta in maternal rubella infection. A vessel in a villous stem is severely narrowed, with a capillary lumen in the place of the usual wide one

with vessels in the villous stems was either impossible because of their absence, or because of the insufficient *vis a tergo*. This shows that the placenta is capable of sustaining the fetus by pure diffusion without formation of syncytio-capillary membranes up to the end of the second trimester, but this immature form cannot nourish the fetus up to term. One possible exception to this statement is the placenta in Rh-isoimmunisation. It remains at the stage of a diffusion placenta, and yet the fetus can be carried to term because the placenta compensates by enlargement.

If avascularity of villi is not equally present in all portions of the placenta, then a fairly large organ may yet be able to supply the fetus. Partial avascularity as a result of endarteritis obliterans during the third trimester is frequently the cause of small-for-dates fetuses, even when this cause is not apparent merely from the weight relationship of fetus and placenta. We found in our own material endarteritis obliterans with avascularity of villi in 30% of macerated stillbirths[17]. Among 126 infants with partial obliteration of vessels in the villous stems there were 100 stillbirths, 5 pre-term infants and 19 term infants.

Occasionally, but much more rarely, one finds extensive vascularisation of the core of the villi without formation of proper syncytio-capillary membranes. This is a disturbance of maturation of the peripheral vessels and may be designated as chorangiosis. The interior of villi is filled with coils of wide capillaries which, however, are not suitable for exchange between maternal and fetal blood. A further disturbance of maturation occurs when the transformation of capillaries into sinusoids is inhibited by very dense collagenous stroma. This occurs, for instance, in congenital syphilis, but also in other infectious diseases and toxemias. Occasionally this collagen transformation of the interior of the villi is also found in pre-eclampsia[18-20]. It is frequently seen in connection with long retained macerated fetuses[21, 22]. In that event the possibility cannot be denied that collagenisation occurred after death of the fetus. In the case of syphilis or non-macerated stillborn infants these findings must be considered as causes of death. The beginning of collagenisation of the stroma of villi is not rare in pre-eclampsia even with birth of surviving infants. When these infants are small-for-dates, the change in the villi must be considered as one component of placental insufficiency.

Fox[23] has summarised his studies of many years to the effect that fibrosis does not occur as a result of ischaemia of the placenta, that it is found more frequently in prolonged pregnancy and in pre-eclampsia, that it is not found associated with fetal death and not as a sign of placental ageing, but rather as the result of reduced blood flow through the fetal vessels. It appears that fibrosis is a non-specific reaction of terminal villi to a variety of conditions (Figure 14.9).

Maturation of fetal vessels (capillaries into sinusoids), the displacement of villous stroma, and the formation of syncytio-capillary membranes are correlated with each other so that the total picture of the mature villus is characterised by a combination of all these processes.

The difficulty in the evaluation of maturity or immaturity of the placenta consists not only in recognition of the normal state of maturity at various stages of pregnancy, but also in determining abnormal maturation at any point during pregnancy. This difficulty is compounded by the fact that various portions of the placenta are not always equally mature so that the significance of abnormalities of maturation may have to be estimated. Various schemes have been devised for the purpose of determining the maturity of placentas.

In Germany, Kloos and co-workers[24-26] have devised a differentiated system of classifying disturbances of maturation. This distinguishes first three main groups according to the timing of the damage:

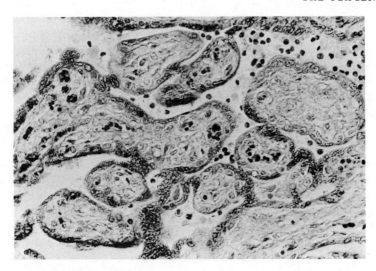

Figure 14.9 Placenta in pre-eclampsia: deficient sinusoid formation and dense stroma. Note numerous syncytial knots

(1) changes secondary to developmental disturbances in the first trimester
(2) the consequences of damage with well marked compensatory changes
(3) latent disturbance of maturation which become manifest only in the late fetal period.

Among damages of villi occurring in the first trimester and recognisable later on, Kloos lists various forms of 'young villi' (arrest of ramification with one- or two-layered trophoblastic lining) and discordant retardation of villi with fibrous stroma and few blood vessels. As attempted compensation, the formation of angiomatous hyperplastic sinusoids is mentioned. This is not true neoplasia in the sense of chorioangioma, but a reaction of the vessels which was described above as the rarely occurring chorangiosis. The third form is characterised by concordant inhibition of maturation of all villi with moderate vascularity and absence of syncytio-capillary membranes (our maturitas retardata, see below.

We have attempted an evaluation of maturity and delayed maturation with very simple criteria[7, 10, 17], and found it expedient to include the following observations:

(1) prenatal diminution in diameter of the villi
(2) transformation of capillaries into sinusoids with displacement of villous stroma
(3) displacement of nuclei in the trophoblast with formation of syncytio-capillary membranes

(4) narrowing and fibrosis of vessels in the villous stems.

When these signs of maturity are taken into consideration, a correlation of maturity of the placenta with that of the fetus is feasible.

Completely mature placentas associated with immature appearing infants do not appear frequently, approximately in 1–2% of cases of pre-term birth. We call this condition *maturitas praecox placentae*. The opposite, *maturitas retardata placentae*, occurs more frequently. It is associated with mature infants, but also prolonged pregnancy by dates. Maturation of the terminal villi is not completed, but obviously often sufficient for maintenance of the fetus. Yet the diminished functional capacity which is the result of this incomplete maturation, occasionally becomes manifest during labour when irregular heart beats, tachycardia, and asphyxia of the fetus, are observed.

Maturitas praecox and *maturitas retardata* of the placenta are states of asynchrony of maturation of placenta and fetus. These fall in the field of chronopathology[17].

The measurements by Gruenwald[27] (his weight curves are shown here in Figure 3.3) show that growth of fetus and placenta do not run parallel during the latter part of gestation. Growth of the placenta falls behind as compared with that of the fetus. This shows the need for improved structural organisation. Asynchronous maturation thus refers not only to weight relationships but also to structural characteristics.

Disturbances of maturation of terminal villi become significant as disease processes in the course of development of the placenta when the fetus demands more of the placenta than its structural condition can offer by way of permeability. A large proportion of functional insufficiency of the placenta is caused by disturbances of maturation. Thus, evaluation of the maturity of the placenta becomes a critical parameter of placental function. This is expressed in the definition of placental insufficiency which can be transferred without difficulty to disturbances of maturation: any change which affects the syncytio-capillary membranes with regard to their area and the distance to be traversed in transfer, leads to placental insufficiency. Disturbances in development of the trophoblastic lining, of the transformation of blood vessels, or of the stroma within the villi interfere with adequate development of terminal villi at the appropriate time, and produce the insufficient immature placenta.

References

1. Hörmann, G. (1958). Zur Systematik einer Pathologie der menschlichen Plazenta. *Archiv Gynäk.*, **191**, 297
2. Amstutz, E. (1960). Beobachtungen über die Reifung der Chorionzotten in der

menschlichen Plazenta mit besonderer Berücksichtigung der Epithelplatten. *Acta anat.*, **42**, 12

3. Getzowa, S. and S. Sadowsky (1950). On structure of human placenta with full time and immature fetus, living or dead. *J. Obstetr. and Gyn. (Brit.)*, **57**, 388

4. Wislocki, G. B. and Dempsey, E. W. (1955). Electron microscopy of the human placenta. *Anat. Rec.*, **123**, 133

5. Bender, H.-G. (1973). Morphometrie der Plazentainsuffizienz. *57. Tagg. Dtsch. Ges. Path., Karlsruhe.* (Stuttgart: G. Fischer) (in press)

6. Bender, H.-G. (1974). Plazenta-Insuffizienz. Morphometrische Untersuchung am Modell der Rhesus-Plazenta. *Archiv Gynäk.* (in press)

7. Becker, V. (1963). Funktionelle Morphologie der Plazenta. *Verhandl. Dtsch. Ges. Gynäkologie*, **34**, 3

8. Wilkin, P. (1965). Pathologie du placenta. Étude clinique et anatomique. (Paris: Masson)

9. Bleyl, U. and Stefek, E. (1965). Zur Morphologie und diagnostischen Bewertung der lockeren jugendlichen Zotten in reifen menschlichen Plazenten. *Beitr. path. Anat.*, **131**, 162

10. Becker, V. (1971). Die Plazenta bei Totgeborenen. In: E. Saling and K. Hüter: *Fortschritte der Perinatalen Medizin*, p. 409 (Stuttgart: Gg. Thieme Verlag)

11. Schuhmann, R. and Wehler, V. (1971). Histologische Unterschiede an Placentazotten innerhalb der materno-fetalen Strömungseinheit. Ein Beitrag zur funktionellen Morphologie der Placenta. *Arch. Gynäk.*, **210**, 425

12. Kloos, K. (1952). Zur Pathologie der Feten und Neugeborenen diabetischer Mütter. *Virchows Arch. path. Anat.*, **321**, 177

13. Emmrich, P. and Gödel, E. (1972). Morphologie der Plazenta bei mütterlichem Diabetes mellitus. Ergebnisse morphologischer Untersuchungen. *Zbl. allg. Path.*, **116**, 56

14. Emmrich, P. and Gödel, E. (1972). Plazentabefunde bei Neugeborenen diabetischer Mütter mit einem Geburtsgewicht unter 3000 g. *Path. et Microbiol. (Basel)*, **38**, 107

15. Emmrich, P. and Gödel, E. (1972). Morphologie der Plazenta bei mütterlichem Diabetes mellitus. *Zentralbl. f. Gynäkologie*, **94**, 881

16. Vogel, M. (1967). Plakopathia diabetica. Entwicklungsstörungen der Placenta bei Diabetes mellitus der Mütter. *Virchows Arch. path. Anat.*, **343**, 51

17. Becker, V. (1971). Die Chronopathologie der Plazenta. Allgemeinpathologische Aspekte der Organreifung. *Dtsch. med. Wschr.*, **96**, 1845

18. Fox, H. (1968). Fibrosis of placental villi. *J. Path. Bact. (Edinb.)* **95**, 573

19. Salvatore, C. A. (1968). The placenta in acute toxaemia. *Amer. J. Obst. Gyn.*, **102**, 347

20. Schuhmann, R. and Geier, C. (1972). Histomorphologische Plazentabefunde bei EPH-Gestose. Ein Beitrag zur Morphologie der insuffizienten Plazenta. *Arch. Gynäk.*, **213**, 31

21. Emmrich, P. (1966). Plazentabefunde bei mazerierten Totgeborenen im Hinblick auf die mögliche Ursache des intrauterinen Fruchttodes. *Z. Geburtsh. u. Gynäk.*, **165**, 185

22. Justus, B., Justus, J. and Holtorff, J. (1968). Plazentaveränderungen bei intrauterinem Fruchttod ohne am Kind erkennbare Ursachen. *Geburtsh. u. Frauenheilk.*, **28**, 70

23. Fox, H. and Langley, F. A. (1973). *Postgraduate Obstetrical and Gynaecological Pathology.* (Oxford: Pergamon Press)

24. Döring, W. and Kloos, K. (1964). Morphologische Routinediagnostik der Plazenta. *Münch. med. Wschr.*, **106**, 1849

25. Frank, G. (1967). Histologische Befunde bei Gestoseplacenten. *Verhandl. Dtsch. Ges. Path.*, **51**, 381
26. Kloos, K. and Vogel, M. (1968). Placentationsstörungen. Histologische Untersuchungen über Placentareifungsstörungen am Routinematerial. *Virchows Arch. path. Anat.*, **343**, 245
27. Gruenwald, P. (1963). Chronic Fetal Distress and Placental Insufficiency. *Biol. Neonat.*, **5**, 215

CHAPTER 15

Placental Manifestations of Malformation and Infection

Shirley G. Driscoll

Among the diverse conditions whose diagnosis or pathogenesis can be clarified by placental studies, those affecting the offspring obviously justify such examinations oftener than do maternal disorders. That placenta and fetus share genes and environment is axiomatic. Congenital malformations— or the broader category 'birth defects' of contemporary idiom—are commonly found or reflected in the associated placentas. The salient features of antenatal and congenital infections call for placental studies to supply unique data relative to their genesis and resolution. This chapter deals with two challenging but disparate circumstances in which the placenta shares grave antenatal disease with the fetus, maldevelopment and infections. Beyond the theoretical interests of associating developmental or infectious lesions of the offspring with abnormalities of the placenta are their practical implications and more than a few challenging, even controversial, problems. Rather than review published reports to date, I have sought to synthesise some valid generalisations concerning feto-placental reactions to disease, and to suggest directions for significant new research.

Successful recent efforts to identify specific fetal disorders long before birth permit antenatal prognostication, an approach to optimal management, or elective termination of pregnancy. Fuller understanding of both normal and aberrant feto-placental physiology is the *sine qua non* of progress in this area. Blanc provided interesting, if partially speculative, insights relating fetal conditions and placental lesions potentially visible *in amnio*[1]. But what are the *functional* implications of the great enlargement of amniotic surface accompanying polyhydramnios? Does a necrotic, inflamed amnion work as well as an intact one—or is it biologically null? Are the circulatory, permeability, and erectile attributes of the umbilical vessels and cord altered when such vessels are narrowed and scarred by fibrous tissue proliferation? What unique and relevant information can be gained from biopsy of the placenta *in situ*? Since malformations and infections 'account for' at least one-fourth of perinatal deaths and inestimable suffering among survivors, the potential beneficiaries of improved understanding of these conditions are legion.

Malformations

Anecdotally and statistically, malformed fetuses and newborns are often associated with anomalous placentas. Such correlations as that of single umbilical artery with fetal anomalies, either non-selectively or as co-constituents of specific syndromes, have empirical value *per se*, especially as diagnostic problems arise following birth. In like fashion, significantly increased risks of fetal maldevelopment accompany abnormal insertions of the umbilical cord and of fetal membranes. How such relationships might evolve is rarely questioned. Also, the *functional* implications of developmental anomalies of umbilical cord, fetal membranes and placental substance are obscure.

Single umbilical artery

Numerous reports document the regular occurrence of single umbilical artery in about 1% of consecutive births, 7% of twin births, and a substantial percentage of the malformed[2]. Large series of cases of single umbilical artery demonstrate its empiric association with fetal maldevelopment. About one-third of infants whose cords contained only one artery were identified as malformed. Limited data suggest that single umbilical artery has the same statistical implications, irrespective of whether the left or the right artery is lacking. Absence of one umbilical artery does not appear to confer selective risks of particular associated anomalies or of consistent trends towards maldevelopment of one system or another. Specific teratological entities, such as the rubella and thalidomide syndromes, some autosomal trisomies, and even diabetic embryopathies often include single umbilical artery among typical constellations of defects. These, plus countless casual occurrences of this vascular lesion, suggest heterogeneous underlying causality. The association of endovasculitis with viral infections of embryo/fetus, notably in rubella, suggests a mechanism for early obliteration of an umbilical artery. Rare observations of unilateral hypoplasia, profound atrophy or necrosis of an umbilical artery support the view that vascular disease may cause a preformed vessel to disappear long before birth. Significantly, Ezaki and co-workers found single umbilical artery to be less frequent in young human embryos than among births late in gestation[3]. Since normally the two umbilical arteries merge prior to their chorionic ramification to placental cotyledons, it seems unlikely that placental function would be impaired as a consequence of single artery in the cord. In view of the rich vascularity of normal developing embryonic tissues, collateral, i.e. alternate, circulatory routes must evolve quite readily.

Accompanying the rare condition of fetal acardia, single umbilical artery is almost always found. In these instances, usually affecting one of diamnionic monochorionic twins but also possible in multiple gestations of higher order, direct continuity is demonstrable from the umbilical vasculature of the reduced, 'parasitic twin' to that of the co-twin 'host'. The single umbilical artery of the acardiac fetus is continuous upon their common chorionic plate through a large chorionic artery with an umbilical artery of the normal twin; conversely, the umbilical vein of the monster communicates directly with a large chorionic vein of his co-twin. Functionally, then, the anomalous twin is perfused by blood from the umbilical artery of the healthy twin and returns blood to the latter's umbilical vein. Concurrent with this profound circulatory disturbance, the recipient twin's development is severely impaired from early gestation. As a result, a bizarre, skin-covered mass of tissue, often axiated, containing abortive vestiges of several viscera, is found attached by a bivascular cord to the shared twin placenta.

Malpositions and other maladies of the umbilical cord

Surveys of malformed births indicate frequent concurrence of abnormal *insertion* of the umbilical cord, either at the placental margin or upon the chorion laeve, i.e. velamentous insertion. Not rarely, such a cord contains a single umbilical artery. Except that malpositioning of the cord may reflect suboptimal placentation, its association with fetal maldevelopment appears to be non-specific. Functional implications of these deviations have not been assessed. Suffice it to cite the hazards of fetal haemorrhage should the associated velamentous vessels occupy the lower uterine segment.

Length and general configuration of the umbilical cord offer few insights relative to fetal development. With grave errors of formation of the body wall and body stalk, a discrete umbilical cord may not be discernible. Instead, short vessels pass from the fetus to the placenta in the walls of a sac of amnion, the latter fusing with the margins of the defect in the body wall. Such defects then permit interadherence of the placenta and the exposed fetal viscera.

Persistence and patency of ductal remnants normally obliterated long before birth, the vitelline and allantoic ducts, is occasionally documented histologically, but is rarely of clinical significance. Larger vestiges may form discrete cysts, blind-ended diverticula or open channels in continuity with intestine or urinary bladder. Symptoms depend on the structure and functional capabilities of the tissues present.

Amniotic adhesions, strings and bands

Rarely amniotic adhesions bind the anomalous fetus to the placenta or the umbilical cord. Defects of fetal integument associated with cranioschisis or visceral eventration (*vide supra*) permit contiguous amnion to adhere to fetal parts. Strands of amnion, avulsed from normal apposition to chorion, sometimes form bridges within the ovisac, potentially threatening the fetus with entanglement. Such strings and bands, like the loops of umbilical cord, have been suspected of playing a role in developmental defects of the fetal extremities. This controversial explanation of antenatal amputations and dysplasias of the limbs is but rarely supported by objective evidence from critical study of the associated placentas and membranes.

Although inherent diseases of the fetal skin, the ichthyoses for example, might also involve the amnion, data relative to such associations are not recorded. In a recent case, amniotic epithelial hyperplasia accompanied epidermal hypertrophy and hyperkeratosis in a premature infant. Profound secondary amnionitis precluded detailed comparison of the amnion with the fetal epidermis.

The placenta per se and fetal maldevelopment

Occasional reports indicate that the placentas associated with a variety of malformational syndromes tend to be light in weight for gestational age and, sometimes, in comparison with fetal weight. Whether these placentas are scale models of normal placentas, i.e. proportionately deficient in all constituents and at all gestational ages, has not been questioned. Does, for instance, autosomal trisomy impair trophoblastic proliferation, villous growth and capillarisation? Is the 300 g of tissue comprising the term placenta in congenital rubella syndrome of similar composition to that of its weight and age peers in, for example, Trisomy 18?

Innumerable observers have characterised a substantial portion of the products of early spontaneous abortion as chromosomally aberrant. Yet the majority of these are karyotypically indistinguishable from surviving individuals, e.g. 45XO and the autosomal trisomies of specific malformational syndromes. Indeed, only a small fraction of the chromosomally anomalous survive birth, their frequency being relatively great among stillbirths. That the mechanism responsible for antenatal lethality in some of these disorders may implicate the placenta has received little attention. The reports of villous 'hydrops' and 'arborising' amniotic polyps in triploid conceptuses suggest that systematic evaluation of chorionic tissues in the chromosomally abnormal may be fruitful[4, 5]. Evaluation of the success of the maternal–chorionic interactions in these syndromes would, of course, require access to the intact conceptus *in situ*, an opportunity rarely accorded the investigator.

Oversized placentas occasionally accompany malformed births. An assortment of fetal anomalies has been associated with feto-placental anasarca, the latter indicating simple edema of the entire conceptus[6]. While a few of these cases seem to be explicable on the basis of a failing malformed heart, such mechanisms cannot always be invoked. On the other hand, the overweight, but bloody, placenta suggests maternal diabetes mellitus. Histologically, these placentas seem to be unusually vascular, with excessive capillarisation of the stem villi as well as the peripheral villi. Systematic evaluation of specific structural constituents, preferably by quantitative means, remains to be undertaken. Similarly, intense villous capillarity, suggesting diffuse chorangiosis, characterised several placentas from Down's syndrome.

The discrete vascular 'tumour' of the placenta, *chorangioma*, rarely accounts for fetal cardiomegaly. These lesions, usually less than two centimetres in diameter and often multiple, appear to occur more frequently in placentas of twins. They are not strongly associated with other fetal anomalies.

Recent reports describe the deposition of masses of pigmented cells within chorionic villi in association with congenital giant pigmented nevi[7]. In rare instances of fetal leukaemia and fetal neuroblastomatosis, villous involvement by the malignant process has been documented.

Fetal malformations and the liquor amnii

Non-specific placental manifestations of fetal malformations are of more than passing interest for the practical reasons that they may aid in diagnosis and clarify pathophysiology. *Oligohydramnios*, irrespective of cause, is accompanied by 'amnion nodosum' ('vernix granulomatosis') (Figure 15.1). Obstructive fetal uropathy, fetal anuria, chronic loss of *liquor amnii*, or fetal death may be the basis of the oligohydramnios. Pulmonary hypoplasia is also a frequent correlate. With marked reduction in amniotic fluid volume, the amniotic epithelial response is one of necrosis, sometimes accompanied by low-grade inflammatory and reparative phenomena[8, 9] (Figure 15.2). Probably in response to trauma, the fragile amniotic epithelium is damaged, particulate matter (vernix, lanugo hairs) may adhere, a few phagocytic cells may gather, and partial healing may ensue. As a result, the amnion is irregularly studded with tan, grey or yellow excrescences, usually liminally visible to diameters of several millimetres. Such lesions tend to be most numerous

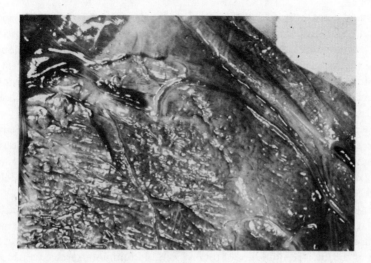

Figure 15.1 Amnion nodosum ('vernix granulomatosis'). Minute, raised, opaque deposits stud the normally smooth, shiny amnion

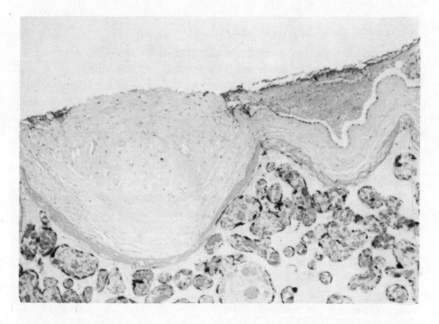

Figure 15.2 Amnion nodosum, microscopic. Normal amniotic epithelium is interrupted and replaced by heaped up debris, including detached squames, in an amorphous matrix

on the placental surface, but may also involve the extraplacental membranes and even the surface of that more mobile target, the umbilical cord. What, if any, amniotic dysfunction accompanies amnion nodosum? Probably none, since the lesions are small and focal, predominantly involving the placental amnion. On the other hand, extensive injury to the extraplacental amnion, apposed along with the chorion to capillarised decidua, might influence fluid transport at this site.

Two other conditions to be distinguished from amnion nodosum are: necrotising amnionitis (q.v.) and squamous 'metaplasia'. The latter term designates the focal pearly-white, semi-opacification of the amnion, found normally at term, as a consequence of keratinising hyperplasia of amniotic epithelium (Figure 15.3).

Polyhydramnios is also commonly associated with fetal anomalies, apparently not implicating placental structure in most instances. The complex and changing geometry of the distended ovisac precludes mathematical estimation of the inter-relationships of total volume and amniotic surface area. How does the amniotic sac accommodate substantial increments in volume of its contents? Is this accomplished by passive stretching and flattening or by proliferation of its epithelial constituents?

Malformations, multiple gestation and placentation

Monozygous twinning, *per se*, constitutes maldevelopment, even when neither twin is overtly deformed. Discordance for anomalies is common among single ovum twins, a circumstance offering significant insights into the formal genesis of such anomalies. Sharing their heritage, the twins are, none the less, often disparate in size, sometimes unequally damaged by suboptimal ante- and intranatal environment, and asymmetrically malformed. Meticulous studies of such twin pairs should contribute substantially to our understanding of polygenic inheritance and the intrauterine factors which may modify gene effects. Of course, the twins and their placenta(s) contribute significantly to each other's environments prior to their births[10,11]. How one fetus may influence the other is dramatically exemplified when intertwined umbilical cords of monoamniotic twins result in fetal death. Twin–twin interactions within the spectrum of altered physiology comprising the twin placenta transfusion syndrome are well known. Subtler instances of deleterious inter-relationships of twins, be they monozygous or dizygous, are probable, although less easily documented.

Malformations are relatively common among twins and discordance is frequent, even in monozygous sets. The placentas of such twins offer considerable potential insight as to the contributions of hereditary and environmental factors in the genesis of the associated fetal anomalies.

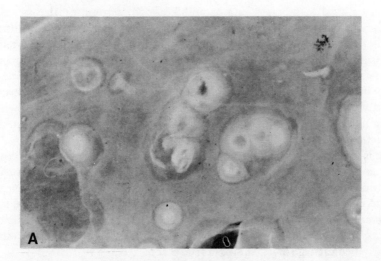

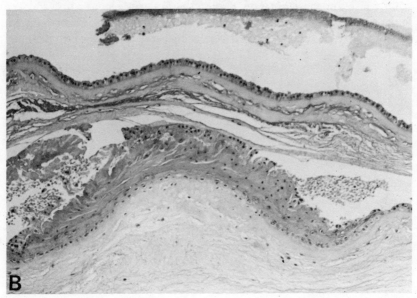

Figure 15.3 A and B Squamous metaplasia of amnion. Translucent to opaque thickening of amnion, produced by proliferation and keratinisation of its epithelium

Infections

Solid documentation can be offered for the occurrence of placental lesions in association with antenatal and congenital infections. Lesions of villous placenta, fetal membranes, and/or umbilical cord accompany the bacterial infections, candidiasis, viral and protozoal diseases, and syphilis present at birth. Indeed, it is probable that every infection of the human embryo/fetus damages these fetal adnexa as it traverses the barriers between host and parasite. Encased in maternal tissues, washed by maternal blood, and in close proximity to the birth canal, the placenta and fetal membranes risk exposure to any pathogen attacking the gravid woman. What practical benefits, what basic biological insights can be anticipated from studies of the placenta in infectious disease?

It is clear that antenatal infections induce two morphologically distinctive placental reactions: (1) inflammation of fetal membranes; (2) inflammation of chorionic villi[12]. The ensuing fetal infections also follow one of two general patterns according to the portals of entry and routes of spread of the offending organisms: (1) transamniotic, to contaminate the respiratory and alimentary tracts, the skin, and conjunctiva; (2) transvillous, with centrifugal and generalised carriage of organisms in fetal blood.

Of course, in some instances a secondary haematogenous phase follows initial transamniotic infections, or the amnion may become contaminated as pulmonary, intestinal or renal lesions discharge organisms into the fluid pool.

Table 15.1

Lesion	Route of entry	Infectious agents
Acute deciduitis Acute chorionitis Acute amnionitis	Ascent and contiguity with lower genital tract	Cervicovaginal flora (various bacteria, *Candida* sp., mycoplasma)
Acute umbilical vasculitis ± perivasculitis	Amniotic fluid	
Acute villous and perivillous inflammation	Haematogenous from gravida	Various bacteria; viruses
Subacute or chronic sclerosing villous inflammation		*T. gondii*; *T. cruzii*; *T. pallidum*; viruses
Subacute or chronic deciduitis	Haematogenous from gravida; ? by direct contiguity	*T. gondii*; viruses
Subacute or chronic umbilical vasculitis ± perivasculitis	? Haematogenous	*Herpes simplex*

- Table 15.1 indicates the typical modes of entry and characteristic distribution of lesions attributable to particular agents. Features serving to distinguish specific infections are dealt with below.

Amnionitis and related conditions

Neutrophilic infiltration of the amniotic membrane is found in about 15% of unselected births. Accompanying, and presumably preceding, this reaction is a similar change in the contiguous chorion (Figure 15.4). Deciduitis is also the

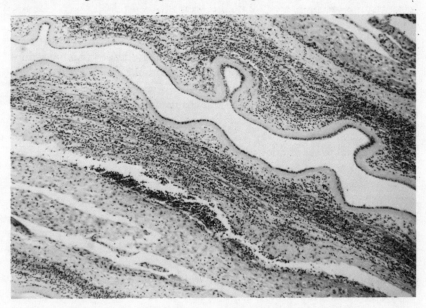

Figure 15.4 Acute chorioamnionitis. Polymorphonuclear leukocytes occupy much of the thickness of amnion and contiguous chorion

rule in such cases. Amnionitis is, of course, the *sine qua non* of transamniotic *fetal* infections—aspiration pneumonia, gastroenteritis, and the like. The topographical and anatomical distribution of the inflammatory infiltrates is consistent with the notion that the process usually begins in the decidua, progresses to involve the apposed chorion and thence the amnion, as *maternal* leukocytes migrate toward the latter membrane. Sometimes the initial stage is seen as neutrophilic margination and migration into the fibrin layer subtending the chorionic plate. Margination followed by emigration of *fetal* leukocytes into the media of umbilical vessels and vessels on the chorionic surface seems to occur in response to a stimulus from within the amniotic cavity.

It is likely that the amniotic epithelium may be damaged by direct spread of micro-organisms and their products upon its surface and within the bathing *liquor*. The degree and extent of epithelial necrosis and the occasional development of necrotising chorionic angiitis, with or without thrombosis, probably reflect particular attributes of the offending pathogens. Discrete macroscopic foci of amniotic epithelial necrosis, dotting the surfaces of umbilical cord and placenta, are typical of placental moniliasis.

The constancy with which acute umbilical vasculitis, with or without perivasculitis, accompanies amnionitis seems to depend on several factors. Most importantly, chorioamnionitis *without* umbilical inflammation is common early in the second trimester; the reverse is seen close to term. Retention of the conceptus, following fetal death, gives rise to mild deciduo-chorionitis, sometimes with amnionitis, but without fetal vasculitis. Conversely, localised injury to the cord, e.g. that occurring with prolapse, may induce umbilical inflammation without change in fetal membrane.

It has repeatedly been demonstrated that most cases of chorioamnionitis are attributable to cervico-vaginal flora. The same organisms that can ascend the birth canal to the amniotic sac may, on other occasions, contaminate the amnion, everted and wrapped around the placenta, as it passes through the cervix and vagina. In the latter event, organisms isolated from the amniotic surface may have been wiped on in transit. To circumvent this confounding source of 'positive' cultures, the amnion should be lifted off the apposed chorion of the placenta suspected of chorioamnionitis, and inocula for culture obtained from their interfacing surfaces, previously shielded from contaminants. Blood-borne agents may be isolated by excising a tissue sample through the unroofed chorionic plate, preferably followed by homogenisation of the sample prior to planting on the appropriate media.

Surveys of unselected births demonstrate the strong association of amnionitis with early delivery[13]. Generally speaking, the more premature the labour, the greater the probability of an associated chorioamnionitis. The obstetric literature perpetuates the myth that apparent physical integrity of the fetal membranes protects the amnion from infection. Contrary to this misconception, intact membranes are often inflamed ones, especially if birth occurs during the second trimester. Clinicians ignore these risks at their own —and their patient's—peril.

Overall, the incidence of inflammation of the fetal membranes and decidua, often accompanied by umbilical and chorionic vasculitis, exceeds any estimate based on morbidity. On the other hand, each year thousands of perinatal deaths are associated with acute chorioamnionitis, a lesion of very premature birth. When the paradox implicit in these observations is explained and the links between prematurity and placental inflammation defined, we can expect progress in prevention of the commonest obstetrical catastrophe.

Mycoplasmas and placental disease

The role of genital *mycoplasmas* in reproductive casualty and, more specifically, in antenatal infections is still problematic. The ubiquity of mycoplasmas in the lower genital tracts of women, their elusory attributes (i.e. direct staining in smears and tissue sections) and the species-specificity that precludes development of animal models frustrate efforts to define their pathogenicity. Yet, mounting evidence implicates these organisms in an occasional instance of congenital infection of the newborn, spontaneous abortion, and especially in a substantial segment of the otherwise cryptogenic acute chorioamnionitis[14]. The inflammatory response provoked by mycoplasmas in the fetal membranes is characterised by neutrophilic infiltration of chorion, amnion, and, of course, contiguous decidua[15]. Often umbilical vessels and those of the chorionic plate are also infiltrated by acute inflammatory cells, seemingly en route from fetal blood to amniotic fluid. Recent studies showed mycoplasmas, especially T-strains, to be present in the vaginas of mothers delivering placentas manifesting chorioamnionitis statistically more often than in association with uninflamed fetal membranes[16].

Except for a predilection for delivery at low birth weights, women colonised by mycoplasmas seem to impose no clear-cut perinatal morbidity on their progeny[17]. Indeed, the associated colonisation of the neonate is unaccompanied by clinical disease in most instances.

Parenchymatous (villous) placentitis

Haematogenous spread of infections to and within the conceptus evokes villous and perivillous inflammatory reactions of different quality[12]. Acute *bacteraemias* elicit acute villous lesions, even abscesses (Figure 15.5). Septic intervillous thrombi may be found. The extent of placental disease varies from case to case. Recent widespread interest in Group B beta haemolytic streptococcal infections of the newborn suggests acquisition of these pathogens in passage through the birth canal. Limited studies indicate that minute villous inflammatory foci may trace the paths of such organisms from gravida to fetus. Of course, the conventional dichotomy which equates neonatal infections to those acquired antenatally and those incurred postnatally may be too simplistic, as it excludes intranatal initiation of infectious disease.

A rare, but significant manifestation of intrauterine infection is that termed 'placental bacteraemia', usually a concomitant of septic abortion. Masses of Gram negative bacilli, essentially colonies growing within chorionic villous vessels, are accompanied by acute inflammation within and

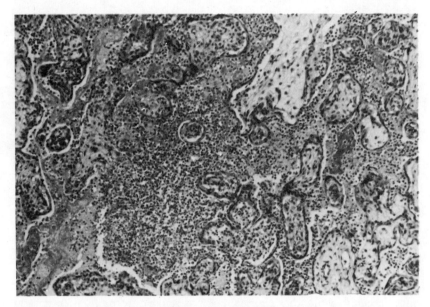

Figure 15.5 Acute villous placentitis with intervillous abscess formation. Villi are necrotic, surrounded and partially replaced by neutrophiles

around the villi[18] (Figure 15.6). Endotoxaemia and systemic collapse of the gravida are clinical expressions of the profusion of bacteria within her uterus.

Viral infections also incite villous inflammation, varying in degree, extent, and cellular characteristics from agent to agent and case to case. In general, such fulminant diseases as variola, vaccinia, varicella, and rubeola provoke intense necrotising and inflammatory phenomena in the villous tissues. More subtle placentitis is likely to be associated with cytomegalovirus, rubella, and *Herpes simplex* infections. Although inclusion bodies typical of the disease in question may be found in placental lesions, positive identification requires other methods than conventional histopathological study.

Placental responses to *Trypanosoma cruzii* and to *Toxoplasma gondii* are similar. In both instances, focal chronic villous inflammation is seen and organisms may be visualised in microscopic sections. Syphilis also induces a low-grade villous reaction, characterised by endovasculitis obliterans and mononuclear infiltration throughout the villous tree. Unselected placentas from large clinics and placentas delivered successively by individual gravidas provide histological evidence of frequent, but silent, chronic villous placentitis. In a morphometric survey of placentas from two urban populations, Guatemalan women of low socio–economic status and middle-class women

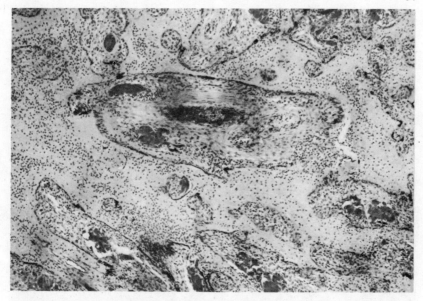

Figure 15.6 Acute villous placentitis with 'fetal bacteremia'. Proliferating bacteria, *Escherichia coli* in this instance, form plug-like masses within villous vessels

living in Boston, Massachusetts, random tissue sections often contained foci of villous inflammation, especially in the Guatemalan group[19]. Low-grade, clinically unapparent antenatal infections, endemic to a population, may bias studies of the effects of other factors, such as perinatal nutrition, on neural and intellectual development. Alford finds 3% of infants to be born with elevated levels of IgM in their sera; in only one in five such instances is this elevation attributable to any of the infections commonly suspected: Toxoplasmosis, Rubella, Cytomegalovirus, *Herpes simplex* or syphilis[20]. Perhaps the remainder will find an explanation in common with the 'incidental' villous placentitis, so unexpectedly frequent among unselected births. The long-term implications of these phenomena for the developing infant and child are presently unknown.

Non-specific evidences of antenatal infection

Feto-placental anasarca is an uncommon but significant manifestation of systemic, usually chronic, antenatal infections[6]. Agents implicated in this bizarre syndrome include Cytomegalovirus, *Toxoplasma gondii*, *Treponema pallidum* and, probably, *Trypanosoma cruzii*. Like the fetus, the chorionic tissues become edematous consequent to hypoproteinaemia and tissue hypoxia. Similarly, many chronic feto-placental infections are associated with fetal anaemia, erythro- and normoblastaemia. Occasionally, the combination of edema, anaemia, and profusion of circulating nucleated cells in the feto-placental vessels is erroneously ascribed to maternal isoimmunisation with fetal haemolytic disease.

In Conclusion

Until recently, the gravid human uterus has been regarded as a sanctuary, its contained conceptus equally inaccessible to direct diagnostic manipulations and to therapeutic attack on antenatal disease. The impressive successes attending the audacious active management of erythroblastosis fetalis encouraged similar approaches to a host of other prenatal conditions. Placentas have been biopsied without interrupting pregnancy. As clinical fetology takes these giant steps, the potential contribution of the pathologist to precision in diagnosis, understanding of feto-placental mechanisms of disease, and recognition of new iatrogenic lesions also grows. Morphologically, the placenta and adnexa comprise the theatre in which the interplay of disease, decompensation, and responses to therapy may be observed. Some of the most challenging problems of perinatology are expressed in these tissues, and keys to their solution may also lie there.

References

1. Blanc, W. A. (1968). The future of antepartum morphologic studies. In *Diagnosis and Treatment of Fetal Disorders* (edited by K. Adamsons), pp. 15–49 (New York: Springer)
2. Benirschke, K. and Driscoll, S. G. (1967). The pathology of the human placenta. *Handbuch der spez. path. Anatomie u. Histologie*. Henke-Lubarsch. Band VII/5, pp. 97–571 (Berlin: Springer)
3. Ezaki, D., Tanimura, T. and Fujikura, T. (1972). Genesis of single umbilical artery. *Teratology*, **6**, 105 (Abstract)
4. Makino, S., Sasaki, M. S. and Fukuschima, T. (1964). Triploid chromosome constitution in human chorionic lesions. *Lancet*, **ii**, 1273
5. Schlegel, R. J., Neu, R., Carneiro Leão, J., Farias, E., Lewczak, P. and Gardner, L. (1966). Arborizing amniotic polyps in triploid conceptuses: A diagnostic anatomic lesion? *Amer. J. Obstet. Gynecol.*, **96**, 357
6. Driscoll, S. G. (1966). Hydrops Fetalis. Current Concepts. *New Engl. J. Med.*, **275**, 1432
7. Demian, S. B. D., Donnelly, W. H., Frias, J. L. and Monif, G. R. G. (1974). Placental lesions in congenital giant pigmented nevi. *Amer. J. Clin. Pathol.*, **61**, 438
8. Bartman, J. and Driscoll, S. G. (1968). Amnion nodosum and hypoplastic cystic kidneys. *Obstet. Gynecol.*, **32**, 700
9. Salazar, H. and Kanbour, A. I. (1974). Amnion nodosum. Ultrastructure and histopathogenesis. *Arch. Pathol.*, **98**, 39

10. Strong, S. J. and Corney, G. (1967). *The Placenta in Twin Pregnancy*. (Oxford: Pergamon Press)
11. Benirschke, K. and Kim, C. K. (1973). Multiple pregnancy. *New Engl. J. Med.*, **288,** 1276
12. Driscoll, S. G. (1967). Fetal infections in man. In *Comparative Aspects of Reproductive Failure* (edited by K. Benirschke) (New York: Springer)
13. Driscoll, S. G. (1965). Pathology and the developing fetus. *Ped. Clin. N. Amer.*, **12,** 493
14. Kundsin, R. B. and Driscoll, S. G. (1970). The role of mycoplasmas in human reproductive failure. *Ann. N.Y. Acad. Sci.*, **174,** 794
15. Kundsin, R. B., Driscoll, S. G. and Ming, P. M. (1967). Strain of Mycoplasma associated with human reproductive failure. *Science*, **157,** 1573
16. Shurin, P. A., Alpert, S., Rosner, B., Driscoll, S. G. and Kass, E. H. (1974). Genital mycoplasmas—association with chorioamnionitis. (In press)
17. Klein, J. O., Buckland, D. and Finland, M. (1969). Colonization of newborn infants by mycoplasmas. *New Engl. J. Med.*, **280,** 1025
18. Studdiford, W. E. and Douglas, G. W. (1956). Placental bacteremia: A significant finding in septic abortion accompanied by vascular collapse. *Amer. J. Obstet. Gynecol.*, **71,** 842
19. Laga, E. M., Driscoll, S. G. and Munro, H. N. (1972). Comparison of placentas from two socioeconomic groups. I. Morphometry. *Pediatrics*, **50,** 24
20. Alford, C. A., Jr (1965). Studies on antibody in congenital rubella infections. I. Physicochemical and immunologic investigations of rubella neutralizing antibody. *Amer. J. Dis. Child.*, **110,** 455

CHAPTER 16

Determination of Maturity and Well-being using Maternal and Amniotic Fluids

Stephen J. DeVoe and Richard H. Schwarz

Introduction

Physicians have speculated on the source, fate, and role of amniotic fluid since the time of Hippocrates. Only in the last few years, however, have the functions and circulatory dynamics been intensively explored and the use of amniotic fluid in assessing fetal maturity and well-being appreciated.

Parameters for estimating fetal maturity are particularly valuable in fetal deprivation syndromes because they highlight the disparity between fetal size and duration of pregnancy. Maturation indices are useful in timing the delivery of high risk patients for the obstetrician who must choose between potential fetal distress and death and the hazards of pre-term birth.

The familiar measurements in amniotic fluid, creatinine, bilirubin, stained fetal cells and pulmonary phospholipids, are assumed to reflect the functional maturity of the fetus as a whole despite obviously uneven maturation of different systems reflected by retardation of his overall growth.

Although we use neonatal evaluation of the skin, neurological and pulmonary functions to substantiate our prenatal estimates of maturity, explicit proof that this evaluation is a reliable check on those estimates is lacking.

Only satisfactory experience seems to validate them. Though impossible to prove, it is conceivable that in the Fetal Deprivation Syndrome, there is occasionally inhibition of integumentary, neurological, and pulmonary development as well as musculo-skeletal lag, making the deprived newborn less mature than would correspond with its gestational age.

Amniotic Fluid Physiology

Many of the homeostatic functions of amniotic fluid are overlooked in the context of fetal evaluation because they are so effective, changing little despite varying degrees of abnormality.

Amniotic fluid serves both as a mechanical cushion against external trauma and as a medium for free fetal mobility as development continues. The fluid also acts as a thermal insulator against temperature extremes as well as a reservoir for fetal wastes. Nutritive elements such as lipids, carbohydrates, and proteins, as well as electrolytes, are probably incorporated from amniotic fluid through swallowing and intestinal absorption[1,2].

Amniotic fluid is elaborated from a number of sources whose relative importance may vary with gestational age and, possibly, from one pregnancy to another. Evidence for fetal micturition as a major source of amniotic fluid is strong but indirect. There is urinary output as early as fourteen weeks of gestation[1] and concentration and excretion of radio-opaque dye by the fetal kidney has been demonstrated by 22 weeks[3]. Fetal urine contains creatinine and urea in increasing amounts late in pregnancy as does amniotic fluid[4], presumably reflecting increasing glomerular function. Amniotic fluid also becomes progressively more hypotonic, probably due to an increasing contribution of hypotonic fetal urine[5]. Other evidence includes inadvertent fetal cystograms showing rapid dilution of dye in the bladder, thought to be due to fetal urine accumulation[6]. These observations all suggest that fetal micturition contributes significantly to amniotic fluid (see also Chapter 17).

The presence of amniotic fluid prior to fetal renal function and the existence of apparently secretory cells on fetal membranes[7] suggest that direct transport across the membranes is also a source of amniotic fluid. It has been hypothesised that the umbilical cord may contribute large amounts of water to amniotic fluid[8], a phenomenon which has been demonstrated with *in vitro* isotope studies[9]. The presence of secretory epithelium in several fetal sites such as the tracheo-bronchial tree and salivary glands raises the possibility that they might add to amniotic fluid production. The recent identification of phospholipids of pulmonary origin in amniotic fluid is good evidence of pulmonary contributions of undetermined size[10].

The effects of various major anomalies on amniotic fluid volume are known[1,11,12]. The presence of even a small amount of fluid with a major fetal malformation such as renal agenesis or total urinary tract obstruction[13] suggests the existence of other sources of production besides the fetal urinary tract.

The major means of disposal of amniotic fluid is thought to be fetal swallowing[14]. There are conflicting estimates of the volume swallowed, ranging from 500 millilitres per day[15] to 1500 millilitres per hour[14]. Much of this fluid is excreted back into the amniotic cavity while some is returned to the mother via the placenta.

The role of the fetal lung in fluid absorption is not clear. Concentration of dye in the fetal lung has been reported by some workers[16] but not confirmed by others[2, 6, 17].

The amnion is a logical and possibly a major route of amniotic fluid disposal but *in vivo* studies have not yet verified this.

As implied by the data on fetal swallowing, the turnover of amniotic fluid is rapid, being complete in approximately three hours[18-20]. Amniotic fluid water has a biological half-life of 90 minutes[20] at term and is exchanged at a rate of 500 millilitres per hour[20]. Approximately 150 millilitres of water per hour are returned through the fetus to the maternal circulation and the remainder diffuses directly across the fetal membranes[8].

Amniotic fluid volumes have been measured by several techniques with fairly comparable results, as summarised by Fuchs in 1966[21]. Although there is some variation, the best evidence is that there are about 50 millilitres of fluid present at 12 weeks and 400 at 20 weeks. The peak volume of one litre occurs at 38 weeks[22, 23] with gradual decreases to as little as 100–500 millilitres at 43 weeks[22, 24].

Amniocentesis

Increased awareness of information to be gained from amniotic fluid studies has led to liberalised indications for amniocentesis. The result is a series of reports of complications such as fetal trauma[25] exsanguination[26-28] feto-maternal haemorrhage[26, 29] premature labour[30], and premature placental separation[31]. Despite these reports, some authors express the thought that complications are 'rare'[32]. Evaluation of risk data is difficult because of sporadic reporting, failure to recognise complications and a poorly defined population at risk.

Obviously, amniotic fluid is a source of valuable information but amniocentesis should not be undertaken casually, the above statement notwithstanding. Patients should be examined thoroughly and the site chosen with care; appropriate studies for placental localisation such as ultrasound should be employed when indicated. The suprapubic route, described by Freda[33] is often overlooked. Procedures should be established for making the diagnosis of fetal injury or haemorrhage and contingency plans for delivery, if appropriate, should be pre-arranged.*

* The presence of fetal blood can be determined most rapidly by making a Wright's stain similar to that used for routine smears of peripheral blood, and looking for nucleated RBCs. The Apt test and Kleihauer–Betke procedures are much more complicated, and generally, take too much time for emergency use.

Amniotic Fluid Studies

Fetal maturity

The most valuable parameter for determining fetal age is the assessment of pulmonary maturity by measurement of amniotic fluid phospholipids, lecithin and sphingomyelin. More precisely, lecithin and sphingomyelin values, expressed as the L/S ratio, reflect the ability of the pulmonary alveolus to maintain low surface tension in late expiration, thus remaining open and avoiding the carnage of respiratory distress syndrome and hyaline membrane disease.

The primary investigator in this area, Louis Gluck, and his co-workers, discovered that stability of the human pulmonary alveolus developed co-incident with a surge in the synthesis of a substance whose primary constituent is dipalmityl phosphatidyl choline (DPC)[10]. This non-acidic phospholipid proved to be the substance earlier referred to by others as pulmonary surfactant. DPC has since been designated choline diphospho-glyceride and is commonly called lecithin.

Lecithin and sphingomyelin both appear in amniotic fluid at 18–20 weeks gestation. The rate of synthesis of both increases as pregnancy progresses but there is an abrupt acceleration of lecithin synthesis at approximately 35 weeks in normal pregnancy. This leads to an increase in the ratio of lecithin to sphingomyelin and is due to augmentation of one to two pathways of lecithin synthesis, choline incorporation. As suggested by Klaus in 1962, Type II pulmonary alveolar cells appear to be the site of synthesis as well as release of this surface-active material[34]. Achievement of alveolar stability occurs rapidly as the choline incorporation pathway accelerates, and is expressed clinically by an L/S ratio of 2:1 or greater. Such a ratio generally suggests that, should Respiratory Distress Syndrome occur, it will be mild and that Hyaline Membrane Disease is unlikely. Babies with Respiratory Distress Syndrome and L/S ratios of 2:1 or greater have been reported although they usually have been born to diabetic mothers or had evidence of asphyxia at birth[35].

Increasing clinical experience with L/S ratios has shown a poor correlation with precise gestational age and, hence, they are not useful in establishing an estimated date of confinement. Gluck has noted that various abnormalities of pregnancy may accelerate lecithin synthesis prior to 35 weeks, leading to a lower than expected incidence of Respiratory Distress Syndrome in infants delivered prematurely of these abnormal pregnancies[36]. He has identified maternal as well as 'primary placental' disease states in this group. Most of these conditions are associated with abnormalities in the maternal supply line. Included are the hypertensive syndromes of pregnancy, and severe gestational diabetes as well as maternal infection, narcotic addiction[37] and sickle haemo-globinopathies. Freeman and his associates, in a larger series of patients, have failed to verify accelerated maturation of the L/S ratio in pregnancies of diabetic or toxaemic patients[35].

'Primary placental' abnormalities such as the so-called 'chronic abruption', circumvallate placenta and placental infarction have been associated with early maturation of L/S ratios in Gluck's experience[36], but the number of cases in each category is small and difficulty is encountered in separating the placental pathology from underlying defects in the maternal supply line which might lead to accelerated lecithin synthesis.

The mechanism whereby pathophysiologically stressful conditions in pregnancy might accelerate lecithin synthesis is unknown but recent evidence suggests that corticosteroids are involved. The steroids might be fetal in origin as suggested indirectly by smaller than normal adrenal glands in neonates dying of Hyaline Membrane Disease[38]. The source might also be maternal, although elevated corticosteroid activity has not been selectively associated with the disease states mentioned and most maternal corticosteroid compounds do not cross the placenta since they are bound in large part to transcortin.

It has been demonstrated that corticosteroids administered to the mother prenatally can prevent Respiratory Distress Syndrome in a controlled double blind study[39]. Increase in lecithin synthesis following exogenous steroids has not yet been shown directly in humans.

Perhaps the placental abnormalities associated with the maternal disease states mentioned give rise to selective permeability to corticosteroids or their precursors without detectable elevation occurring in the maternal circulation.

Gluck has reported delayed maturation of L/S ratios in two fetal conditions, hydrops fetalis and the smaller of monochorionic non-parabiotic twins[36]. However, again, the number of patients is small and the findings have not been substantiated by others. In a larger series of patients, Gluck reports delayed maturation of the L/S ratio in cases of mild maternal diabetes[36]. Although Polishuk et al. reported that their diabetic patients tended to exhibit decreasing L/S ratios in late pregnancy, the ratios remained above 2:1, and R.D.S. did not occur[40]. Freeman and associates, on the other hand, found no alteration in lecithin synthesis in their diabetic patients[35].

An association between premature rupture of fetal membranes of greater than 24 hours duration and a lower incidence of respiratory distress syndrome compared with infants with a duration less than 12 hours was noted by Yoon and Harper[41]. At about the same time, Gluck demonstrated an acceleration in lecithin synthesis in these patients associated with a decrease in incidence of R.D.S.[36] He, therefore, cautions against aggressive management of the uninfected pre-term infant *in utero* with premature rupture of membranes. Some might add a short course of corticosteroids in accordance with the preliminary evidence of Liggins[39]. Management of these patients must be carefully individualised, however, weighing the risks of neonatal sepsis and the morbidity and mortality of puerperal infection[42] against the threat of the Respiratory Distress Syndrome.

Though detailed discussions of technique are beyond the scope of this chapter, a simplified method of pulmonary phospholipid measurement, the 'Shake Test', has been reported by Clements *et al.*[43] It can be done with a minimum of equipment and technical experience. Subsequent clinical evaluations[44-46] of the 'Shake Test' have generally confirmed its usefulness though there appears to be a small but significant rate of falsely mature results in most studies[44, 45].

Though the L/S ratio has shown no consistent relationship to fetal weight, it has been noted that small-for-gestational-age fetuses undergo normal pulmonary maturation and develop Respiratory Distress Syndrome much less frequently than weight-matched pre-term infants. Thus, determination of the L/S ratio offers some aid to the obstetrician in deciding whether a given small fetus is premature or victimised by a growth retarding Deprivation Syndrome. In addition, the study enables him to avoid the hazards of premature delivery of patients in whom pre-term delivery is indicated because of maternal or fetal disease.

The L/S ratio is a valuable tool in total fetal assessment because it provides more than a passive parameter of the fetus' length of residence *in utero*. It forecasts his ability to survive in the extrauterine environment and can be used to determine his moment of entry into that environment.

The remaining measures of fetal maturity also reflect progressive maturation of organ systems, but because immaturity of these systems is rarely threatening to the neonate, they are viewed with less interest by obstetricians.

Amniotic fluid creatinine, fetal cell counts and bilirubin concentration are the markers most widely used. Of these, creatinine determination is the most reliable. Pitkin and Zwirek, the first in the English literature to consider creatinine concentration as a function of maturity, reported that 94% of 120 patients studied had amniotic fluid creatinine values of 2 milligrams per 100 ml or greater after 37 weeks gestation[47]. Subsequent investigators have suggested that a value of 1·8 milligrams per 100 ml, at 36 weeks[48] and 1·5 milligrams at 35 weeks[49] gestation can be used clinically. Droegemueller *et al.* found that amniotic fluid creatinine concentration did not correlate with fetal size, and, indeed, included in their series several small-for-gestational-age newborns with 'mature' creatinine concentrations[48]. They suggested that the creatinine concentration reflects glomerular maturation, not muscle mass.

At least one investigator contends[50], however, that birth weight and amniotic fluid creatinine correlate closely in late gestation. It is likely that both birth weight and fetal glomerular maturation play a role in creatinine concentration with the latter having the major influence.

In contrast to pulmonary maturation, renal functional maturity appears to occur at a fixed rate regardless of associated pregnancy-pathology, allowing approximation of gestational age and not just the functional capacity of a single organ system. An additional advantage is that the determination is technically easy.

Problems in interpretation arise in the occasional patient who has an abnormal fluid volume; polyhydramnios, for example, leads to lowered concentration of creatinine and underestimation of fetal age. The opposite situation is seen with oligohydramnios. Most series have included a small percentage of patients (usually less than ten) with 'mature' creatinine concentration prior to 36 weeks[47, 48, 51]. There is little speculation as to whether this is accelerated maturation, minor undetected degrees of oligohydramnios, or 'normal scatter'. The latter is probably the case, illustrating the danger inherent in relying on laboratory values, particularly a single one, in making clinical decisions.

Estimation of fetal maturity using the staining characteristics of amniotic fluid cells was first suggested by Brosens and Gordon[52, 53]. Using Nile Blue Sulfate, a vital stain for lipid, they noted two populations of cells, one which stained blue and the other orange. The latter, which contain lipid, are markedly increased in percentage by 38 weeks of gestation and were felt to originate from mature fetal sebaceous glands. Skin biopsies stained with Nile Blue Sulfate confirmed this impression[51, 54] although some still feel that the orange cells are precornified squames or degenerating epithelial cells[55]. The blue staining cells are clearly mature fetal squames.

Several groups have reported satisfactory results using stained fetal cells to estimate maturity[51, 56, 57]. In general, more than 10% orange-positive cells indicates 36 or more weeks of gestation and 20% or more indicates a 40 week gestation. The presence of orange cells in clumps and/or free lipid droplets also denote a term pregnancy[54].

At least two groups have reported less satisfactory correlations between percentages of orange staining cells and gestational age[48, 58]. Droegemueller et al. felt that staining of fetal cells was less reliable than amniotic fluid creatinine since they occasionally found 10% or more orange staining cells earlier than 36 weeks[48]. Of particular importance is the finding of Anderson and Griffiths[57] that the Fetal Deprivation Syndromes do not invalidate this test for estimation of gestational age. This finding has been confirmed in several small series[54, 55, 59].

Analysis of fetal fat-containing cells is a valuable tool, usually giving a satisfactory estimate of gestational age, and is the simplest and most rapid study to perform.

Analysis of bilirubin pigments in amniotic fluid was explored in the late 1950s and early 1960s by many investigators[60-62] who were attempting to unravel the pathophysiology of Rhesus isoimmunisation. Coincidentally, Liley[61] realised that the optical density peak of amniotic fluid attributable to bilirubin diminished as normal pregnancy progressed. Mandelbaum and co-workers subsequently demonstrated the disappearance of the bilirubin peak (ΔOD 450) in non-Rh affected fetuses often occurred at 36 weeks gestation[63]. This was interpreted as evidence of hepatic maturation and it was noted that 85% of such infants weighed more than six pounds. Accordingly, they suggested that the ΔOD 450 could be used to assess fetal maturity. Subsequent experience has shown that many pregnancies progress well beyond 36 weeks with a persistent 450 peak[48, 51] and, therefore, cannot be dated by this method. A positive result alone (disappearance of the ΔOD 450) is useful. Obviously, this approach is not helpful in estimating maturity in cases of Rh isoimmunisation. Experience has shown that elevated bilirubin concentrations are seen with maternal diabetes, while most investigators feel that the various hypertensive syndromes do not have an effect. Effects of the Fetal Deprivation Syndromes on hepatic maturation, as reflected by amniotic fluid bilirubin densities, have not been worked out.

A number of other factors in amniotic fluid have been identified, but at present, none seems useful in assessing fetal maturity. Among them are osmolality, urea, creatine, uric acid, and adrenal steroids. An association has been noted, however, between fetal adrenal hypoplasia and prolonged pregnancy[64] while fetal adrenal hyperplasia has been identified in cases of pre-term birth[65]. A causal relationship between the adrenal pathology and gestational length has been speculated upon[64, 65]. Perhaps more intensive serial studies will identify a correlation between steroid concentration and length of gestation and conceivably, lead to the ability to anticipate premature labour.

Fetal well-being

Assessment of fetal well-being has logically turned to amniotic fluid. A number of substances have been assayed but none has found widespread clinical application. Among them are estriol and its congeners, meconium, human placental lactogen (HPL or HCS (human chorionic sommatomammotropin)), pH and partial pressures of oxygen and carbon dioxide, osmolality and protein.

Interested readers might pursue information about amniotic fluid osmolality[51, 66], proteins[67-69] and pH and partial pressures from these sources[70-72].

The presence of meconium in amniotic fluid at the onset of labour has been associated with a marked increase in perinatal morbidity and mortality of vaginally delivered infants; hence, knowledge of its presence is valuable. Difficulties arise, however, in interpretation, particularly when prompt delivery is not desirable. For example, one cannot tell if the observed meconium remains from a transient severe insult or is present due to chronic, ongoing fetal stress. Its presence merely designates that patient as one requiring prompt, thorough evaluation of fetal well-being and careful followup should the pregnancy be allowed to continue.

Technical difficulties with transcervical amnioscopy and risks of repeated amniocentesis obviate routine, prospective use, even in high risk patients.

Pregnancy estrogens or estriol determination offers another means of fetal evaluation. With widespread use of maternal urinary estriol determinations that followed Greene's work in the early 1960s[73, 74], interest inevitably turned to assessment of amniotic fluid estriol. The familiar normal curves showing rising urinary estriol values in late pregnancy were duplicated for amniotic fluid determinations in amounts one millionth as large. Correlation between urinary and amniotic fluid estriol values was thus established[75, 76]. The greater technical difficulty of amniotic fluid estriol determinations and the eventual realisation that little additional information was gained has restricted the clinical application of the procedure. In addition, clinical experience with urinary estriol determination has repeatedly shown that serial values are required to make any interpretation; thus, multiple amniocenteses would be required. The area in which amniotic fluid estriols are probably useful is the management of severe Rh isoimmunisation[77, 78]. Fortunately, serial amniocentesis are required in management of this disease. Amniotic fluid estriol might also prove useful in management of patients with compromised renal function but little experience has been accumulated to substantiate this.

Maternal Fluids

Blood

The ease of collecting serial specimens of maternal blood has led to a plethora of tests attempting to evaluate fetal welfare as well as fetal age. All mirror some aspect of the placenta's enzymatic or endocrinological functions; some unfortunately reflect the adequacy of placental function only, or merely just the size of the placenta. Few give information about the fetus and none has been found to give more than a rough estimate of fetal age.

Evaluation of enzymatic and endocrinological placental functions as a reflection of fetal well-being presumes that these functions parallel the critical respiratory function. The error of this presumption is demonstrated by the all too frequent loss of a carefully monitored fetus. At present, however, there is no direct assessment of the respiratory function of the placenta utilising maternal blood.

As a result, although estriol, human placental lactogen (HPL) diamine oxidase, cystine aminopeptidase (CAP) and heat-stable alkaline phosphatase (HSAP) can be measured in plasma or serum, none has proved valuable enough to find its way into routine care of high risk patients at more than a few centres.

Plasma estriol determination holds the greatest potential, particularly if simplification in methodology becomes widely available[79]. Plasma estriol determination eliminates the necessity for 24-hour urine collections and guarantees adequacy and completeness of samples. In addition, the time-lag between availability of the test results and the point in time reflected by the test would diminish.

The effects of diurnal variation[80, 81] appear avoidable by measurement of unconjugated plasma estriol[82]. Confirmation of this is awaited. Remaining to be worked out are the values of plasma estriols in abnormal pregnancies as well as the effects of maternal hepatic disease on unconjugated estriol concentrations.

There are suggestions that diabetic nephropathy results in falsely high values[83, 84] while evaluation of plasma estriols in the hypertensive syndromes of pregnancy and other conditions associated with diminished renal function has not been carried out. Low plasma concentrations, despite poor renal function, however, certainly suggest fetal compromise. Calculation of estriol clearance might also prove useful in difficult cases[84]. Plasma estriols can be helpful in the management of patients with fetal deprivation syndromes and mild gestational diabetes where there is little or no compromise in renal function.

Following the determination of the structure and source of human placental lactogen (HPL), numerous investigators sought to correlate serum values with various clinical abnormalities of pregnancy[85-89]. The only consistent conclusion emerging from the resulting data is that serum levels of HPL correlate directly with placental size[86, 89, 91, 93]. Studies suggesting the HPL levels are inconsistently related to fetal welfare have been confirmed by the observation that HPL levels often remain normal after fetal death[92]. Because of the positive correlation of placental size to fetal size, HPL levels indirectly reflect fetal weight. The association is not close enough to supplant other estimations of fetal weight, however[88, 91, 93] HPL determination is of little use in estimating fetal maturity, even with frequent serial samples, because of the wide range of normal values.

Consistently low values have been seen in pathological pregnancies associated with small placentas, i.e. chronic hypertension and fetal growth retardation syndromes[85, 94-97]. Some investigators feel that low HPL values can be predictive of fetal death in hypertensive pregnancies[95-97]; as yet, no such claim has been made for pregnancies complicated by fetal growth retardation of unknown cause. It is in these areas where there is marginal placental growth and function that serum HPL determinations may eventually prove valuable in improving fetal salvage. As yet, clinical experience is insufficient to establish critical levels of HPL which would suggest that intervention is required.

Plasma diamine oxidase (DAO) levels were recommended in 1968 as a means of identifying and following high risk patients, especially those with diabetes[98]. Subsequent experience, however, has not verified the earlier report. In fact, satisfactory (rising) DAO levels have been reported simultaneously with fetal distress and subsequent demise[99, 100].

A more promising measure of placental function and, indirectly, of fetal well-being, is the measurement of the placental fraction of alkaline phosphatase. This enzyme, known as heat-stable alkaline phosphatase (HSAP), seems to be released from damaged placental tissue[101]. Hence, increasing levels correlate with diminishing amounts of functional placenta available to the fetus. Current experience suggests that it is most useful in pregnancies of hypertensive diabetics. Carrington et al. have verified Hunter's report that sudden elevations of already abnormal values can precede imminent fetal death by several weeks[100]. She feels that it is useful in selecting patients that require extremely close monitoring by urinary estriols. Others feel that diabetics at high risk for fetal loss have low HSAP[102, 103] and that a sudden drop of HSAP precedes fetal death by as little as twenty-four hours[102]. Though there are conflicting reports of HSAP patterns in abnormal pregnancy, its low cost and technical ease warrant more evaluation.

An assay for an oxytocinase, cystine aminopeptidase, has been developed and early reports suggest that it may be useful in pregnancies complicated by diabetes[104] as well as fetal growth retardation[105].

Determinations of estetrol (15α hydroxy-estriol) concentrations in plasma[106] as well as in urine[107] and amniotic fluid[108] have been suggested as a more direct reflection of fetal well-being than estriol[107]. The accumulated information to date has failed to confirm this suggestion and the clinical value of estetrol is uncertain[108, 109].

Attempts are currently being made to develop an assay for 16α hydroxy-dehydroepiandrosterone, an estriol precursor of fetal origin. If successful, this would theoretically represent a more direct assessment of fetal welfare than is currently available. Clinical experience would be necessary to determine its value.

Maternal urine

Analysis of maternal urine to assess placental function and/or fetal well-being has been utilised since the 1920s when Smith[110] and Aschheim and Zondek[111] discovered rising titres of estrogen activity through the course of pregnancy. Subsequently, measurement of urinary chorionic gonadotrophin (UCG) and pregnanediol have also been carried out. Persistent high levels of UCG have been noted in pregnancies delivering prematurely[112].Also a correlation has been noted between elevated chorionic gonadotrophin, in serum, and the development of hydrops in severe isoimmunisation[113]. Numerous other studies attempting to correlate chorionic gonadotrophin concentration with fetal outcome have met with little success.

Pregnanediol excretion was first measured in 1937[114]. Shortly thereafter two groups noted that falling pregnanediol excretion might be a reliable warning of fetal death[115, 116]. Subsequent experience has shown that pregnanediol excretion reflects only placental function, however, and numerous reports of stable and normal pregnanediol excretion accompanied by fetal death have eliminated its use as a measure of fetal well-being[117-119].

Nearly 35 years elapsed before the ability to measure urinary estrogens became clinically useful to obstetricians. Development of the laboratory procedure gradually evolved from a complicated painstaking bioassay to a simplified chemical assay that can be done quickly and reproducibly. Following a preliminary report in 1961[73], Greene and Touchstone published a series of 2015 determinations in 279 pregnancies, establishing the normal ranges for estriol values at various points in gestation as well as guidelines for management of various abnormalities[74]. Since that report, the technique has been modified in many laboratories so that total estrogens are measured by the Brown method[120]. In the years following publication of the initial series, estriol measurement has formed the cornerstone for objectifying the management of many types of high risk pregnancy. Its use is now routine in the care of patients with hypertensive syndromes, prolonged pregnancy[121], and diabetes[122, 123]. Out of the enormous experience accumulated in many centres, several conclusions have been reached. First, estriol (or total estrogen) excretion is subject to marked daily variation, even in the same patient. Second, a series of determinations at frequent intervals is much more valuable than a single isolated result. Third, one or even a small series of determinations does not enable the clinician to estimate fetal maturity accurately. In addition, exogenous factors such as corticosteroids[124, 125], ampicillin[126], urinary tract antiseptics[74], infections[127] and the patient's posture[128] can diminish estriol values. Urinary estriol values bear little correlation to fetal welfare in cases of Rh sensitisation. Most importantly, the clinician cannot depend on results unless he is thoroughly familiar with the reliability of his own laboratory in terms of reproducibility, percentage of estriol or total estrogens retrieved by the assay and the normal ranges of that laboratory.

Many investigators have reported depressed estriol excretion in fetal deprivation syndromes[129-132]. Accumulated results suggest that 70%[133] to 90% of these deprived fetuses[134, 135] will have persistently low estriol values. An additional 10% of infants with low-normal birth weight will have estriol values that fall in the normal range but consistently below average[136, 137]. The range of birth weights and estriol values undoubtedly reflects both varying degrees of severity and diverse aetiologies.

The diagnostic use of serial estriol determinations in suspected fetal deprivation syndromes is supplanted to some extent by increasingly available B mode ultrasound scans for determining fetal growth rates (see Chapter 17). Serial estriols retain their value, however, as the most important tool for monitoring fetal well-being and determining when increased fetal jeopardy mandates delivery.

Indirect evaluation of the functional capacity of the maternal supply line has been attempted through a variety of 'stress tests' in recent years[138, 139]. The most recent of these, the Oxytocin Challenge Test (O.C.T.), appears to be the most rewarding[140, 141]. By electronically recording fetal heart rate responses to induced uterine contractions, Ray and his associates feel they can assess the degree of 'fetoplacental respiratory reserve'[140]. In their hands, a negative test has not been followed by intrauterine death or fetal distress within seven days. They feel the O.C.T. is particularly valuable in following patients with chronically low estriols. They noted, however, that positive O.C.T.'s appear before estriol excretion decreases. The overall experience of Ray et al. has been duplicated by others[141-144] confirming that the O.C.T. is a valuable clinical tool in monitoring high risk patients. Difficulty in standardising the intensity of contractions by external means remains a problem, however.

The ability to measure urinary estriol followed by definition of its value and limitations opened a new era in clinical obstetrics and perinatology. Not only can we estimate the age of a fetus and measure his rate of growth, but we can also determine when he is in jeopardy, when he should be delivered and what his chances of survival are.

Though the aetiology for fetal deprivation syndromes can be discovered in the neonatal period in a number of cases and obstetricians are increasingly able to appreciate fetal growth retardation, the majority of cases remain unexplained. The placental histopathology associated with this syndrome is well covered elsewhere in this book. Remaining undiscovered are the precise pathophysiological alterations in the maternal supply line, their causes and potential modes of therapy. At present, we do not know what determines which fetuses will be affected, which will escape despite similar circumstances, what requirement for proper growth of the feto-placental unit is lacking, or, indeed, what deleterious influence might be operative.

In recent years, we have increased our diagnostic sophistication impressively without improving our therapeutic ability. With the increasing realisation of the amount of human potential lost both by the individual and by society, increasingly broad research efforts will inevitably be undertaken, eventually uncovering answers to these questions.

References

1. Jeffcotte, T. N. A. and Scott, J. S. (1959). Polyhydramnios and Oligohydramnios. *Can. M.A.J.*, **80,** 77

2. Liley, A. W. (1963). Amniotic Fluid. In: *Modern Trends in Human Reproduction Physiology.* (Carey, A. M., editor) (London: Butterworth)

3. Thomas, C. R., Lang, E. K. and Lloyd, F. P. (1963). Fetal Pyelography—A method for detecting fetal life. *Obstet. Gynecol.*, **22,** 335

4. Poulsen, H. (1955). Uric acid in blood and urine of infants. *Acta Physiol. Scand.*, **33,** 372

5. Pitkin, R. M., Reynolds, W. A. and Burchell, R. C. (1968). Fetal contribution to amniotic fluid. A preliminary report. *Amer. J. Obstet. Gynecol.*, **100,** 834

6. Liley, A. W. (1965). Physiological observations in foetal transfusion. In: *Studies in Physiology.* (Berlin: Springer-Verlag)

7. Danforth, D. N. and Hull, R. W. (1958). The microscopic anatomy of the fetal membranes with particular reference to the detailed structure of the amnion. *Amer. J. Obstet. Gynecol.*, **75,** 536

8. Hutchinson, D. L., Gray, M. J., Plentl, A. A., Alvarez, H., Caldeyro-Barcia, R., Kaplan, B. and Lind, J. (1959). The role of the fetus in the water exchange of the amniotic fluid of normal and hydramniotic patients. *J. Clin. Invest.*, **38,** 971

9. Plentl, A. A. (1961). Transfer of water across the perfused umbilical cord. *Proc. Soc. Exper. Biol. Med.*, **107,** 622

10. Gluck, L., Kulovich, M. V., Borer, R. C., Jr., Brenner, P. H., Anderson, G. G. and Spellacy, W. N. (1971). Diagnosis of respiratory distress syndrome by amniocentesis. *Amer. J. Obstet. Gynecol.*, **109,** 440

11. Benirschke, K. and McKay, D. G. (1953). The antidiuretic hormone in fetus and infant. *Obstet. Gynecol.*, **1,** 638

12. Wagner, M. L., Rudolph, A. J. and Singleton, E. B. (1968). Neonatal defects associated with abnormalities of the amnion and amniotic fluid. *Radiol. Clin. N.A.*, **6,** 279

13. Taussig, F. J. (1927). The amniotic fluid and its quantitative variability. *Amer. J. Obstet. Gynecol.*, **14,** 505

14. Ostergard, D. R. (1970). The physiology and clinical importance of amniotic fluid. A review. *Obstet. Gynecol. Surv.*, **25,** 297

15. Pritchard, J. A. (1966). Fetal swallowing and amniotic fluid volume. *Obstet. Gynecol.*, **28,** 606

16. Davis, M. E. and Potter, E. L. (1946). Intrauterine respiration of the human fetus. *J. Amer. Med. Ass.*, **131**, 1194

17. Sauvigmac, E. M. (1953). Roentgen amniography. A valuable and safe aide to obstetrical diagnosis. *Radiology*, **60**, 545

18. Cox, L. W. and Chalmers, T. A. (1953). The transfer of sodium to the amniotic fluid in normal and abnormal cases, determined by Na^{24} tracer methods. *J. Obstet. Gynaecol. Brit. Commonw.*, **60**, 222

19. Plentl, A. A. and Hutchinson, D. L. (1953). Determination of deuterium exchange rates between maternal circulation and amniotic fluid. *Proc. Soc. Exper. Biol. Med.*, **82**, 681

20. Hutchinson, D. L., Hunter, C. B., Neslen, E. D. and Plentl, A. A. (1955). The exchange of water and electrolytes in the mechanism of amniotic fluid formation and the relationship to hydramnios. *Surg. Gynecol. Obstet.*, **100**, 391

21. Fuchs, F. (1966). Volume of amniotic fluid at various stages of pregnancy. *Clin. Obstet. Gynecol.*, **9**, 449

22. Charles, D., Jacoby, H. E. and Burgess, F. (1965). Amniotic fluid volumes in the second half of pregnancy. *Amer. J. Obstet. Gynecol.*, **93**, 1042

23. Charles, D. and Jacoby, H. E. (1966). Preliminary data on the use of sodium amniohippurate to determine amniotic fluid volumes. *Amer. J. Obstet. Gynecol.*, **95**, 266

24. Elliot, P. M. and Inman, W. H. W. (1961). Volume of liquor amnii in normal and abnormal pregnancy. *Lancet*, **ii**, 835

25. Berner, H. W., Seisler, E. P. and Barlow, J. (1972). Fetal cardiac tamponade. A complication of amniocentesis. *Obstet. Gynecol.*, **40**, 599

26. Crystle, C. D. and Rigsby, W. C. (1970). Amniocentesis: Experience and complications. *Amer. J. Obstet. Gynecol.*, **106**, 310

27. Ryan, G. T., Ivy, R. and Pearson, J. W. (1972). Fetal bleeding as a major hazard of amniocentesis. *Obstet. Gynecol.*, **40**, 702

28. Goodlin, R. C. and Clewell, A. H. (1974). Sudden fetal death following diagnostic amniocentesis. *Amer. J. Obstet. Gynecol.*, **118**, 285

29. Wang, M. Y. W., McCutcheon, E. and Desforges, J. F. (1967). Fetomaternal hemorrhage from diagnostic transabdominal amniocentesis. *Amer. J. Obstet. Gynecol.*, **97**, 1123

30. Liley, A. W. (1960). Technique and complications of amniocentesis. *N.Z. Med. J.*, **59**, 581

31. Mayer, M., Gueritat, P., Ducas, P. *et al.* (1961). Examination of amniotic fluid: Essential element of antenatal prognosis of fetal erythroblastosis. *Presse. Med.*, **69**, 2493

32. Gluck, L. (1974). Symposium on preventability of perinatal injury. New York, March 21

33. Freda, V. J. (1967). The control of Rh disease. *Hospital Practice*, **2**, 54

34. Klaus, M., Reiss, O. K., Tolley, W. H., Piel, C. and Clements, J. A. (1962). Alveolar epithelial cell mitochondria as a cause of the surface active lung lining. *Science*, **137**, 750

35. Donald, I. R., Freeman, R. K., Goebelsman, U., Chan, W. H. and Nakamura, R. M. (1973). Clinical experience with the amniotic fluid lecithin/sphingomyelin ratio. I. Antenatal prediction of pulmonary maturity. *Amer. J. Obstet. Gynecol.*, **155**, 547

36. Gluck, L. and Kulovich, M., V. (1973). Lecithin/sphingomyelin ratios in amniotic fluid in normal and abnormal pregnancy. *Amer. J. Obstet. Gynecol.*, **115**, 539

37. Glass, L., Rajegowda, B. K. and Evans, H. E. (1971). Absence of respiratory distress syndrome in premature infants of heroin addicted mothers. *Lancet*, **ii**, 685

38. Naeye, R. L., Harcke, H. T. and Blanc, W. A. (1971). Adrenal gland structure and the development of hyaline membrane disease. *Pediatrics*, **47**, 650

39. Liggins, G. C. and Howie, R. N. (1972). A controlled trial of antepartum gluco-corticoid treatment for prevention of the respiratory distress syndrome in premature infants. *Pediatrics*, **50**, 515

40. Polishuk, W. Z., Anteby, S., Stein, Y. and Baro-On, H. (1974). Lecithin/sphingomyelin ratio in amniotic fluid of diabetic and latent diabetic pregnancies. *Int. J. Gynaecol. Obstet.*, **12**, 49

41. Yoon, J. J. and Harper, R. G. (1973). Observations on the relationship between duration of rupture of the membranes and the development of idiopathic respiratory distress syndrome. *Pediatrics*, **52**, 161

42. Gibbs, R. S. (1974). Puerperal infection in the antibiotic era. (In press)

43. Clements, J. A., Platzker, A. C. G., Tierney, D. F. *et al.* (1972). Assessment of the risk of the respiratory-distress syndrome by a rapid test for surfactant in amniotic fluid. *New Engl. J. Med.*, **286**, 1077

44. Shephard, B., Buhi, W. and Spellacy, W. (1974). Critical analysis of the amniotic fluid shake test. *Obstet. Gynecol.*, **43**, 558

45. Goldstein, A. S.. Fukunaga, K., Malachowski, N. and Johnson, J. D. (1974). A comparison of the lecithin/sphingomyelin ratio and shake test for estimating fetal pulmonary maturity. *Amer. J. Obstet. Gynecol.*, **118**, 1132

46. Merola, J. G. L., Johnson, L. M., Bolognese, R. J. and Corson, S. L. (1974). Determination of fetal pulmonary maturity by amniotic fluid lecithin/sphingomyelin ratio and rapid shake test. *Amer. J. Obstet. Gynecol.*, **119**, 243

47. Pitkin, R. M. and Zwirek, S. J. (1967). Amniotic fluid creatinine. *Amer. J. Obstet. Gynecol.*, **98**, 1135

48. Droegemueller, W., Jackson, C., Makowski, E. L. and Bataglia, F. C. (1969). Amniotic fluid examination as an aid in the assessment of gestational age. *Amer. J. Obstet. Gynecol.*, **104**, 424

49. White, C. A., Doorenbos, D. E. and Bradbury, J. T. (1969). Role of chemical and cytological analysis of amniotic fluid in determination of fetal maturity. *Amer. J. Obstet. Gynecol.*, **104**, 664

50. Roopnarinesingh, S. (1970). Amniotic fluid creatinine in normal and abnormal pregnancies. *J. Obstet. Gynecol. Brit. Commonw.*, **77**, 785

51. Andrews, B. F. (1970). Amniotic fluid studies to determine maturity. *Ped. Clin. N. Amer.*, **17**, 49

52. Brosens, I. A. (1966). Cytological study of amniotic fluid with Nile blue sulfate staining. *Acta Cytol.*, **10**, 159

53. Brosens, I. A. and Gordon, H. (1966). The estimation of maturity by cytological examination of the liquor amnii. *J. Obstet. Gynaecol. Brit. Commonw.*, **73**, 88

54. Gordon, H. and Brosens, I. (1967). Cytology of amniotic fluid: A new test for fetal maturity. *Obstet. Gynecol.*, **30**, 652

55. Huisjes, H. J. and Arendzen, J. H. (1970). Estimation of fetal maturity by cytological evaluation of liquor amnii. *Obstet. Gynecol.*, **35**, 725

56. Bishop, E. H. and Corson, S. (1968). Estimation of fetal maturity by cytological examination of amniotic fluid. *Amer. J. Obstet. Gynecol.*, **102**, 654

57. Anderson, A. B. M. and Griffith, A. D. (1968). Estimation of duration of gestation by amniotic fluid cytology. *J. Obstet. Gynaecol. Brit. Commonw.*, **75**, 300

58. Huisjes, H. J. (1968). Cytologic features of liquor amnii. *Acta Cytol.*, **12**, 42

59. Sharp, F. (1968). Estimation of fetal maturity by amniotic fluid extoliative cytology. *J. Obstet. Gynaecol. Brit. Commonw.*, **75**, 812

60. Bevis, D. C. A. (1953). The composition of liquor amnii in hemolytic disease of the newborn. *J. Obstet. Gynaecol. Brit. Emp.*, **60**, 244

61. Liley, A. W. (1961). Liquor amnii analysis in the management of the pregnancy complicated by Rhesus sensitization. *Amer. J. Obstet. Gynecol.*, **82**, 1359

62. Freda, V. J. (1965). The Rh problem in obstetrics and a new concept of its management using amniocentesis and spectrophotometric scanning of amniotic fluid. *Amer. J. Obstet. Gynecol.*, **92**, 341

63. Mandelbaum, B., La Croix, G. C. and Robinson, A. R. (1967). Determination of fetal maturity by spectrophotometric analysis of amniotic fluid. *Obstet. Gynecol.*, **29**, 471

64. Roberts, G. and Cawdery, J. E. (1970). Congenital adrenal hypoplasia. *J. Obstet. Gynaecol. Brit. Commonw.*, **77**, 654

65. Anderson, A. B., Lawrence, K. M., Davies, K. *et al.* (1971). Fetal adrenal weight and the cause of premature delivery in human pregnancy. *J. Obstet. Gynaecol. Brit. Commonw.*, **78**, 481

66. Goodlin, R. C. and Kresch, A. J. (1968). Amniotic fluid osmolality following intra-amniotic injection of saline. *Amer. J. Obstet. Gynecol.*, **100**, 839

67. Cherry, S. H., Kochwa, S. and Rosenfield, R. E. (1965). Bilirubin–protein ratio in amniotic fluid as an index in the severity of erythroblastosis fetalis. *Obstet. Gynecol.*, **26**, 826

68. Andrews, B. F., Wolfe, W. M., Jr., Hoffman, J. H. and Thomas, P. P. (1968). Significance of protein and bilirubin–protein ratio in amniotic fluid from Rh-isoimmunized mothers. *J. Kentucky Med. Assoc.*, **66**, 363

69. Andrews, B. F. (1968). Significance of pigment, protein, immune globulin G and osmolality in amniotic from Rh isoimmunized mothers. *Proc. XII Int. Cong. Pediat. Mexico City*, **3**, 98

70. Quilligan, E. J. (1962). Amniotic fluid gas tensions. *Amer. J. Obstet. Gynecol.*, **84**, 20

71. Rooth, G. and Sjoval, A. (1966). Acid–base status of amniotic fluid during delivery. *Lancet*, **ii**, 371

72. Vasicka, A. and Hutchinson, H. T. (1964). Oxygen tension in amniotic fluid and fetal distress. Preliminary report of clinical findings. *Amer. J. Obstet. Gynecol.*, **88**, 530

73. Greene, J. W., Jr., Touchstone, J. C. and Fields, H. F. (1961). Urinary estriol as an index of placental function. A Preliminary report. *Obstet. Gynecol.*, **17**, 349

74. Greene, J. W., Jr. and Touchstone, J. C. (1963). Urinary estriol as index of placental function. A study of 279 cases. *Amer. J. Obstet. Gynecol.*, **85**, 1

75. Bolognese, R. J., Corson, S. L., Touchstone, J. C. and Lakoff, K. M. (1971). Correlation of amniotic fluid estriol with fetal age and well-being. *Obstet. Gynecol.*, **37**, 437

76. Klopper, A. (1972). Estriol in liquor amnii. *Amer. J. Obstet. Gynecol.*, **112**, 459

77. Schindler, A. E. and Herrman, W. L. (1966). Estriol in pregnancy urine and amniotic fluid. *Amer. J. Obstet. Gynecol.*, **95**, 301

78. Schindler, A. E., Ratanasopa, V., Lee, T. Y. and Herrman, W. L. (1967). Estriol and Rh-isoimmunization: A new approach to the management of severely affected pregnancies. *Obstet. Gynecol.*, **29**, 625

79. Kempers, R. D. in discussion of Sciarra, J. J., Tagatz, G. E., Notation, A. D. and Depp, R. (1974). Estriol and estetrol in amniotic fluid. *Amer. J. Obstet. Gynecol.*, **118**, 626

80. Selinger, M. and Levitz, M. (1969). Preliminary communication. Diurnal variation of total plasma estriol levels in late pregnancy. *J. Clin. Endo. Metab.*, **29,** 995

81. Macourt, D., Corker, C. S. and Naftolin, F. (1971). Plasma estriol in pregnancy. *J. Obstet. Gynaecol. Brit. Commonw.*, **78,** 335

82. Tulchinsky, D., Hobel, C. and Horenman, S. G. (1971). A radioligand assay for plasma unconjugated estriol in normal and abnormal pregnancies. *Amer. J. Obstet. Gynecol.*, **III,** 311

83. Levitz, M. and Selinger, M. (1970). Plasma estriols in Class D diabetes of pregnancy. *Amer. J. Obstet. Gynecol.*, **108,** 82

84. Carrington, E. R., Oesterling, M. J. and Adams, F. M. (1970). Renal clearance of estriol in complicated pregnancies. *Amer. J. Obstet. Gynecol.*, **106,** 1131

85. Josimovich, J. B., Kosor, B., Bocella, L. *et al.* (1970). Placental lactogen in maternal serum as an index of fetal health. *Obstet. Gynecol.*, **36,** 244

86. Singer, W., Desjardins, P. and Friesen, H. G. (1970). Human placental lactogen— An index of placental function. *Obstet. Gynecol.*, **36,** 222

87. Selenkow, H. A., Varma, K., Younger, D. *et al.* (1971). Patterns of serum immuno-reactive human placental lactogen (IR–HPL) and chorionic gonadotropin (R–HCG) in diabetic pregnancy. *Diabetes,* **20,** 696

88. Letchworth, A. T., Boardman, R. J., Bristowe, C. *et al.* (1971). A rapid semi-automated method for the measurement of human chorionic somatomammo-trophin. The normal range in the third trimester and its relation to fetal weight. *J. Obstet. Gynaecol. Brit. Commonw.*, **78,** 542

89. Cramer, D. W., Beck, P. and Makowski, E. L. (1971). Correlation of gestational age with maternal human chorionic somatomammotropin and maternal and fetal growth hormone plasma concentrations during labor. *Amer. J. Obstet. Gynecol.*, **109,** 649

90. Josimovich, J. B. (1969). Severity of erythroblastosis fetalis determined by hormone measurement. *J. Amer. Med. Ass.*, **208,** 2005

91. Saxena, B. N., Emerson, K., Jr. and Selenkow, H. A. (1969). Serum placental lactogen (HPL) levels as an index of placental function. *New Engl. J. Med.*, **281,** 225

92. Spellacy, W. N. (1973). Human placental lactogen in high risk pregnancy. *Clin. Obstet. Gynecol.*, **16,** 298

93. Spellacy, W. N., Buhi, W. C., Schram, J. D. *et al.* (1971). Control of human chorionic somatomammotropin levels during pregnancy. *Obstet. Gynecol.*, **37,** 567

94. Samman, N. A., Bradbury, J. T. and Goplerud, C. P. (1969). Serial hormonal studies in normal and abnormal pregnancy. *Amer. J. Obstet. Gynecol.*, **104,** 781

95. Spellacy, W. N., Teoh, E. S. and Buhi, W. C. (1970). Human chorionic somato-mammotropin (HCS) levels prior to fetal death in high risk pregnancies. *Obstet. Gynecol.*, **35,** 685

96. Spellacy, W. N., Teoh, E. S., Buhi, W. C. *et al.* (1971). Value of human chorionic somatomammotropin in managing high-risk pregnancies. *Amer. J. Obstet. Gynecol.*, **109,** 588

97. Samman, N. A., Gallagher, H. S., McRoberts, W. A. and Faris, A. M., Jr. (1971). Serial estimation of human placental lactogen, estriol and pregnanediol in preg-nancy correlated with whole organ section of placenta. *Amer. J. Obstet. Gynecol.*, **109,** 63

98. Southren, A. L., Weingold, A. B., Kobayashi, Y. *et al.* (1968). Plasma diamine oxidase in pregnancy complicated by diabetes mellitus. *Amer. J. Obstet. Gynecol.*, **101,** 899

99. Carrington, E. R., Frishmuth, G. J., Oesterling, M. J. *et al.* (1972). Gestational and postpartum plasma diamine oxidase values. *Obstet. Gynecol.*, **39,** 426

100. Carrington, E. R. (1973). Diabetes in pregnancy. *Clin. Obstet. Gynecol.*, **16,** 78

101. Hunter, R. J. (1969). Serum heat stable alkaline phosphatase: An index of placental function. *J. Obstet. Gynecol. Brit. Commonw.*, **76,** 1057

102. Curzen, P., Morris, I. (1968). Heat stable alkaline phosphatase in maternal serum. *J. Obstet. Gynecol. Brit. Commonw.*, **75,** 151

103. McEvoy, D., DeCherney, A., Martin, M. J., Morgan, V. *et al.* (1972). Heat stable alkaline phosphatase in pregnancy. *Int. J. Gynecol. Obstet.*, **10,** 229

104. Fort, A. T., Ragland, J. B., Morgan, B. S., Koiken, L. and Roberts, A. S. (1973). Maternal serum oxytocinase, diamine oxidase, heat stable alkaline phosphatase and urinary estriol applied simultaneously and serially for fetal assessment in pregnancy complicated by diabetes mellitus. *Int. J. Gynecol. Obstet.*, **11,** 96 ·

105. Petrucco, O. M., Chellier, K., Fishtall, A. (1973). Diagnosis of intrauterine growth retardation by serial serum oxytocinase, urinary estrogen and heat stable alkaline phosphatase in uncomplicated and hypertensive pregnancies. *J. Obstet. Gynaecol. Brit. Commonw.*, **80,** 499

106. Fishman, J. and Guzik, H. (1972). Radioimmunoassay of 15α hydroxyestriol in pregnancy plasma. *J. Clin. Endocrinol.*, **35,** 892

107. Heikkila, J. and Luukkainen, T. (1971). Urinary excretion of estriol and 15α hydroxyestriol on complicated pregnancies. *Amer. J. Obstet. Gynecol.*, **110,** 509

108. Sciarra, J. J., Tagatz, G. E., Notation, A. D. and Depp, R. (1974). Estriol and estetrol in amniotic fluid. *Amer. J. Obstet. Gynecol.*, **118,** 676

109. Greene, J. W., Jr. in discussion of Sciarra, J. J., Tagatz, G. E., Notation, A. D. and Depp, R. (1974). Estriol and estetrol in amniotic fluid. *Amer. J. Obstet. Gynecol.*, **118,** 676

110. Smith, M. G. (1927). A study of ovarian follicular hormone in the blood of the pregnant woman. *Bull. Johns Hopkins Hosp.*, **41,** 62

111. Aschheim, S. and Zondek, B. (1928). Die schwanger schafts diagnose aus den harn durch nachweis des hypophysenvoroderlappen hormons. *Klin. Wchnschr.*, **2,** 1453

112. Hughes, E. C. (1959). The relationship of the chorion to the fetal liver in normal and abnormal pregnancy. *Amer. J. Obstet. Gynecol.*, **77,** 880

113. Bradbury, J. T. and Goplerud, C. P. (1963). Serum chorionic gonadotrophin studies in sensitized Rh negative patients. *Obstet. Gynecol.*, **21,** 330

114. Venning, E. H. and Browne, J. S. L. (1937). Urinary excretion of sodium pregnanediol glucoronidate in the menstrual cycle. *Amer. J. Physiol.*, **119,** 417

115. Browne, J. S. L., Henry, J. S. and Venning, E. H. (1939). The significance of endocrine assays in threatened and habitual abortion. *Amer. J. Obstet. Gynecol.*, **38,** 297

116. Cope, C. L. (1940). The diagnostic value of pregnanediol excretion in pregnancy disorders. *Brit. Med. J.*, **2,** 545

117. Coyle, M. G., Greig, M. and Walker, J. (1962). Blood progesterone and urinary pregnanediol and oestrogens in foetal death from severe pre-eclampsia. *Lancet*, **ii,** 275

118. Appleby, J. L. and Norymberski, J. K. (1957). The urinary excretion of 17-hydroxycorticosteroids in human pregnancy. *J. Endocrinol.*, **15,** 310

119. Cassmer, O. (1959). Hormone production of the isolated human placenta. Studies on the role of the foetus in the endocrine functions of the placenta. *Acta Endocrinol. Suppl.* 45

120. Brown, J. B. (1955). A clinical method for the determination of oestriol, oestrone and oestradiol in human urine. *Biochem. J.*, **60**, 185

121. Smith, K., Greene, J. W., Jr. and Touchstone, J. C. (1966). Urinary estriol determination in the management of prolonged pregnancy. *Amer. J. Obstet. Gynecol.*, **96**, 901

122. Greene, J. W., Jr., Smith, K., Kyle, G. C., Touchstone, J. C. and Duhring, J. L. (1965). The use of urinary estriol excretion in the management of pregnancies complicated by diabetes mellitus. *Amer. J. Obstet. Gynecol.*, **91**, 684

123. Schwarz, R. H. and Fields, G. A. (1971). The management of the pregnant diabetic. *Obstet. Gynecol. Survey*, **26**, 277

124. Scommegna, A., Nedoss, B. R. and Chattoraj, S. C. (1968). Maternal urinary estriol excretion after dehydroepiandrosterone-sulfate infusion and adrenal stimulation and suppression. *Obstet. Gynecol.*, **31**, 526

125. Wray, P. M. and Russell, C. S. (1964). Maternal urinary oestriol levels before and after death of the foetus. *J. Obstet. Gynaecol. Brit. Commonw.*, **71**, 97

126. Willman, K. and Pulkkinen, M. O. (1971). Reduced maternal plasma and urinary estriol during ampicillin treatment. *Amer. J. Obstet. Gynecol.*, **109**, 893

127. Taylor, E. S., Hassner, A., Bruns, P. D. and Drose, V. E. (1963). Urinary estriol excretion of pregnant patients with pyelonephritis and Rh isoimmunization. *Amer. J. Obstet. Gynecol.*, **85**, 10

128. Dickey, R. P., Carter, W. T., Besch, P. K. and Ullery, J. C. (1966). Effect of posture on estrogen excretion during pregnancy. *Amer. J. Obstet. Gynecol.*, **96**, 127

129. Zondek, B. and Pfeifer, V. (1959). Further studies on urinary oestriol during pregnancy and its significance for the estimation of placental function and dysfunction in advanced pregnancy. *Acta Obstet. Gynecol. Scandinav.*, **38**, 742

130. Banerjea, S. K. (1962). Index of placental function by endocrine assay and its clinical application in obstetrical practice. *J. Obstet. Gynaecol. Brit. Commonw.*, **69**, 963

131. Bell, E. T., Loraine, J. A., McEwan, H. P. and Charles, D. (1967). Serial hormone assays in patients with uteroplacental insufficiency. *Amer. J. Obstet. Gynceol.*, **97**, 562

132. Galbraith, R. S., Low, J. A. and Boston, R. W. (1970). Maternal urinary estriol excretion patterns in patients with chronic fetal insufficiency. *Amer. J. Obstet. Gynecol*, **106**, 352

133. Michie, E. (1967). Urinary oestriol excretion in pregnancies complicated by suspected intra-uterine growth, toxemia, or essential hypertension. *J. Obstet. Gynaecol. Brit. Commonw.*, **74**, 896

134. Klopper, A. (1965). A critical review of urinary oestriol excretion in the assessment of placental function. Abhamdlungen der deutchen akademia der Wissenshaften Zu Berlin akademie, Verlag, Berlin, p. 247

135. Yousem, H., Seitchik, J. and Solomon, D. (1966). Maternal estriol excretion and fetal dysmaturity. *Obstet. Gynecol.*, **78**, 491

136. Klopper, A. (1965). Assays of urinary oestriol as a measure of placental function in *Research on Steroids*, Vol. 2, p. 63 (C. Cassano, editor) (Rome: Il Pensiero Scientifico)

137. Coyle, M. G. and Brown, J. B. (1963). Urinary excretion of oestriol during pregnancy. *J. Obstet. Gynaecol. Brit. Commonw.*, **70**, 225

138. Hon, H. E. and Wohlgemuth, R. (1961). The electronic evaluation of the fetal heart rate: Effect of maternal exercise. *Amer. J. Obstet. Gynecol.*, **81**, 361

139. Štembera, Z. K. (1968). Intra-uterine danger to the fetus. (Amsterdam: Excerpta Med. Found.)

140. Ray, M., Freeman, R., Pine, S. and Hesselgesser, R. (1972). Clinical experience with the oxytocin challenge test. *Amer. J. Obstet. Gynecol.*, **114,** 1

141. Pose, S. V., Castillo, J. B., Mora-Rojas, E. D., Soto-Yances, A. and Caldeyro-Barcia, R. (1970). Test of fetal tolerance to induced uterine contractions for the diagnosis of chronic fetal distress. *Int. J. Gynaecol. Obstet.*, **8,** 93

142. Christie, G. B. and Cudmore, D. W. (1974). The oxytocin challenge test. *Amer. J. Obstet. Gynecol.*, **118,** 327

143. Ewing, D. E., Farina, J. R. and Otterson, W. N. (1974). Clinical application of the oxytocin challenge test. *Obstet. Gynecol.*, **43,** 563

144. DeVoe, S. J. and Schwarz, R. H. (unpublished data)

CHAPTER 17

Ultrasonic and Radiological Examination

S. Campbell

Introduction

Both X-ray and ultrasonic diagnostic techniques involve the imaging of body structures by means of waves of energy from an external source. Here, however, the similarity ends. X-ray visualisation depends on the shadow phenomenon in which the image is displayed on a photographic plate on the side of the body distal to the energy source while diagnostic ultrasound being an echo technique has the energy source and receiver on the same side of the body. X-rays are a part of the electro-magnetic spectrum and have profound biological effects due to the production of ionising radiation. In pregnancy these effects undoubtedly constitute a hazard to the fetus although with modern radiological techniques the risk of a single X-ray examination performed after 12 weeks is very small. For example, the chance of developing leukaemia in childhood from two standard radiographs in pregnancy is raised by about 10% or one in 12 000 examinations[1,2]. However, as the risks are cumulative, serial X-rays to assess fetal growth cannot be justified. While ultrasonic examination can cause cell damage at high intensity, current experimental evidence indicates that at diagnostic power levels there is no hazard to the fetus[3-5]. Furthermore, because its biological effects are mechanical, the effects of ultrasonic examination are not cumulative and serial measurements to assess the fetal growth rate can be safely made. For this reason, and because of its superior ability to demonstrate soft tissue boundaries, ultrasound has become a better method of assessing fetal well-being than radiology.

Ultrasound

Diagnostic ultrasound is a relatively young discipline, being introduced into obstetrics by Donald and his co-workers in Glasgow as recently as 1958[6]. By definition it employs sound frequencies above the upper auditory range (20 000 cycles per second) and in practice frequencies in the region of $2\frac{1}{2}$ megacycles per second (mHz are used). High frequencies are necessary to provide a narrow beam with good directional control and fine echo resolution. The sound waves are transmitted from a piezo-electric cystal (transducer) which is in contact with the patient's skin.

Imaging techniques

These employ the use of pulsed ultrasonic waves in which very short pulses in the region of 2 microseconds in length are transmitted through the maternal abdomen. This has the advantage that the same transducer can be used to transmit the sound wave and receive the returning signal during the silence between pulses. The sound pulse passes down through maternal and fetal tissues being gradually attenuated in intensity in the process. As it crosses the junction (interface) between different tissues it encounters an acoustic mismatch and partial reflection of the sound wave occurs. The remainder of the ultrasonic pulse passes on to the next interface where the process is repeated. The reflected sound waves are detected by the transducer which converts the acoustic signals into electric signals which are then amplified and processed by a cathode ray tube into visual signals. Strong echoes are obtained when the ultrasonic beam is at right-angles to the interface or when the acoustic mismatch between the tissues of each side of the interface is great. The transducer can also receive weak signals from interfaces that are not at right-angles to the ultrasonic beam, due to minor irregularities of the surfaces; in the past this diffuse backscatter was eliminated by signal processing in order to facilitate interpretation of the echograms, but nowadays these echoes can be displayed by grey-scaling techniques[7, 8] and can thus aid the visualisation of many organs which could previously not be detected. There are two display systems commonly employed in antenatal measurement. In the first (A-scan) the echoes are shown as vertical deflections on a horizontal time base (Figure 17.5). The interval between any two deflections represents the time taken by the sound wave to pass between the relevant interfaces and if we know the sound velocity in this tissue the distance between the two interfaces can be exactly determined. This is usually done by means of electronic caliper markers which, when placed in the A-scan deflections give the measurement to the nearest 0·1 mm. On the B-scan display the echoes from each interface are shown on the time base as a bright spot. As the transducer is moved over the maternal abdomen the time base starting point and direction move in a corresponding manner so that the movements of the time base on the screen correspond to the movements of the ultrasonic beam in the body. To obtain optimal information the transducer is moved at different angles to the skin surface so that the ultrasonic beam crosses all possible interfaces at right-angles (compound scanning) and as the bright spots coalesce a two-dimensional outline of abdominal structures is produced (Figures 17.1, 2 and 4).

Doppler ultrasound

This ultrasonic technique is used in obstetrics principally for monitoring fetal heart movements. For this purpose the doppler devices do not emit a pulsed ultrasonic wave as used in imaging techniques but send a low intensity continuous wave through the maternal abdomen; moving surfaces will cause a variation in the frequency of the returning signal (doppler effect) which is detected by a receiving crystal and transformed into an audible signal or continuous tracing. For continuous monitoring technical difficulties have arisen because the narrow ultrasonic beam will sometimes lose track of the fetal heart if movements occur. Various technical innovations to overcome this problem, such as having a rosette of receivers in the transducer, have been devised and with the latest instruments it is unusual not to get a satisfactory continuous tracing of the fetal heart rate.

Range gating of a pulsed doppler signal can also be used to assess blood flow. With these instruments a gate can be placed on the signals from a particular blood vessel allowing estimation of vessel size and the flow profile within it[9].

Placentography

Assessment of placental function by estimation of placental volume or by studying the echo patterns from the substance of the placenta have not yet been achieved but studies in this field are under way[10, 11]. Likewise, measurement of uterine blood flow with range gated doppler instruments, although theoretically a means of assessing placental perfusion is beset with technical problems and has not yet been successfully accomplished. ·Ultrasonic scanning of the placenta can, however, help indirectly in the assessment of utero-placental function. Firstly, it can assist in the differential diagnosis of placenta praevia and abuptio placentae for while both conditions can result in impaired utero-placental function, abruptio placentae has invariably the more severe effect and has a significantly higher perinatal loss.

Placental localisation by ultrasound is highly successful and in many ways comes nearest to the ideal technique in that it is simple, rapid and causes no discomfort to the mother. Both the edge of the placenta and the cervix can be visualised so that the degree of placenta praevia can be determined. Placental tissue is recognised as an area of speckling, confluent with a length of uterine wall; when a placenta is on the anterior wall the fetal surface can be recognised as a distinct line which is less apparent with the posteriorly situated placenta. Nevertheless, when there is an interface between liquor amnii and placental tissue, the fetal surface of the posterior placenta can be easily seen. Trouble arises in the case of the posterior placenta when the fetal body 'shadows' the placenta which means that the placental tissue does not speckle and the fetal surface cannot be identified. (Figure 17.1a). The problem

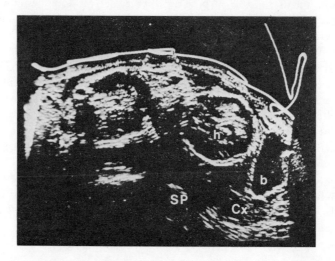

Figure 17.1a Echogram showing longitudinal section of a 36-week fetus. There is 'shadowing' of a posterior type III placenta praevia by the fetal head and trunk. Suspicion of placenta praevia is raised by the space between the fetal head and the sacral promontory. h = Fetal head, b = bladder, SP = Sacral Promontory, Cx = Cervix

of the posterior placenta can be illustrated by the major studies of Donald and Abdulla[12], Morrison *et al.*[12] and Kobayashi *et al.*[14]. Taking these studies together, in 72 cases of placenta praevia, there were 6 failures (8·3%); one was in the anterior wall, one was central, and 4 were on the posterior wall. These difficulties with the posterior placenta can be overcome if the technique of Campbell[15] is employed; when there is a space between the presenting part and the sacral promontory, the scanning couch is tilted 20% 'head down' thus causing upward displacement of the head. If placenta praevia exists the lower edge can now be identified and the distance to the cervix determined (Figure 17.1b).

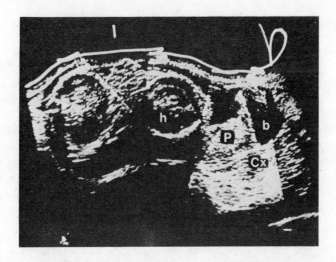

Figure 17.1b Echogram of the same case illustrated in Figure 17.1a with a 20° foot up tilt of the scanning couch; there has been upward displacement of the fetal head thus allowing good visualisation of the placenta and placental edge which can be seen to cover the cervix. P = Placenta

The diagnosis of abruptio placentae is usually made by excluding placenta praevia in a case of antepartum haemorrhage. The suspicion is of course heightened if an area of uterine tenderness lies over the placental site. Kobayashi et al.[15] believe that retro-placental clots can be recognised on echograms of the placenta but it is unlikely that these will be recognised in the majority of cases of abruptio placentae.

There is a further way in which ultrasonic placentography can indirectly assist in the assessment of fetal well being, that is in the localisation of the placenta and fetus prior to amniocentesis for prenatal diagnosis. Even when the placenta is anteriorly situated, it is usually possible to find a space on the anterior wall where the placenta does not lie and therefore obtain amniotic fluid without traversing the placenta. Campbell[17] describes how in Queen Charlotte's Hospital amniocentesis is performed in the laboratory immediately after ultrasonic scanning to preclude the possibility of the fetus moving into the amniocentesis site. In a comparison between 44 cases of amniocentesis performed 'blind' by suprapubic tap and 41 cases of amniocentesis in which prior localisation of the placenta was carried out, there was a fourfold decrease in the incidence of significant feto-maternal transfusions and also a reduction in the number of 'bloody taps' in the ultrasonic group.

Embryonic Growth in the First Trimester

The fetal gestation sac and embryonic echo can first be recognised at 6 weeks menstrual age on the B-scan display. Embryonic maturity and growth assessment during the first trimester were originally made by measurement of the gestation sac[18, 19] but more accurate results can now be achieved by making Crown–Rump measurements of the embryonic echo[20]. These measurements have been facilitated by the newer ultrasonic machines (e.g. Diasonograph 4102) which can give life-size images of the embryonic echo. Robinson makes his measurements from a transverse abdominal scan following several initial longitudinal scans which identify the axis of the embryo. The measurements are made either directly from the face of the cathode ray tube or from an echogram (Figure 17.2). Robinson's graph (Figure 17.3) shows a gradual

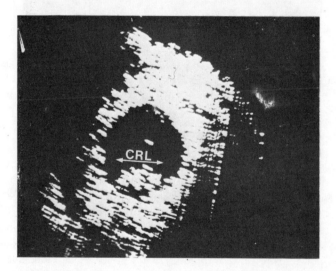

Figure 17.2a Echogram taken at 8 weeks menstrual age illustrating Crown–Rump length (CRL) measurement of the embryo. The fetal heart pulsations can always be detected at this stage

acceleration of embryonic growth from 6 to 14 weeks menstrual age. Predictions of maturity during this period in 34 patients who were certain of the date of their last menstrual period were found to be remarkably

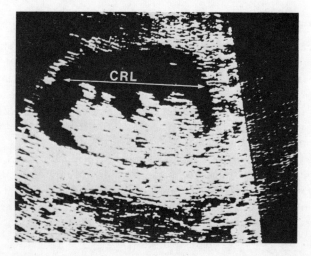

Figure 17.2b CRL measurement at 12 weeks menstrual age showing the remarkable increase in embryonic size over this 4-week period

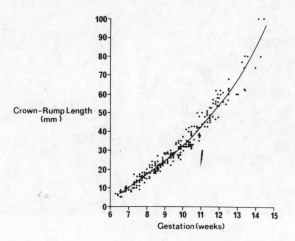

Figure 17.3 Robinson's graph showing the relationship between embryonic CRL growth and menstrual age from the 6th to the 14th week of normal pregnancy

accurate; in 33 cases the prediction was within 3 days of the true maturity and in 25 the prediction was within 2 days. Arrest of growth at this stage inevitably results in embryonic death; this can immediately be diagnosed from 7 weeks onwards for under normal circumstances fetal heart pulsation can always be recognised from A-scan display[21].

Cephalometry

Ultrasonic cephalometry employs the combined use of the A- and B-scan display as described by Campbell[22]. The measurement of the fetal biparietal diameter is the most accurate measurement that can be obtained antenatally. This is firstly because the midline structures of the fetal skull allow the operator to locate and measure the same diameter on each occasion and secondly because the skull bone reflections are very sharply defined, thus permitting precise measurement.

The technique involves scanning the fetal head in two planes. The first longitudinal scan determines the angle of the head to the vertical axis; the second transverse scan is made with the transducer inclined at this angle so that the ultrasonic beam passes through the fetal parietal eminences. If the correct transverse section has been obtained a well defined midline echo can be observed bisecting the cephalic outline (Figure 17.4). The ultrasonic beam

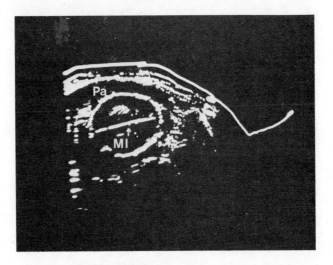

Figure 17.4 Echogram taken at 28 weeks menstrual age showing the correct transverse section of the fetal head for accurate cephalometry. A strong continuous midline echo (Ml) must be observed. The biparietal diameter is the widest diameter orthogonal to the midline echo. Pa = Parietal bone

is then placed at right-angles to this midline echo and across the parietal bones and an A-scan measurement taken (Figure 17.5). Further scans are then made to ensure that the widest transcoronal diameter (biparietal) has been measured. Cephalometry is a difficult technique which demands experience and care.

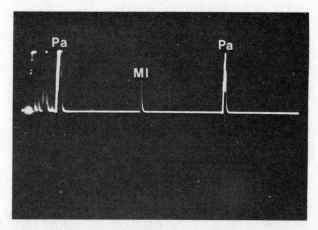

Figure 17.5 A-scan tracing of the fetal head illustrated in Figure 17.4 showing measurement of the biparietal diameter. Measuring caliper markers are placed on the leading edges of the parietal bone (Pa) echoes and a direct reading obtained to the nearest 0·1 mm

Some of the difficulties and the various methods of overcoming them are discussed by Campbell[23]. With experience, however, the average time for cephalometry should not be longer than 10 minutes and good midline echoes should be obtained in 98% of examinations. When properly performed the variance between successive measurements should be within 0·7 mm in 95% of cases.

Normal values

The fetal biparietal diameter can be accurately measured from 13–14 weeks menstrual age. There are now several published charts in which biparietal diameter values taken in normal pregnancy have been plotted against the menstrual age of the fetus. All of them show a similar growth pattern, i.e. linear growth during the middle trimester and early third trimester with a gradual reduction in the growth rate from 36 weeks onwards. There is, however, a disparity between the various published studies in the absolute size of the biparietal diameter for a particular week of gestation. This cannot be completely explained by technical, social or ethnic factors for even if we compare studies where these factors were equal this disparity remains. For example, the mean values of Campbell and Newman[24] are about 5 mm greater at each week of gestation when compared with those of Flamme[25]. The probable explanation is that different ultrasonic velocities are being used to determine the distance between the A-scan deflections, the higher velocities giving the largest readings. For fetal growth and maturity assessment it is unimportant which ultrasonic velocity is used (as long as an appropriate chart for a particular velocity is used) for it is the *relative* increase in head size that determines the growth rate. Where the absolute value is important, for example in cases of suspected cephalopelvic disproportion, the calibrating velocity of 1600 metres per second determined by Willocks *et al.*[25] would appear to be the optimum figure for determining the true unmoulded head size[27].

Campbell and Newman[24] describe the two 'normal data' graphs which are required in the antenatal assessment of the fetus. In the first (Figure 17.6a) the

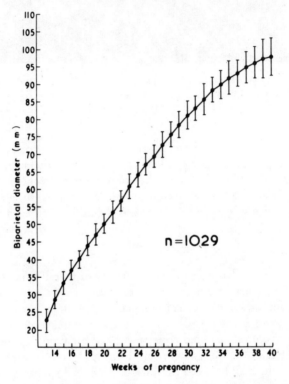

Figure 17.6a Mean biparietal diameter values ±2 standard deviations for each week of pregnancy from 13 weeks to term; 1029 individual readings taken during normal pregnancy. This graph is used to assess fetal maturity and size

individual biparietal diameter values are plotted against the menstrual age of the fetus. It can be seen that the mean weekly increase in the biparietal diameter is rapid and linear from 13 until 30 weeks gestation (3·5 mm per

week), slows slightly between 30 and 34 weeks (2·2 mm per week) and thereafter falls rapidly until 40 weeks at which time the increase is less than 1 mm
per week. The range of head size for a particular week of gestation is confined within narrow limits during the middle trimester and widens gradually
after 30 weeks maturity. This graph is used to assess fetal size and maturity.
In the second (Figure 17.6b) longitudinal data is used to give the growth rate

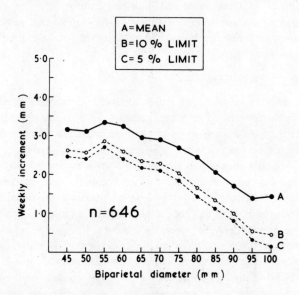

Figure 17.6b Mean weekly growth rate of the biparietal diameter with lower tolerance
limits according to the size of the biparietal diameter. This graph is constructed from
longitudinal measurements obtained from normal pregnancies and is used to assess the
fetal growth rate

of the fetal biparietal diameter in relation to maturity and the actual size of the
biparietal diameter. This latter graph is the most useful in assessing the fetal
growth rate.

Fetal weight

To assess the value of any technique in fetal weight prediction it is important
to assess a significant number of babies at the extremes of the birth weight
range. This is illustrated by the study of Loeffler[28] who assessed the accuracy
of antenatal abdominal palpation in fetal weight prediction; while overall the
growth weight could be predicted to within 454 g of the actual weight in
80% of estimates, the success rate fell to 43% when the weight of the fetus was

less than 2·27 kg. Campbell[23] studied the accuracy of fetal weight prediction from a single biparietal diameter measurement made on 781 patients within 1 week of delivery; 211 of these patients had a birth weight below 2·5 kg while 23 were over 4 kg. The birth weight was predicted to within 405 g in 68% of cases and furthermore ultrasonic prediction of birth weight was as accurate at the extremes of the birth weight range as in the middle. Thus while a single measurement of the fetal biparietal diameter cannot compare with serial measurements in the assessment of the small-for-dates fetus, nevertheless a single measurement near term is of more value in fetal weight prediction than abdominal palpation.

Fetal maturity

The prediction of fetal maturity is a successful and valuable application of ultrasonic cephalometry. The most accurate predictions are made when measurements are taken before 30 weeks menstrual age (or equivalent head size) because of the rapidity and uniformity of fetal growth during this period. Campbell[29] made maturity predictions between 20 and 30 weeks menstrual age on 170 antenatal patients in whom the fetal maturity was in doubt; delivery occurred within 9 days of the date predicted from the ultrasonic measurement in 84% of patients in whom labour began spontaneously and who were delivered of mature babies. Varma[30] in a similar study achieved more striking results by taking two measurements and excluding those cases that had retarded growth rates; 91·2% of 274 patients with unknown dates went into spontaneous labour within 9 days of the ultrasonic prediction. Certainly serial measurements should give greater reliability because they will establish whether fetal growth is normal or not; maturity predictions are unreliable if growth is already retarded when the measurement is taken. An alternative is to take single measurements before 20 weeks menstrual age (or equivalent head size) for fetal growth retardation is extremely rare at this time. This is the present policy in our department.

Because the growth rate of the biparietal diameter is still rapid between 30 and 34 weeks menstrual age, predictions of maturity during this period are still useful. After 34 weeks maturity predictions become increasingly unreliable due to the slower more variable growth rate of the fetal biparietal diameter. Serial measurements however can be useful in determining whether the maturity is mistaken or not, and this is discussed in the next section.

Fetal growth

Willocks *et al.*[26] pioneered the use of serial measurements in the assessment of fetal growth. While it is possible to make assessments of the fetal growth rate from two measurements one week apart there is no doubt that the more numerous the measurements and the earlier in pregnancy they are started the more accurate and useful will be the diagnostic predictions. To measure the fetal growth rate reference should be made to the graphs of Campbell and Newman[24]. When the first measurement is taken it is compared with the graph of the biparietal diameter v. menstrual age (Figure 17.6a) to determine whether the reading is in the normal range for the particular week of gestation; subsequent growth is then assessed using the graph of weekly growth rate v. biparietal diameter (Figure 17.6b). For example, if a fetus whose maturity is supposed to be 34 weeks and has a biparietal diameter of 80 mm then this measurement is well below two standard deviations for that particular week of pregnancy. Excluding some cranial abnormality there are only two possible explanations for this small head size, either the maturity is in error or fetal growth is retarded. If a further measurement is taken one week later and the biparietal diameter measures 83 mm then fetal growth is normal and the probability is that the maturity is in error. It is our practice to allow these patients to proceed past term providing fetal growth continues to be normal. On the other hand, if the biparietal diameter reading is only 81 mm then this indicates growth retardation and the patient is admitted for further studies.

Campbell and Dewhurst[31] studied 406 cases who were referred because they were clinically small-for-dates or had a pregnancy complication; 149 were found to be normal, 117 had a maturity problem and 140 had retarded growth rates. In the latter group 68% of babies were below the 5th centile weight for gestation. The fetuses with retarded growth rates also had a significant increase in low Apgar scores, perinatal deaths and fetal abnormalities when compared with the other groups. Campbell and Kurjak[32] compared the value of serial ultrasonic cephalometry and urinary estrogen estimations in the assessment of a similar group of 284 'at risk' babies. All patients had at least 3 in-patient urinary estrogen estimations which were continued to within one week of delivery. Ultrasonic cephalometry was found to be significantly better at diagnosing the small-for-dates fetus, although there was no significant difference between the two methods in predicting perinatal asphyxia. In a similar study Varma[32] confirmed the superiority of ultrasonic cephalometry in predicting growth retardation and demonstrated that cephalometry was significantly superior to estrogen assay in predicting perinatal asphyxia. Campbell[23] from analysis of the cephalometry charts in cases of growth retardation describes different patterns of intrauterine growth which may be of importance in the short and long term prognosis of the fetus. These patterns can be considered to fall into two main groups. In the first group there is a lengthy period of normal growth and then at a variable time, though usually in the third trimester there is a sudden reduction of the growth rate (Figure 17.7); the later in pregnancy the abnormal growth develops the larger will be the baby which accounts for a number of babies who have retarded ultrasonic growth rates but who are above the 5th centile

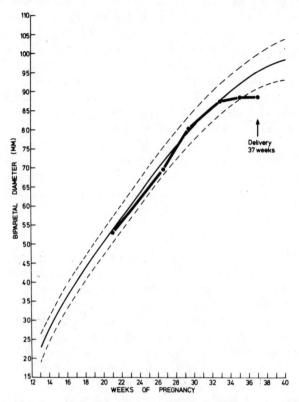

Figure 17.7 Cephalometry chart showing typical 'late flattening' growth retardation pattern. The patient was a 37-year-old primigravida with essential hypertension. Labour was induced at 37 weeks. An emergency Caesarean section was performed for fetal distress and the Apgar score was 2 at 1 minute. The birth weight was 1·80 kg which is below the 5th centile weight for gestation

weight for gestation. This 'late flattening' growth retardation pattern is frequently associated with conditions causing reduced placental perfusion such as pre-eclampsia. Furthermore these babies have a high incidence of perinatal asphyxia, may develop postnatal hypoglycaemia and usually have an increased head to liver ratio. In the other growth pattern group the chart shows a persistently low growth rate usually from early in the second trimester, without any tendency to cessation of growth (Figure 17.8). This 'low profile' growth retardation pattern is usually associated with a very small baby whose biparietal diameter is smaller in relation to birth weight than

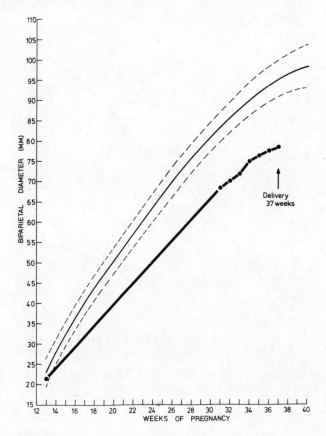

Figure 17.8 Cephalometry chart showing typical 'low profile' growth retardation pattern. The patient was a 19-year-old primigravida. Pregnancy labour and delivery were uneventful and the Apgar score was 7 at 1 minute. The birth weight was 1·35 kg which is below the 5th centile weight for gestation

that of the 'late flattening' group; pregnancy is usually unassociated with toxaemia while the Apgar score and brain to liver ratio are usually normal. About 20–30% of small-for-dates babies referred for ultrasonic examination conform to this growth pattern. Some of these low profile growth retardation babies have some genetic or chromosomal abnormality and are examples of reduced growth potential (Figure 17.9). Studies are at present

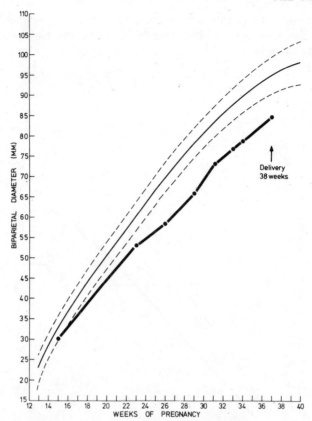

Figure 17.9 Cephalometry chart of a case of fetal abnormality showing the typical 'low profile' pattern that is obtained when there is low growth potential. The patient wàs a 36-year-old primigravida. Labour was induced at 38 weeks. The baby weighed 2·42 kg at birth and had a trisomy 13/15.

being carried out to determine whether postnatal growth and development is determined by the duration and severity of intrauterine growth retardation.

Fetal Trunk Measurements

Measurements of the fetal trunk can also be made during the second and third trimesters of pregnancy[34-37]. Linear measurements to determine the fetal growth rate are less reliable than measurements of the biparietal diameter, firstly because slight alterations in a particular diameter can occur with changes in the fetal position and secondly because of difficulties in determining the same diameter on each occasion. Area or circumference measurements of the fetal trunk can, however, be useful, especially in determining fetal weight. As with fetal head measurements a longitudinal scan is first performed to determine the angulation of the fetal spine to the vertical axis and a series of transverse scans is subsequently made with the transducer inclined to this angle. This ensures that true transverse sections of the fetal body are obtained. A particular problem, however, is to determine the exact level of the section. The fetal chest can always be identified from the pulsations and outline of the fetal heart, but the widest chest circumference lies at a level immediately caudal to the heart pulsations in the region of the diaphragm. The widest and most reproducible measurement is a transverse section of the fetal abdomen in the region of the liver; this can be recognised by the typical configuration of the umbilical vein (Figure 17.10). A section at this level in

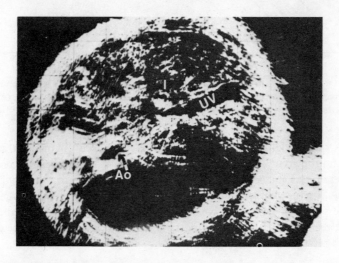

Figure 17.10 Echogram showing transverse section of the upper fetal abdomen. The umbilical vein (UV), fetal abdominal aorta (Ao) and fetal liver (l) can be clearly identified. A circumference measurement at this level is used to make birth weight predictions

our experience will permit prediction of fetal weight to within 280 g of the actual birth weight in 68% of cases (Figure 17.11). Another measurement of value may be the head to abdomen circumference ratio especially if the section is taken through the fetal liver. Towards term the circumference of the head is almost invariably less than that of the upper fetal abdomen, the ration being on average 1 : 1·1. In many cases of fetal growth retardation this

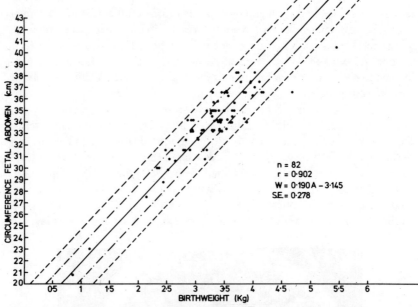

Figure 17.11 Correlation between the fetal abdomen circumference measurement and birth weight in 82 cases measured within 3 days of delivery (linear regression, 68% and 95% confidence limits); the birth weight can be predicted to within 280 g in 68% of cases

ratio is reversed and ratios as high as 3 : 2 have been obtained in cases of severe uteroplacental vascular insufficiency. In cases of low growth potential or where ultrasonic cephalometry growth rates conform to the 'low profile' pattern then normal or near normal ratios are frequently observed. This work is still at an early stage but it is possible that the fetal head to abdomen circumference ratio will yield important information as to the nature of fetal growth retardation.

Fetal Urine Production

A new ultrasonic technique for estimating the hourly fetal urine production rate (HFUPR) was described by Campbell et al.[38]. The bladder is demonstrated on a B mode display and measured in three dimensions (Figure 17.12) and the volume calculated from a formula. In 33 cases studied throughout a complete fetal bladder cycle, the length of the cycle varied from 50 to 155 minutes (mean 110 minutes). Filling of the bladder occurred at a constant rate indicating that intermittent voiding of urine during the process of bladder filling was most unlikely. Emptying of the bladder usually occurred in a few

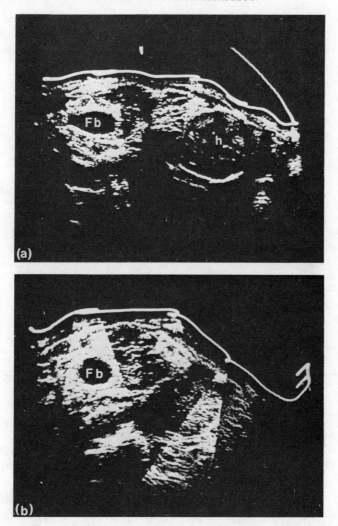

Figure 17.12 Echograms showing longitudinal (a) and transverse (b) sections of the fetal bladder (Fb) at 36 weeks menstrual age. Three bladder diameters are measured and the fetal bladder volume calculated from the formula $4/3\pi\left(\dfrac{d_1}{2}\times\dfrac{d_2}{2}\times\dfrac{d_3}{2}\right)$

seconds although frequently it was a gradual process covering a period of 30 minutes. Measurement of the HFUPR was made by taking two fetal bladder volume measurements at intervals of $\frac{1}{2}$ or 1 hour during the process of bladder filling and calculating the rate of increase over this period.

Wladimiroff and Campbell[39] studied HFUPR values in 92 normal antenatal patients; there was a rapid and linear rise in the mean HFUPR values from 9·6 ml at 30 weeks to 27·3 ml at 40 weeks menstrual age. No circadian variation was demonstrated. In 62 antenatal patients with complicated pregnancies 29 (47%) had HFUPR values below the 5th percentile tolerance limit (Figure 17.13) and of these 62% were delivered of babies whose birth

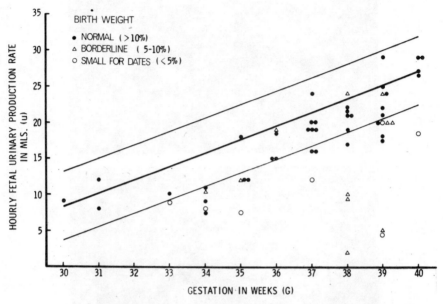

Figure 17.13 Relationship between the hourly fetal urinary production rate (HFUPR) in complicated pregnancies and the normal range (linear regression line and 95% confidence limits) from 30 to 40 weeks menstrual age. All the small-for-dates babies had HFUPR values below the normal range

weight was below the 10th centile weight for gestation. All the small-for-dates babies had HFUPR values below the normal range. There thus appears to be a strong correlation between a reduced HFUPR and fetal growth retardation. From this study, however, there was no evidence that the test was useful in indicating which babies would be liable to develop perinatal hypoxia.

Fetal Respiratory Movements

It is now recognised that the human fetus makes respiratory movements during the second and third trimesters of pregnancy. An A-scan ultrasonic method for recording these movements was described by Boddy and Robinson[40]. In this technique a strobe gate pulse is used to isolate the chest wall echo and movement of this echo in the gate is converted into an electric signal to drive a pen recorder. Since chest movement can be as little as 2 mm, considerable sensitivity is required (Figure 17.14).

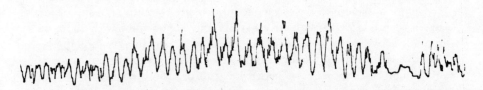

Figure 17.14 Human fetal respiratory movements as detected by an A-scan ultrasonic technique; this continuous tracing shows that the rate of respiratory movements in this mature fetus is 45 per minute. By kind permission of D. J. Farman, University College Hospital, London

The normal mature fetal respiratory pattern consists of 30–90 movements per minute for approximately 80% of the time; breaking up this rhythmic movement are very short periods of inspiratory apnoea. This normal respiratory pattern is disturbed under certain adverse circumstances, notably hypoxia and hypoglycaemia; these are associated with extended periods of apnoea which contain episodes of gasping movements, each lasting for more than 2 seconds. In these cases the amount of normal respiratory movement is severely reduced. When the fetus is in extremis and in imminent danger of intrauterine death, respiratory movement is not observed, the pattern consisting of prolonged apnoea interspersed with gasping. (Boddy, personal communication.)

Fetal Stress Tests

It has long been recognised that when there is incipient utero-placental respiratory failure, the contractions of labour will further compromise the utero-placental circulation and changes in the fetal heart rate will occur, the earliest abnormality being a baseline tachycardia with the superimposition in severe cases of late decelerations and loss of baseline variability (beat to beat variation). Monitoring of the fetal heart during labour is most reliably made with a continuous fetal ECG tracing obtained from a scalp electrode, a technique which is clearly unsuitable during the antenatal period and before rupture of the membranes. Continuous monitoring of the fetal heart, therefore, before the onset of labour is generally performed with the ultrasonic Doppler devices which produce a satisfactory tracing of the 'instantaneous' heart rate but unfortunately do not provide a true measurement of beat to beat variation.

Attempts to simulate the stress of labour during the antenatal period and thus produce similar changes in cases of utero-placental insufficiency have been made by means of the oxytocin stress or challenge test. Although there are minor variations in the technique from centre to centre, the aim of the test is to produce approximately 8–10 uterine contractions with about 90 seconds between two contractions by means of a titration oxytocin infusion and to simultaneously monitor any changes in the fetal heart rate. Kubli *et al.*[41] found that the test was a better predictor of a low Apgar score at birth than urinary estriols or ultrasonic cephalometry while Ray *et al.*[42] found a strong correlation between a positive test and depressed urinary estriols, low Apgar scores and fetal death *in utero*. Patients with negative tests did uniformly well in the absence of congenital abnormality or cephalo-pelvic disproportion. These initial enthusiastic reports have not however been reproduced in recent studies. Boyd *et al.*[43] found no correlation between a positive test and the development of intra-partum fetal distress or depressed Apgar score and described a case of intrauterine death which occurred 7 days after a negative test. Christie and Cudmore[44] similarly found no correlation between a positive test and low estriols, the occurrence of fetal distress in labour or low Apgar scores, but considered that a negative test in a high risk pregnancy may justify allowing the pregnancy to continue. Baillie[45] only found the test reliable when after producing 8 uterine contractions at the threshold of maternal pain, the oxytocin infusion rate was doubled to produce a prolonged uterine contraction lasting between 3 and 7 minutes. Clearly such a stress must be considered potentially dangerous especially to the already compromised fetus and on present evidence the oxytocin stress test would appear to have limitations as a means of assessing utero-placental respiratory reserve.

A more rapid and potentially more useful test is a hypoxic stress test in which the fetal heart response to maternal inhalation of 12% oxygen for 15 minutes is monitored. Baillie[44] investigated the effects of this test on both mother and fetus. Maternal changes included a slight increase in the respiratory rate, a lowered PCO_2 and a small increase in PH. The maternal P_aO_2 fell from a mean of 99 mm to 44 mmHg. The maternal cardiovascular system was unaffected and there was no maternal subjective distress. Baillie[45] considered that the stress was safe for the mother in the absence of cardiac and severe respiratory disease. An abnormal fetal heart response to this test was a rise in the heart rate of 10 beats per minute or more over the baseline with failure to return to baseline levels within 5 minutes of cessation of the test. Great care was taken to achieve a stable fetal state (by administering intravenous pethidine 50 mg to the mother) before the test was commenced. Baillie[45] claimed outstanding precision for the test; when the fetal heart rate took longer than 8 minutes to settle, all cases were in poor condition at birth and conversely when the tachycardia settled in less than 5 minutes, all babies had normal Apgar scores. In 4 cases where the fetal heart took longer than 10 minutes to settle, all suffered intra-uterine death within 72 hours of the test. Unfortunately Baillie does not give a detailed statistical breakdown of these results and more evidence is clearly required to establish the value of the hypoxic stress test as a predictor of placental respiratory functional reserve.

Radiology

While with ultrasonic diagnosis the earlier the measurement the more accurate the prediction of maturity, the contrary rule applies in radiology. After 36 weeks a single X-ray is probably of more value than a single ultrasonic measurement in fetal maturity prediction, for although ultrasound can assess fetal size more precisely, the visualisation of the developing ossification centres by radiology offers an index of physiological development which is of definite value in the prediction of fetal maturity. The development of these centres is well described by Russell[2]. The ankle centres are the first to appear, the calcaneum appearing at about 26 weeks and the talus at 28 weeks menstrual age. The centres grow and maintain their spherical shape until 34 weeks when the talus widens coronally and by 36 weeks both the calcaneum and talus develop angulations. Interest now moves from the ankle to the knee centres. At 37 weeks the lower femoral centre is clearly visible and grows rapidly over the following three weeks. The upper tibial centre can be identified at 38 weeks and frequently the cuboid centre can also be seen. By 42 weeks the two knee centres are equal in size. Russell[46] analysed the accuracy of radiological predictions of maturity in over 3000 patients by projecting forward an 'X-ray EDD' and comparing this with the actual date of spontaneous delivery. He found that the radiological prediction was more accurate than the prediction from the menstrual history at all stages in pregnancy and that the accuracy of the radiological prediction improved with increasing maturity. For example, the standard deviation of error of the radiological prediction was 19·4 days between 31 and 35 weeks, but fell to 9·9 days between 38 and 39 weeks. This stresses the importance of the knee centres in making maturity predictions. Good correlation has been shown by Schreiber et al.[47] between the development of the knee centres and the state of neurological development of the newborn. They found that when the tibial centre was visible all 39 infants were neurologically mature, while if only the femoral centre was visible 169 of 173 infants were considered mature.

Growth retardation

Severe fetal growth retardation is associated with impaired development of the epiphyseal centres. Scott and Usher[48] found the lower femoral epiphysis in 63% and the upper tibial in 16% of 30 growth retarded infants, compared with 100% and 83% respectively in a group of controls. Croall and Grech[49] showed that it was only in the most severely growth retarded infants that significant ossification delay occurred. In their study only 5% of mildly growth retarded infants had ossification delay of 2 weeks or more; this rose, however, to 20% with moderate growth retardation and 47% when growth retardation was severe (defined as a birth weight of 200 g or more below the 5th percentile). Hyperflexion of the fetal spine is another radiological finding in growth retardation. Croall and Grech[50] observed hyperflexion in 10 out of 47 grossly small-for-dates fetuses; of these, three died during labour and one was born severely asphyxiated. Hyperflexion thus indicates a particularly high risk of intrapartum hypoxia.

References

1. Stewart, A. and Kneale, G. W. (1970). Radiation Dose Effects in relation to obstetric X-rays and childhood cancers. *Lancet*, **i,** 1185
2. Russell, J. G. B. (1973). *Radiology in Obstetrics and Antenatal Paediatrics*, (London: Butterworths)
3. Taylor, K. J. W. and Dyson, M. (1972). Possible hazards of diagnostic ultrasound. *Brit. J. Hosp. Med.*, **8,** 571
4. Taylor, K. T. W. and Pond, J. B. (1972). Experimental ultrasonic injury and safety limits in its use. *Acta Radiologica*, **13,** 743
5. Ulrich, W. D. (1974). Ultrasonic dosage for non-therapeutic use on human beings— extrapolations from a literature survey. *I.E.E.E. Transactions on Biomedical Engineering, January*, p. 48
6. Donald, I., MacVicar, J. and Brown, T. G. (1958). Investigation of abdominal masses by pulsed ultrasound. *Lancet*, **i,** 1188
7. Kossoff, G. (1972). Improved techniques in ultrasonic cross sectional echoscopy. *Ultrasonics*, **10,** 221
8. Kossoff, G., Garrett, W. J. and Radovanovich, G. (1973). Grey scale echography in obstetrics and gynaecology. C.A.L. Report No. 59. (Sydney, Australia: Commonwealth Acoustic Laboratories)
9. Yao, S. T. (1972). Ultrasound in the transcutaneous assessment of blood flow. *Brit. J. Hosp. Med.*, **8,** 521

10. Hellman, L. M., Kobayashi, M., Tolles, W. E. and Cromb, E. (1970). Ultrasonic studies on the volumetric growth of the human placenta. *Amer. J. Obstet. Gynecol.*, **108**, 740

11. Donald, I. (1974). New problems in sonar diagnosis in obstetrics and gynecology. *Amer. J. Obstet. Gynecol.*, **118**, 299

12. Donald, I. and Abdulla, U. (1968). Placentography by sonar. *J. Obstet. Gynaecol. Brit. Commonw.*, **75**, 993

13. Morrison, J., Kohorn, E. I., Ashford, C. and Fredgold, C. (1969). Ultrasonic scanning in obstetrics. 2. The diagnosis of placenta praevia. *Aust. N.Z. J. Obstet. Gynaec.*, **9**, 206

14. Kobayashi, M., Hellman, L. M. and Fillisti, L. P. (1970). Placental localisation by ultrasound. *Amer. J. Obstet. Gynecol.*, **106**, 279

15. Campbell, S. (1972). Ultrasound in obstetrics. *Brit. J. Hosp. Med.*, **8**, 541

16. Kobayashi, M., Hellman, L. M. and Cromb, E. (1972). Atlas of Ultrasonography in Obstetrics and Gynecology. (New York: Appleton-Century-Crofts)

17. Campbell, S. (1974). The antenatal detection of fetal abnormality by ultrasonic diagnosis. In: *Birth Defects*, p. 240 (Molulsky, A. G. and Lentz, W., editors) (Amsterdam: Excerpta Medica)

18. Donald, I. (1969). Sonar as a method of studying prenatal development. *J. Pediat.*, **75**, 326

19. Hellman, L. M., Kobayashi, M., Fillisti, L. P. and Lavenhar, M. (1969). Growth and development of the human fetus prior to the twentieth week of gestation. *Amer. J. Obstet. Gynecol.*, **103**, 789

20. Robinson, H. D. (1973). Sonar measurement of fetal crown-rump length to assess maturity in first trimester of pregnancy. *Brit. Med. J.*, **4**, 28

21. Robinson, H. D. (1972). Detection of fetal heart movement in the first trimester of pregnancy using pulsed ultrasound. *Brit. Med. J.*, **4**, 466

22. Campbell, S. (1968). An improved method of fetal cephalometry by ultrasound. *J. Obstet. Gynaecol. Brit. Commonw.*, **75**, 568

23. Campbell, S. (1974). Fetal Growth. Clinics in Obstetrics and Gynaecology. In: *Fetal Medicine*. Ch. 3. (Beard, R. W., editor) (London: W. B. Saunders & Co.)

24. Campbell, S. and Newman, G. B. (1971). Growth of the fetal biparietal diameter during normal pregnancy. *J. Obstet. Gynaecol. Brit. Commonw.*, **78**, 513

25. Flamme, P. (1972). Ultrasonic fetal cephalometry—percentiles curve. *Brit. Med. J.*, **3**, 384

26. Willocks, J., Donald, I., Duggan, T. C. and Day, N. (1964). Foetal cephalometry by ultrasound. *J. Obstet. Gynaecol. Brit. Commonw.*, **71**, 11

27. Campbell, S. (1970). Ultrasonic fetal cephalometry during the second trimester of pregnancy. *J. Obstet. Gynaecol. Brit. Commonw.*, **77**, 1057

28. Loeffler, F. E. (1967). Clinical foetal weight prediction. *J. Obstet. Gynaecol. Brit. Commonw.*, **74**, 675

29. Campbell, S. (1969). The prediction of fetal maturity by ultrasonic measurement of the biparietal diameter. *J. Obstet. Gynaecol. Brit. Commonw.*, **76**, 603

30. Varma, T. R. (1973). Prediction of delivery date by ultrasound cephalometry. *J. Obstet. Gynaecol. Brit. Commonw.*, **80**, 316

31. Campbell, S. and Dewhurst, C. J. (1971). Diagnosis of the small-for-dates fetus by serial ultrasonic cephalometry. *Lancet*, **ii**, 1002

32. Campbell, S. and Kurjak, A. (1972). Comparison between urinary oestrogen assay and serial ultrasonic cephalometry in assessment of fetal growth retardation. *Brit. Med. J.*, **4**, 337

33. Varma, T. R. (1973). A comparison between serial cephalometry and maternal urinary oestrogen excretion in assessing fetal prognosis. *Aust. N.Z. J. Obstet. Gynaecol.*, **13,** 191

34. Thompson, H. E., Holmes, J. H., Gottesfeld, K. R. and Taylor, E. S. (1965). Fetal development as determined by ultrasonic pulse echo techniques. *Amer. J. Obstet. Gynecol.*, **92,** 44

35. Garrett, W. J. and Robinson, D. E. (1971). Assessment of fetal size and growth rate by ultrasonic echoscopy. *Obstet. Gynecol.*, **38,** 525

36. Levi, S. (1972). Diagnostic Pur Ultrasons en Gynecologie et en Obstetrique; (Paris: Masson et Cie)

37. Hansmann, M., Voigt, U., and Backer, H. (1973). Die Wertigkeit intrauterin mit Ultraschall messbarer Parameter für Gewichtsklassenschützung des Feten. *Arch. Gynäk.*, **214,** 314

38. Campbell, S., Wladimiroff, J. W. and Dewhurst, C. J. (1973). The Antenatal measurement of fetal urine production. *J. Obstet. Gynaecol. Brit. Commonw.*, **80,** 680

39. Wladimiroff, J. W. and Campbell, S. (1974). Fetal urine production rates in normal and complicated pregnancy. *Lancet*, **i,** 151

40. Boddy, K. and Robinson, J. S. (1971). External method for detection of fetal breathing in utero. *Lancet*, **ii,** 1231

41. Kubli, F. W., Kaeser, O. and Hinselmann, M. (1969). In: *The Feto-placental Unit*, p. 323 (Pecile, A. and Finzie, C., editors) (Amsterdam: Excerpta Medica)

42. Ray, M., Freeman, R., Pine, S. and Hesselgesser, R. (1972). Clinical experience with the oxytocin challenge test. *Amer. J. Obstet. Gynecol.*, **114,** 1

43. Boyd, I. E., Chamberlain, G. V. P. and Fergusson, I. L. C. (1974). The oxytocin stress test and the isoxsuprine placental transfer test in the management of suspected placental insufficiency. *J. Obstet. Gynaecol. Brit. Commonw.*, **81,** 120

44. Christie, G. B. and Cudmore, D. W. (1974). The oxytocin challenge test. *Amer. J. Obstet. Gynecol.*, **118,** 327

45. Baillie, P. (1974). Non-hormonal methods of antenatal monitoring. Clinics in Obstetrics and Gynaecology. In: *Fetal Medicine*. Ch. 6. (Beard, R. W., editor) (London: W. B. Saunders & Co.)

46. Russell, J. G. B. (1969). Radiological assessment of fetal maturity. *J. Obstet. Gynaecol. Brit. Commonw.*, **76,** 208

47. Schreiber, M. H., Nichols, M. M. and McGarity, W. J. (1963). Epiphyseal ossification centre visualisation. Radiological diagnosis in paediatrics. *J. Amer. Med. Assoc.*, **184,** 504

48. Scott, K. E. and Usher, R. (1966). Fetal Malnutrition: Its incidence, causes and effects. *Amer. J. Obstet. Gynecol.*, **94,** 951

49. Croall, J. and Grech, P. (1970). Radiological maturity of the small-for-dates fetus. *J. Obstet. Gynaecol. Brit. Commonw.*, **77,** 802

50. Croall, J. and Grech, P. (1970). Hyperflexion of the small-for-dates fetus. *J. Obstet. Gynaecol. Brit. Commonw.*, **77,** 808

CHAPTER 18

Intrauterine Growth and Maturation in Relation to Fetal Deprivation

Yves W. Brans and George Cassady

Introduction

A monograph on the placenta would be incomplete without considering the life it supports. The fetus is in perpetual flux as evidenced by the changes in body composition which occur between conception and birth[1]. The nutrients which provide energy substrate and basic material for these changes reach the baby with either active participation or passive permission of the placenta. It is no wonder that disturbances of the supply line may have profound repercussions on fetal development and maturation. While 7–20% of all neonates are of low birth weight (less than 2500 grams)[2-5], one-third of these are actually mature (37 or more weeks gestational age)[3, 6] and can be clearly distinguished from their premature weight peers on clinical[1, 3, 6-57], chemical[3, 40, 45, 58-73], metabolic[45, 50, 51, 69, 74-87], histological[12, 15, 17, 57, 88-111], and developmental grounds. More importantly, the very biochemical substrates of life are altered in these undergrown newborns[17, 112-134]. Through the careful observations of some and inquisitive research of others, the unresolved questions concerning intra-uterine growth retardation are slowly being unravelled. Certain of these observations, reviewed in the present chapter, concern a comparative analysis of current methods proposed for assessing gestational age at birth and the altered body composition which accompanies fetal growth retardation in both human and laboratory animals.

Estimation of Gestational Age

Gestational age is usually expressed as time elapsed since the first day of the mother's last normal menstrual period. This estimate, although at best uncertain as a consequence of the variability of the pre-ovulatory phase, remains at present *the best single* clinical estimate of fetal maturity available. Consequently, menstrual age is generally accepted as *the standard of reference* for all other methods.

A wide variety of objective parameters have been shown to correlate with gestational age (Table 18.1). The medical world has been divided concerning the value of these parameters both historically and geographically; the French school relies heavily on neurological parameters while the Anglo-Saxon school appears to prefer observation of external physical body characteristics. The former is best exemplified by the scheme of Amiel-Tison which selects such variables as passive and active tone and reflex activity to predict gestational age[33]. Electroencephalograms[27, 31, 34, 35], often employing evoked responses to sensorial stimuli[37, 38, 154] as well as measurements of nerve conduction velocity[36, 135, 149, 152, 153] have been used in an attempt to quantify neurological maturity. Electroencephalographic patterns of intra-uterine growth retarded neonates have been shown by all these studies to be comparable, with some minor discrepancies, to those of their normally grown gestational peers[27, 34, 35]. Unfortunately, these sophisticated laboratory techniques require rare expertise in interpretation and are therefore of limited everyday clinical value.

Physical observations are easily available in every patient but have definite limitations. Anthropometric measurements, taken singly or in combinations are of limited value as they are all affected in varying degrees by the quality of intra-uterine growth. Head circumference is least affected and is therefore the best of these in predicting fetal maturity[19, 140]. The biparietal diameter as determined ultrasonically (Chapter 17), although little used by pediatricians, is extensively employed by obstetricians to determine maturity. A potential hazard of this technique, poorly documented to date, is that the maturity of intra-uterine growth retarded fetuses may be underestimated while that of macrosomic babies may be overestimated. A number of external somatic characteristics have been carefully studied. These include skin texture, colour, opacity and edema, hair texture, skull hardness, number of plantar skin creases, formation and firmness of external ear cartilage, breast size and nipple formation, and character and pigmentation of external genitalia[13, 26, 142, 146-148]. Taken separately, these characteristics correlate only moderately with gestational age[25] but, except for breast size, are little affected by quality of intra-uterine growth[9, 12, 13, 24-26]. Combinations of several taken together,

Table 18.1 Parameters used to estimate gestational age

Parameters	Correlation with gestational age estimated from menstrual history		References
	r	95% Confidence limits (days)	
Physical:			
birth weight	0·34–0·80	21–36	19, 24, 135–142
crown-heel length	0·34–0·78	29–36	19, 138, 140, 143, 144
crown-rump length	0·60		136
head circumference	0·58–0·87	26	19, 140
occipito-frontal diameter	0·65		19
biparietal diameter	0·56	35	19, 25
skinfold thickness	0·18–0·84	52	17, 145
external characteristics	0·75–0·84	7–24	13, 26, 142, 146–148
Neurological:		24	18, 28–33, 38, 137, 149
Physical and Neurological:	0·93	14–21	24, 149
Radiological:			
epiphyses (femur, tibia, calcaneum)	0·14	28–33	10, 149, 150
skull		14	27, 151
Nerve Conduction Velocities:	0·64–0·83	29–37	36, 135, 149, 152, 153
Electroencephalogram:			27, 31, 34, 35
auditory evoked response			38
photic evoked response	– 0·59		37, 154
Laboratory:			
fetal haemoglobin	– 0·37 — – 0·77	14–53	138, 139, 155
fetal haemoglobin/birth weight	– 0·54 — – 0·87	18–23	138, 139
total serum proteins		42	62, 156–158
albumin	0·58–0·67	43	61, 62, 159
alpha-1-fetoprotein	– 0·81 — – 0·89	16–30	61, 62, 157, 160
alpha-2-macroglobulin	– 0·68		159
immunoglobulin G	0·72–0·88		61, 63, 64, 159, 161, 162
immunoglobulin G/alpha-1-fetoprotein ratio	0·86		61
immunoglobulin M	0·64		159
transferrin	0·51		159
carbonic anhydrase activity		21	174
SGPT, SGOT			163
Pepsinogen 7 (urine)			164
alkaline phosphatase (meconium)			165
reticulocyte count	0·88		59
coagulation factors II, VIII			166

however, allow estimation of gestational age with an accuracy of about 3 weeks[13, 26, 142, 146]. The careful studies of Dubowitz and associates have provided a classic, widely used, and highly valuable clinical scheme which uses both neurological and external characteristics[24]. Each observation is assigned a score of 0 to 4 and, when performed with precision and care, the resulting total score correlates highly with gestational age ($r = 0.93$).

Roentgenological evidence of epiphyseal maturity, a long time favourite of obstetricians, is a poor predictor of gestational age[10, 149, 150]. Though presence of the distal femoral epiphysis indicates maturity, its absence has no meaning. Moreover, bone maturity is retarded in intra-uterine growth retardation[10, 39]. A number of laboratory chemical parameters correlate with gestational age but none, taken separately, can better the prediction obtained from an accurate clinical examination using the Dubowitz scheme. Alpha-1-fetoprotein level[61, 62, 157, 160] and reticulocyte counts[59] are potentially interesting since they seem to be independent of the quality of intra-uterine growth.

In summary, the schemes developed by Amiel–Tison and by Dubowitz and associates appear to be the most useful and precise in clinically estimating gestational age. The degree of precision increases with the clinician's proficiency. Gestational age, estimated from a careful, accurate menstrual history, remains the single most valuable clinical tool in estimating fetal maturity and is the standard of reference for all other techniques. A final word of caution is appropriate concerning these techniques. It is commonly overlooked that, for the most part, these studies have involved white babies. Extension of the results to black infants must be made tenuously. Recently, the number of skin creases on the sole of the foot has been shown to be different at similar gestations in white and black babies[148]. Other observations suggest that the black fetus may 'mature faster', both neurologically and physically[4, 18]. A great deal of work is required to clarify these questions and extend these observations.

Clinical Characteristics of Intra–uterine Growth Retarded Neonates

The 'typical' intra-uterine growth retarded infant, presenting with evidence of muscle wasting, prominent ribs and depressed abdomen, a dry, wrinkled, peeling skin, meconium staining of skin and umbilical cord, and widening of the skull sutures is in fact uncommon and represents only one end of a spectrum[6-12]. More common is a baby who, though normal at first glance, reveals on detailed examination a discrepancy between maturity and weight (Table 18.2). Length, head, chest, and abdominal circumferences are often less affected by fetal deprivation than weight[1, 8, 11-23]. Subcutaneous fat deposits, as measured by skinfold thickness[12, 17, 92], and muscle mass as

Table 18.2 Clinical characteristics of intra-uterine growth retarded babies contrasted to those of gestational and weight peers

Parameter	Gestational peers	Weight peers	References
General appearance:	Varies from normal to marasmic: emaciation; loose, dry, peeling skin; meconium staining; prominent ribs and scaphoid abdomen		6–12
Anthropometric measurements at birth:			1, 8, 11–23
weight	lower		
length	normal or lower	higher or normal	
head circumference	normal or lower	higher or normal	
chest circumference	normal or lower	higher or normal	
abdominal circumference	lower or normal	higher or normal	
weight/length	lower	normal	
weight/head circumference	lower	normal	
thigh girth	lower	normal or lower	
skinfold thickness	lower	normal or lower	
foot length	lower	normal	
biparietal diameter	lower	normal	
occipito-frontal diameter	lower	normal	
Maturity parameters:			9, 12, 13
skin creases on sole of foot	similar	more numerous	24–26
breast size	normal or smaller	larger	
hair texture	similar	more mature	
ear cartilage	similar	more mature	
Neurological maturity:			
examination	similar	greater	7–9, 18, 20 27–33
electroencephalogram	some abnormalities	more mature	27, 34, 35
nerve conduction velocity	normal	greater	24, 36
photic evoked responses	normal	more mature	37
auditory evoked responses	normal	more mature	38
Skeletal maturity:			
bone age	similar or delayed		9, 20
epiphyseal ossification	delayed		10, 39
Neonatal morbidity:			
perinatal asphyxia	increased frequency	similar frequency	3
fetal anomalies	increased frequency	increased frequency	3, 23, 40, 41
hypoglycaemia	increased frequency	increased frequency	3, 42–49
hyperbilirubinaemia	similar frequency	decreased frequency	50, 51
hyaline membrane disease	similar frequency	decreased frequency	3
Neonatal mortality:	increased	decreased	3, 11, 14, 23, 41, 52–57

reflected by thigh girth[12, 92] may be unusually low for maturity and often lower than expected for weight in the fetal growth retarded infant. Neurological examination may confirm the baby's maturity[7-9, 18, 20, 24, 27-38] while bone age is commonly retarded[9, 10, 20, 39].

Blood chemistry may be altered in many respects compared to either gestational or weight peers (Table 18.3). These changes essentially reflect fetal

Table 18.3 Chemical findings in intra-uterine growth retarded babies contrasted to those of gestational and weight peers (from blood obtained at or within 12 hours of birth)

Parameter	Gestational peers	Weight peers	References
Haematocrit	higher	higher	3, 58
Haemoglobin	higher	higher	40, 58
Fetal/total haemoglobin	higher	normal	58
Erythrocyte count	higher	higher	40, 58
Mean corpuscular volume	normal	normal	58
Mean corpuscular haemoglobin	normal	normal	58
Mean corpuscular haemoglobin			
concentration	normal	normal	58
Reticulocyte count	normal	normal	58
Erythropoietin	higher		60
Albumin	normal	higher	61, 62
Alpha-1-fetoprotein	normal	lower	61, 62
Immunoglobulin G	normal or lower	higher	61, 63, 64
Immunoglobulin M	normal or increased		63
Urea	higher		65
Ammonia	higher		65, 66
Uric acid	normal		65
Amino acids:			64, 69–71
glycine, alanine, cystine and			
tyrosine	higher		
others	normal		
non-essential/essential			
concentration ratio	higher	higher	
Lactate	higher		69
Free fatty acids:			45, 67, 68
at birth	normal	normal	
postnatal increase	greater	greater	
Glycerol:			68
at birth	higher	normal	
postnatal increase	greater	greater	
Cortisol	higher		69
Growth hormone	higher		69
	normal	normal	72, 73

deprivation of food and oxygen resulting in a catabolic state. Chronic oxygen deprivation may be reflected by elevated erythropoietin levels at birth[60] with consequently higher haemoglobin concentration and erythrocyte count[40, 58]. A rapid increase in free fatty acids and glycerol following birth suggests greater reliance on lipid catabolism than on glycolysis[68] in the growth retarded neonate. Elevated levels of urea and ammonia may indicate an unusual and excessive reliance on protein substrates in energy metabolism, but they may also be explained by transient hepatic dysfunction[65, 66]. It is interesting to note that growth hormone levels are normal to high[69, 72, 73], thus suggesting that diminished levels are not causative in fetal growth retardation. Extrapolation of Whitehead's findings in older infants and children[167-169] suggests that observations at birth of a non-essential/essential amino acid ratio higher than in either normally grown gestational or weight peers may indicate fetal protein-calorie malnutrition[71]. Observations in discordant twins are particularly interesting in this regard. Twins born before 32 weeks, grown at a normal intra-uterine rate have a non-essential/ essential amino acid ratio which corresponds to that of a singleton fetus of similar gestation. In twins born after 32 weeks gestation with discordance in growth rates, the amino acid ratio in the smaller twin increases at a more rapid rate than that of the larger, better-grown twin[71]. Though still speculative, the concept that changes in non-essential/essential amino acid ratios are detectable in fetal urine and consequently in amniotic fluid[185], thus permitting an early prenatal diagnosis of intra-uterine growth retardation, is most exciting[170-173].

Serious metabolic differences have emerged but little definitive information is available (Table 18.4). Collagen turnover, measured by peptide-bound hydroxyproline excretion in urine, is normal for maturity on the first post natal day but low for weight in the growth retarded neonate[74, 136]. On the third postnatal day, however, collagen turnover appears to actually surpass that of gestational peers[74, 75, 126]. Urinary excretion of glycosaminoglycan, another index of collagen turnover, supports these observations[76]. Overall metabolic activity (oxygen consumption) is greater on a per kilo basis than in normally grown weight peers but is similar to that of normally grown gestational peers[77, 78]. In fact, if intra-uterine growth retardation is severe, oxygen consumption may even surpass that of gestational peers. The meaning of the decreased energy capacity of leukocytes is yet to be explained, especially since similar findings in maternal leukocytes have also been observed[79]. Asphyxial stress may induce a diminished adrenal response[80], while hypoglycaemic stress is sometimes better tolerated[45, 81]. Gluconeogenesis is impaired, in both human[69, 82] and rat[86, 87] growth retarded neonates, suggesting that the higher incidence of hypoglycaemia is not due solely to lower glycogen stores[175, 176]. Placental oxygen consumption is diminished[84],

Table 18.4 Metabolic characteristics of intra–uterine growth retarded neonates (human and rat) contrasted to those of gestational and weight peers

Parameter	Gestational peers	Weight peers	References
HUMAN:			
Collagen turnover:			
—urinary peptide-bound hydroxyproline (mg/kg/day)			
day 1	normal	lower	74
day 3	higher	normal	74, 75
—urinary glycosaminoglycan (μM/kg/day)			
day 3	higher	higher	76
Oxygen consumption (ml/kg)	similar or higher	higher	77, 78
Leukocyte energy capacity	lower	lower	79
Response to asphyxial stress (urinary steroids)	decreased	normal	80
Response to hypoglycaemic stress (urinary catecholamines)	normal, decreased		45, 81
Glucuronyl-transferase activity	normal	higher	50, 51
Gluconeogenesis	decreased		69, 82
Placenta:			
—energy capacity	normal		83
—oxygen consumption	decreased		84
—glucose utilisation	normal		85
RAT:			
Gluconeogenesis (production of glucose from alanine)	decreased		86
Liver fructose-1, 6-diphosphatase activity	slower postnatal increase		87

whereas glycogen utilisation[85] and energy capacity[83] are similar to that in placentas of normal infants.

Organ histology has been carefully studied in intra–uterine growth retarded humans and animals. In Figure 18.1, mean weight for each organ in each species in intra–uterine growth retarded offspring has been calculated from all the data available in the literature and expressed as percentage of weight in normally grown matures (full bars) and normally grown pre–terms (dotted bar) of the same body weight. It is clear that organs are variably affected according to species. The brain is the least affected of all organs. Weight of heart, kidneys, and adrenals are generally appropriate for body weight, but all organs are lighter when compared to either normally grown gestational or weight peers. Histologically, organ maturity is appropriate for gestational

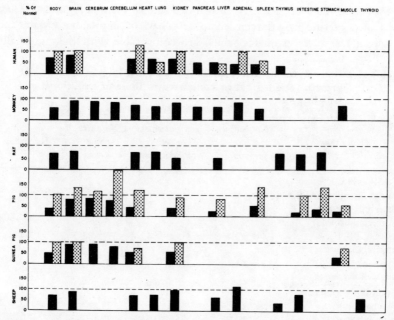

Figure 18.1 Weight of organs in intra-uterine growth retarded neonates (human and animal) compared with normally grown gestational (solid bars) and weight (stippled bars) peers[12, 15, 17, 57, 88-111]

age, but the cells are smaller[12, 15, 17, 57, 88-111, 177, 178]. In the pancreas, islets of Langerhans are decreased in size. In growth retarded rats, enzymatic activities are normal in brain, but diminished in most other organs[97].

Body and Organ Chemical Composition

The 'metabolic mass' (oxygen consumption/kg) relative to body weight in growth retarded neonates is similar to that of their gestational peers[77, 78]. Compared with their normally grown weight peers, however, growth retarded infants are hypermetabolic. Several explanations have been proposed: (1) metabolic mass is greater in intra-uterine growth retarded infants than in their weight peers (due to *reduced* extracellular water)[77], (2) recovery from malnutrition increases metabolic potential as a function of cell number rather than cell mass[78], (3) as brain has a high metabolic rate relative to other organs and the brain weight is least affected in intra-uterine growth retardation, a disproportionate excess of highly active 'metabolic tissue' is present in the growth retarded newborn[78], and/or (4) loss of metabolically-inactive intracellular water occurs[112]. As shown in Table 18.5 and in Figures 18.2 and 18.3, intra-uterine growth retarded neonates have mean total body water and extracellular water estimates which are comparable with their normally

Table 18.5 Body water estimates (mean ± 1 S.E., in ml/kg) in intra-uterine growth retarded babies contrasted to those of gestational and weight peers

Water space	Normally-grown premature	Intra-uterine growth retarded mature	Normally-grown mature	References
Total body water (antipyrine space, APS)★	809 ± 10.6	750 ± 13.0	688 ± 16.2	112
Extracellular water (corrected bromide space, CBS)★	432 ± 6.2	433 ± 8.1	371 ± 6.1	113, 114
Intracellular water (APS minus CBS)★	375 ± 15.1	379 ± 21.9	324 ± 17.1	112
$\dfrac{\text{Intracellular water}}{\text{Total body water}} \times 100$	46 ± 1.3	46 ± 2.0	47 ± 1.6	112
Plasma volume (albumin space)†	47 ± 0.8	48 ± 1.5	43 ± 1.5	115
	39 ± 2.7	53 ± 3.2	47 ± 2.3	116

★ Estimated within 24 hours of birth
† Estimated within 12 hours of birth

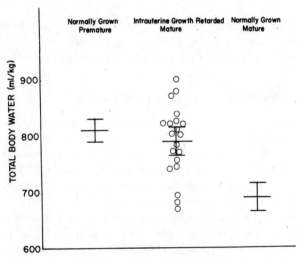

Figure 18.2 Total body water (ml per kg; mean ± 2 S.E.) in intra-uterine growth retarded neonates compared with normally grown gestational and weight peers[112]

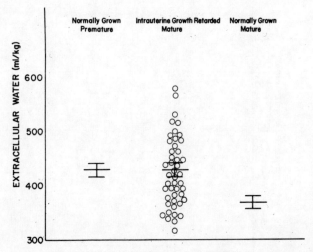

Figure 18.3 Extracellular water (ml per kg; mean ± 2 S.E.) in intra-uterine growth retarded neonates compared with normally grown gestational and weight peers[113, 114]

grown weight peers and significantly *higher* than their normally-grown gestational peers[112-114]. This contradicts theory (1) above—that intra-uterine growth retardation is accompanied by a decrease in extracellular water. Intracellular water estimates, whether expressed in reference to total body weight or in reference to total body water, vary neither with maturity nor with quality of growth[112] (Figure 18.4). Therefore, no loss of non-metabolising intracellular water occurs and Theory 4 is unlikely to be correct. Brain weight has been shown to be relatively normal in intra-uterine growth retarded infants[15, 57, 88-90] as well as in most animal models (Figure 18.1)[93-98, 101, 105-109, 111] and could certainly contribute to the increased metabolic rate. Too little data on total body cell number exist in both humans and animals to do more than speculate on the 'recovery effect'.

Dynamic changes after birth in certain portions of the extracellular compartment are of interest. Mean plasma volume (ml/kg) is identical to that for normal mature and premature peers if all measurements taken within 12 hours of birth are considered[115] (Figure 18.5). If measurements within four hours of birth are analysed alone, however, growth retarded neonates have significantly higher plasma volumes than their weight peers ($52 \cdot 0 \pm 2 \cdot 1$ *v.* $46 \cdot 2 \pm 1 \cdot 2$ ml/kg; $P < 0 \cdot 02$). A rather dramatic decline in plasma volume within four hours of birth therefore characterises the growth retarded newborn.

Total extracellular water is significantly increased in growth retarded

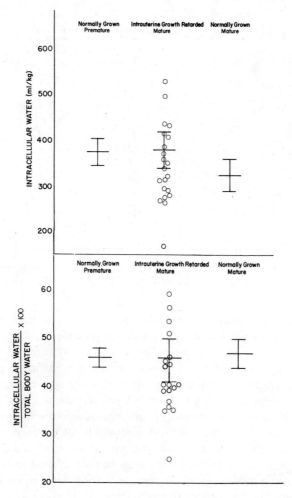

Figure 18.4 Intracellular water in ml/kg (upper graph) and intracellular water/total body water ratios (lower graph) in intra-uterine growth retarded neonates compared with normally grown gestational and weight peers[112] (mean ±2 S.E.)

newborns[113]. Skinfold measurements have been used not only to assess subcutaneous fat deposits but also to assess the amount of expressible material present in the skin[17, 179]. It has been theorised that expressible material was subcutaneous interstitial water. Recent work from our laboratory suggests that intra-uterine growth retarded neonates have the same amount of sub-cutaneous interstitial water as their gestational peers[17]. This finding is sup-

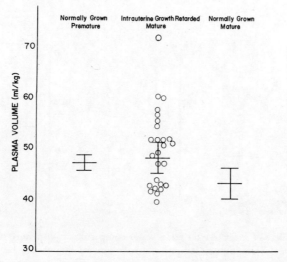

Figure 18.5 Plasma volume (ml/kg; mean ± 2 S.E.) in intra-uterine growth retarded neonates compared with normally grown gestational and weight peers[115]

ported by the work of Lugo *et al.* who found no differences in the proportion of water between eviscerated carcasses of intra-uterine growth retarded and normally grown rats[125]. On the other hand, analysis of *whole carcass* in the same animal model has revealed an increased proportion of total body water[122]. This suggests that selective water retention occurs in the visceral organs. Confirmation of this hypothesis was suggested by Younoszai and associates who showed that intra-uterine growth retarded rats indeed have an increased intestinal water content[102-103] while other organs show no difference.

Figure 18.6 summarises the effect of study age on body water compartments in normally grown and intra-uterine growth retarded mature neonates. It is provocative to note that in intra-uterine growth retarded infants values return to normal within 6 to 24 hours of birth.

The many similarities between intra-uterine growth retardation and post-natal malnutrition have been discussed at length, and the increased water spaces are not the least argument for similitude. This rapid return toward normal in extracellular water, however, is quite dissimilar to the more sluggish return toward normal (weeks to months) of the expanded water compartments which characterise postnatal protein-calorie malnutrition. It is well known that intra-uterine growth retarded newborns are more prone than others to perinatal asphyxia and their relative lack of subcutaneous fat increases the risk of cold stress at birth. The fact that a more rapid redistribution of water compartments toward normal occurs in growth retarded infants

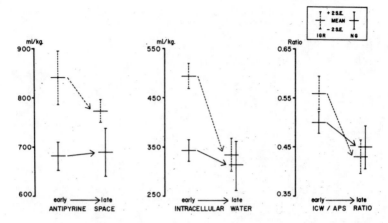

Figure 18.6 Effect of study age on body water compartments in mature study infants (mean ±2 S.E.). Solid figures indicate normally grown infants and broken figures indicate growth retarded infants. Studies within 6 hours of birth were considered 'early' while studies 6 to 24 hours after birth were considered 'late'. (Reproduced from[112]—with permission from the editor)

but not in their normally grown peers suggests that these postnatal changes are compatible with asphyxial impairment of cellular metabolism (so called 'sick-cell syndrome'). This reasoning can only remain speculative until concurrent body water and acid-base studies are performed.

Aside from information on water spaces in intra-uterine growth retarded neonates, little tissue data are currently available for fetal growth retarded babies. On the assumption that fingernail nitrogen reflects muscle or total body nitrogen and protein economy, we have analysed samples from a variety of neonates[123, 124]. Interestingly, normally grown infants, whether mature or pre-term, have a significantly higher mean fingernail nitrogen content than their intra-uterine growth retarded peers ($13 \cdot 3 \pm 1 \cdot 34$ v. $12 \cdot 3 \pm 1 \cdot 46$ gN/100 g sample; $P < 0 \cdot 005$). The difference seems to disappear after the third post-natal week. Further speculations concerning these results must await demonstration of a correlation between fingernail nitrogen and muscle proteins as well as qualitative identification and quantitation of these nitrogenous products.

Harpenden caliper measurements have also been used in neonates to estimate the amount of subcutaneous and total body fat[17]. Values for intra-uterine growth retarded infants deviate markedly from the mean expected for their gestational age but are normal for weight. Other authors[12, 92] have found that intra-uterine growth retarded neonates often have less subcutaneous fat than their normally grown weight peers.

For more detailed data on body composition we must turn toward animal models. Interest has recently emerged to biochemically determine cell number and cell size. The ground work for such determinations was performed by Enesco and Leblond who discovered that, in a given animal species, the nucleus of each cell contains the same amount of DNA[180]. Total DNA, therefore, provides a useful approximation of total cell number and the protein/DNA ratio allows an estimate of cell size. Figures 18.7 through 18.10 indicate the weight and composition of various organs in several

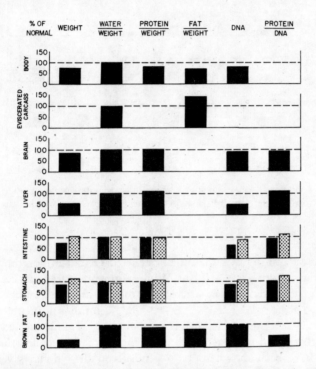

Figure 18.7 Whole body and individual chemical composition in intra-uterine growth retarded rats compared with normally grown gestational (solid bars) and weight (stippled bars) peers[87, 93, 95, 96, 99, 100, 102–104, 118, 122, 125, 127, 181]

animal species. Water, protein and fat are expressed in proportion to body weight. Total DNA content and protein/DNA ratio are also indicated. The most striking fact which emerges from these figures is the tremendous variability from species to species, indicating once again the hazards of extrapolation from animal to human. Of all organs studied, the brain arouses the

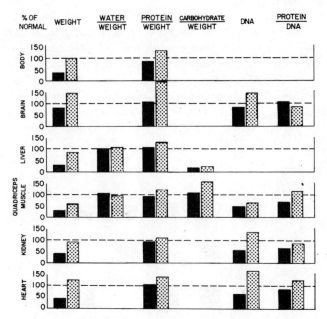

Figure 18.8 Body and organ chemical composition in intra-uterine growth retarded piglets compared with normally grown gestational (solid bars) and weight (stippled bars) peers[107, 109, 110]

most interest as it involves the future intellectual and neurological development of the growth retarded infant. While in most animal species brain is one of the least affected organs in intra-uterine malnutrition, cell number is often diminished[95, 96, 105, 107, 108, 111, 118, 127, 181] while cell size is normal[93, 95, 99, 105, 107, 108, 111, 127] and the cerebellum is commonly more severely affected than the cerebral cortex and brain stem[105, 108, 111]. The degree and the location of this damage have been shown to be dependent on the timing, severity and duration of the insult[111, 118, 119, 121, 130]. The faster the rate of cell division when the insult occurs, the more severe the reduction of brain cells is likely to be. Human data are extremely sparse but one study suggests that infants under-grown at birth have a 15% reduction in brain cell number[118, 182]. If we add to this intra-uterine insult a degree of postnatal malnutrition, the number of brain cells may be reduced as much as 60%. The importance of adequately feeding intra-uterine growth retarded neonates early after birth is obvious although we do not know whether the hoped-for recovery in cell number may occur in the human. Experiments in rats, however, suggest that adequate nutrition may lead to complete recovery if rehabilitation is begun before the end of the

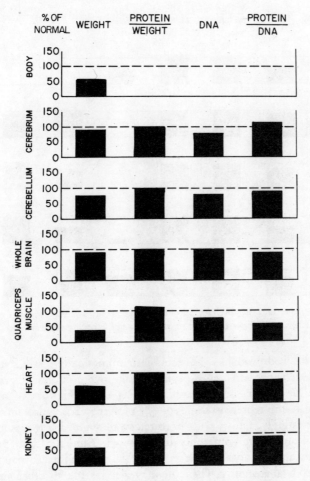

Figure 18.9 Whole body and individual organ chemical composition in intra-uterine growth retarded, newly-born guinea-pigs compared with normally grown gestational peers[108, 111]

normal cell division period[118, 131]. In the human, this would be about 14 months after conception[129, 182].

Fetal Nutrition and Malnutrition

Current knowledge concerning normal fetal nutrition has been summarised elsewhere[1]. One point is worth emphasising—swallowing and digestion of amniotic fluid protein by the human fetus have both been demonstrated.

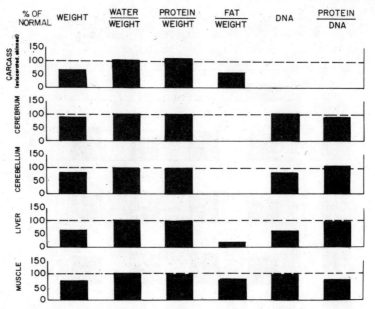

Figure 18.10 Body and organ chemical composition in intra-uterine growth retarded, newly-born Rhesus monkeys compared with normally grown gestational peers[105]

When ^{131}I-labelled proteins are injected into amniotic fluid, radioactivity is found in the fetal gut and tagged protein breakdown products are present in urine[183, 184]. Near term, the fetus swallows 0·24–0·30 g/kilo/day of amniotic fluid proteins—this represents some 10–15% of the newborn's protein requirements. Interestingly, fetuses with impaired swallowing due to oesophageal or intestinal atresia are commonly undergrown. Amniotic fluid proteins, though contributing only a small fraction of fetal protein intake, may well be important to fetal economy. The same may well be true for other nutrients. Although in the final analysis all nutrients must come from the mother, direct maternal–fetal transport via placenta may not be the sole source of fetal nutrition[1, 173]. The therapeutic implications of these facts demand intense, systematic investigation of this area.

Conclusions and Summary

The purpose of this chapter has been to review our present knowledge concerning intra-uterine growth and maturation of the deprived fetus. An even more important aspect of the discussion has been to reveal how little we really know about the undergrown fetus and how many important basic facts we have yet to uncover. The dangers of extrapolating animal data to humans have been stressed, but there are methods available or which could be developed to permit *in vivo* study of body composition in human neonates. Similarities between pre- and postnatal malnutrition have been pointed out[114], but basic differences are beginning to appear as more precise data are obtained. The contraction of cell size due to reduction of intracellular water as well as diminished total body solids in postnatal malnutrition have not been shown to be present in intra-uterine growth retardation. Furthermore, the rapid recovery of water compartments toward normal between 6 and 24 hours after birth pleads against simple protein-calorie malnutrition as the primary insult. The insight that amniotic fluid provides a significant fetal source of proteins as well as other nutrients, combined with the likely possibility of developing methods to allow prenatal diagnosis of impaired fetal growth, raise fascinating therapeutic possibilities. Prenatal nutrition of the fetus by injection of various nutrients into the amniotic fluid is no more impossible than treatment of haemolytic disease by intra-uterine transfusion. The number of intra-uterine growth retarded neonates born each year as well as the potential neuro-intellectual compromise in these children certainly justifies an intense commitment to research in this direction. But first and foremost we need more basic data.

References

1. Brans, Y. W. and Cassady, G. (1974). Fetal nutrition and body composition. In *Total Parenteral Alimentation: Premises and Promises* (Ghadimi, H., editor) (Philadelphia: J. Wiley and Sons)
2. Butler, N. R. and Bonham, D. G. (1963). *Perinatal Mortality: The First Report of the 1958 British Perinatal Mortality Survey* (London: E. and S. Livingstone Ltd.)
3. Lugo, G. and Cassady, G. (1971). Intrauterine growth retardation: clinicopathologic findings in 233 consecutive infants. *Amer. J. Obstet. Gynecol.*, **109**, 615
4. Vincent, M. and Hugon, J. (1962). Relationships between various criteria of maturity at birth. *Biol. Neonat.*, **4**, 223
5. Brans, Y. W. (Unpublished data)
6. Warkany, J., Monroe, B. B. and Sutherland, B. S. (1961). Intrauterine growth retardation. *Amer. J. Dis. Child.*, **102**, 249
7. Pick, W. (1954). Malnutrition of the newborn secondary to placental abnormalities. *New Engl. J. Med.*, **250**, 905
8. Wigglesworth, J. C. (1966). Foetal growth retardation. *Brit. Med. Bull.*, **22**, 13
9. Minkowski, A. and Lardinois, R. (1970). Détermination postnatale de l'âge gestationnel: âges cliniques, osseux, biologiques. In: *Journées Parisiennes de Pédiatrie*, p. 337 (Paris: Editions Médicales Flammarion)
10. Scott, K. E. and Usher, R. (1964). Epiphyseal development in foetal malnutrition syndrome. *New Engl. J. Med.*, **27**, 822

11. Scott, K. E. and Usher, R. (1966). Fetal malnutrition: its incidence, causes, and effects. *Amer. J. Obstet. Gynecol.*, **94,** 951

12. Usher, R. H. (1970). Clinical and therapeutic aspects of fetal malnutrition. *Pediat. Clin. N. Amer.*, **17,** 169

13. Usher, R., McLean, F. and Scott, K. E. (1966). Judgment of fetal age: II. Clinical significance of gestational age and an objective method for its assessment. *Pediat. Clin. N. Amer.*, **13,** 835

14. North, A. F. (1966). Small-for-dates neonates. I. Maternal, gestational, and neonatal characteristics. *Pediatrics*, **38,** 1013

15. Naeye, R. L. (1965). Malnutrition: probable cause of fetal growth retardation. *Arch. Path.*, **79,** 284

16. Silverman, W. A. and Sinclair, J. C. (1966). Infants of low birth weight. *New Engl. J. Med.*, **274,** 450

17. Brans, Y. W., Sumners, J. E., Dweck, H. S. and Cassady, G. (1974). A non-invasive approach to body composition in the newborn: dynamic skinfold measurements. *Pediat. Res.*, **8,** 215

18. Brett, E. M. (1965). The estimation of foetal maturity by the neurological examination of the neonate. In: *Clinics in Developmental Medicine*, Vol. 19, p. 105 (Dawkins, M. and McGregor, W. G., editors) (Lavenham: The Lavenham Press Ltd.)

19. Finnströmm, O. (1971). Studies on maturity in newborn infants. I. Birth weight, crown-heel length, head circumference and skull diameters in relation to gestational age. *Acta Paediat. Scand.*, **60,** 685

20. Holt, K. (1965). Age, growth, and maturity of the neonate. In: *Clinics in Developmental Medicine*, Vol. 19, p. 100 (Dawkins, M. and McGregor, W. G., editors) (Lavenham: The Lavenham Press Ltd.)

21. Lubchenco, L. O. (1970). Assessment of gestational age and development at birth. *Pediat. Clin. N. Amer.*, **17,** 125

22. Urrusti, J., Yoshida, P., Velasco, L., Frenk, S., Rosado, A., Sosa, A., Morales, M., Yoshida, T. and Metcoff, J. (1972). Human fetal growth retardation. I. Clinical features of sample with intrauterine growth retardation. *Pediatrics*, **50,** 547

23. Dylikowska-Gadomska, L. (1969). Zastosowanie polaczenia wagi urodzeniowej i wieku plodowego jako kryterium umownej dojrzalosci w praktycznej klasyfikacji noworodkow. *Ped. Pol.*, **44,** 1337

24. Dubowitz, L. M. S., Dubowitz, V. and Goldberg, C. (1970). Clinical assessment of gestational age in the newborn infant. *J. Pediat.*, **77,** 1

25. Finnström, O. (1972). Studies on maturity in newborn infants. II. External characteristics. *Acta Paediat. Scand.*, **61,** 24

26. Petrussa, I. (1971). A scoring system for the assessment of gestational age of newborn infants. In: *Proc. 2nd Eur. Cong. Perinat. Med.*, Huntingford, p. 247 (P. J. Beard, R. W. Hytten, F. E. and Scopes, J. W., editors) (Basel: S. Karger)

27. Minkowski, A., Saint-Anne Dargassies, S., Dreyfus-Brissac, C., Larroche, J. Cl., Vignaud, J. and Amiel, C. (1968). The assessment of foetal age by examination of the central nervous system. In: *Aspects of Praematurity and Dysmaturity*, p. 46 (Jonxis, J. H. P., Visser, H. K. A., Troelstra, J. A., editors) (Springfield: Charles C. Thomas)

28. Saint-Anne Dargassies, S. (1955). La maturation neurologique du prématuré. *Et. Néonat.*, **4,** 71

29. Saint-Anne Dargassies, S. (1970). Détermination neurologique de l'âge foetal néonatal. In: *Journées Parisiennes de Pédiatrie*, p. 311 (Paris: Editions Médicales Flammarion)

30. Robinson, R. J. (1966). Assessment of gestational age by neurological examination. *Arch. Dis. Childh.*, **41**, 437

31. Koenigsberger, M. R. (1966). Judgment of fetal age: neurological evaluation. *Pediat. Clin. N. Amer.*, **13**, 823

32. Amiel-Tison, C. (1968). Neurological evaluation of the maturity of newborn infants. *Arch. Dis. Childh.*, **43**, 89

33. Amiel-Tison, C. (1971). Neurological evaluation of the maturity of newborn infants. In: *Status of the Fetus*, p. 274 (Hellegers, A., editor). Report of the 2nd Ross Conference on Obstetric Research. (Columbus, Ohio: Ross Laboratories)

34. Dreyfus-Brisac, C. (1970). Maturation électroencéphalographique et âge conceptionnel. In: *Journées Parisiennes de Pédiatrie*, p. 327 (Paris: Editions Médicales Flammarion)

35. Dreyfus-Brisac, C., Flescher, J. and Plassart, E. (1962). L'électroencéphalogramme: critère d'âge conceptionnel du nouveau-né à terme et prématuré. *Biol. Neonat.*, **4**, 154

36. Schulte, J. F., Michaelis, R., Linke, I. and Nolte, R. (1968). Motor nerve conduction velocity in term, preterm and small-for-dates newborn infants. *Pediatrics*, **42**, 17

37. Engel, R. and Butler, B. V. (1963). Appraisal of conceptual age of newborn infants by electroencephalographic methods. *J. Pediat.*, **63**, 386

38. Graziani, L. T., Weitzman, E. D. and Velasco, M. S. A. (1968). Neurologic maturation and auditory evoked responses in low birth weight infants. *Pediatrics*, **41**, 483

39. Wilson, M. E., Myers, H. I. and Peter, A. H. (1967). Postnatal bone growth of infants with fetal growth retardation. *Pediatrics*, **40**, 213

40. Dylikowska-Gadomska, L. (1969). O Niektorych roznicach miedzy noworodkami z niska waga urodzeniowa donoszonymi a przedwczesnie urodzonymi. *Ped. Pol.*, **44**, 1347

41. Van den Berg, B. J. and Yerushalmy, J. (1966). The relationship of the rates of intra-uterine growth of infants of low birth weight to mortality, morbidity, and congenital anomalies. *J. Pediat.*, **69**, 531

42. Neligan, G. A., Robson, E. and Watson, J. (1963). Hypoglycaemia in the newborn: a sequel of intra-uterine malnutrition. *Lancet*, **i**, 1282

43. Lubchenco, L. O. and Bard, H. (1971). Incidence of hypoglycemia in newborn infants classified by birth weight and gestational age. *Pediatrics*, **47**, 831

44. Haworth, J. C., Dilling, L. and Younoszai, M. K. (1967). Relation of blood glucose to haematocrit, birth weight and other body measurements in normal and growth-retarded newborn infants. *Lancet*, **ii**, 901

45. Anagnostakis, D. E. and Lardinois, R. (1971). Urinary catecholamine excretion and plasma NEFA concentration in small-for-date infants. *Pediatrics*, **47**, 1000

46. Blum, D., Dodium, J., Loeb, H., Wilkin, P. and Hubinont, P. O. (1969). Studies on hypoglycaemia in small-for-dates newborns. *Arch. Dis. Childh.*, **44**, 304

47. Cornblath, M., Odell, G. B. and Levin, E. Y. (1959). Symptomatic neonatal hypo-glycaemia associated with toxemia of pregnancy. *J. Pediat.*, **55**, 545

48. Cornblath, M., Wybregt, S. H., Baens, G. S. and Klein, R. I. (1964). Symptomatic neonatal hypoglycemia: studies of carbohydrate metabolism in newborn infant. *Pediatrics*, **33**, 388

49. Scott, K. E., Usher, R. and McLean, F. (1963). Postnatal study of fetal malnutrition syndrome. *J. Pediat.*, **63**, 734, (abstract)

50. Trolle, D. (1965). A comparison between the incidence of jaundice of unknown

aetiology in premature and in underweight, full-term infants. *Danish Med. Bull.*, **12,** 35

51. Friis-Hansen, B. (1971). Care and hazards of the small-for-date infant. In: *Proc. 2nd Eur. Cong. Perinat. Med.*, p. 223 (Huntingford, P. J., Beard, R. W., Hytten, F. E. and Scopes, J. W., editors) (Basel: S. Karger)

52. Colman, H. I. and Rienzo, J. (1962). The small term baby. *Obstet. Gynecol.*, **19,** 87

53. Rumboltz, W. L. and McGoogan, L. S. (1953). Placental insufficiency and the small undernourished full-term infant. *Obstet. Gynecol.*, **1,** 294

54. McBurney, R. D. (1947). The undernourished full-term infant: a case report. *Western J. Surg.*, **55,** 363

55. Lubchenco, L. O., Searls, D. T. and Brazie, J. V. (1972). Neonatal mortality rate: relationship to birth weight and gestational age. *J. Pediat.*, **81,** 814

56. Yerushalmy, J., Van den Berg, B., Erhardt, C. L. and Jacobziner, H. J. (1965). Birth weight and gestation as indices of immaturity. *Amer. J. Dis. Childh.*, **109,** 43

57. Gruenwald, P. (1963). Chronic fetal distress and placental insufficiency. *Biol. Neonat.*, **5,** 215

58. Humbert, J. R., Abelson, H., Hathaway, W. E. and Battaglia, F. C. (1969). Polycythemia in small-for gestational age infants. *J. Pediat.*, **75,** 812

59. Lochridge, S., Pass, R. and Cassady, G. (1971). Reticulocyte counts in intra-uterine growth retardation. *Pediatrics*, **47,** 919

60. Finne, P. H. (1966). Erythropoietin levels in cord blood as an indicator of intra-uterine hypoxia. *Acta Paediat. Scand.*, **55,** 478

61. Hyvarinen, M., Zeltzer, P., Oh, W. and Stiehm, E. R. (1973). Influence of gestational age on serum levels of alpha-1-fetoprotein, IgG globulin and albumin in newborn infants. *J. Pediat.*, **82,** 430

62. Bergstrand, C. G., Karlsson, B. W., Lindberg, J. and Ekelund, H. (1972). Alpha-1-fetoprotein, albumin and total protein in serum from pre-term and term infants and small for gestational age infants. *Acta Paediat. Scand.*, **61,** 128

63. Papadatos, C., Papaevangelou, G., Alexiou, D. and Mendris, J. (1969). Immunoglobulin levels and gestational age. *Biol. Neonat.*, **14,** 365

64. Yeung, Y. C. and Hobbs, R. J. (1968). Serum gamma-G-globulin levels in normal premature, postmature and small-for-dates newborn babies. *Lancet*, **i,** 1167

65. Rubaltelli, F. F., Formentin, P. A. and Tato, L. (1970). Ammonia nitrogen urea and uric acid blood levels in normal and hypodystrophic newborns. *Biol. Neonat.*, **15,** 129

66. Rubaltelli, F. F. and Peratonen, L. (1969). Ammonia nitrogen in small-for-dates newborn babies. *Lancet*, **i,** 208

67. Robertson, A. F., Sprecher, H. W. and Wilcox, J. P. (1969). Total lipid fatty acid patterns of umbilical cord blood in intra-uterine growth failure. *Biol. Neonat.*, **14,** 28

68. Melichar, V. and Wolf, H. (1968). Glycerin und freie Fettsäuren im Blutplasma bei hypotrophen Neugeborenen. *Klin. Wchnschr.*, **46,** 549

69. Haymond, M., Karl, I. and Pagliara, A. (1973). Defective gluconeogenesis in small for gestational age infants. *J. Pediat.*, **83,** 153 (abstract)

70. Lindblad, B. S., Rahimtoola, R. J. and Khan, N. (1970). The venous plasma free amino acid levels during the first hours of life. II. In a lower socio-economic group of refugee area in Karachi, West Pakistan, with special reference to the small-for-dates syndrome. *Acta Paediat. Scand.*, **59,** 21

71. Mestyan, J., Fekete, M., Jarai, I., Sulyok, E., Imhof, S. and Soltesz, G. Y. (1969). The postnatal changes in the circulating free amino acid pool in the newborn

infant. II. The plasma amino acid ratio in intrauterine malnutrition (small-for-dates full-term, pre-term and twin infants). *Biol. Neonat.*, **14**, 164

72. Humbert, J. R. and Gotlin, R. W. (1971). Growth hormone levels in normo-glycaemic and hypoglycaemic infants born small for gestational age. *Pediatrics*, **48**, 190

73. Cornblath, M., Blankenship, W. J., Joassin, G., Parker, M. L. and Swiatek, K. R. Intrauterine growth and growth hormone.

74. Younoszai, M. K. and Haworth, J. C. (1968). Excretion of hydroxyproline in urine by premature and normal full-term infants and those with intra-uterine growth retardation during the first three days of life. *Pediat. Res.*, **2**, 17

75. Klujber, L., Mestyan, J., Sulyok, W. and Soltesz, G. (1972). Urinary hydroxy-proline excretion in normally-grown and growth retarded newborn infants. *Biol. Neonat.*, **20**, 196

76. Klujber, L. and Sulyok, E. (1972). Urinary glycosaminoglycan excretion in normally-grown and growth retarded neonates. I. Total glycosaminoglycan excretion. *Acta Paediat. Acad. Sci. Hung.*, **13**, 81

77. Sinclair, J. C. and Silverman, W. A. (1966). Intrauterine growth in active tissue mass of the human fetus with particular reference to the undergrown baby. *Pediatrics*, **38**, 48

78. Sinclair, J. C. (1970). Heat production and thermoregulation in the small-for-date infant. *Pediat. Clin. N. Amer.*, **17**, 147

79. Yoshida, T., Metcoff, J., Morales, M., Rosado, A., Sosa, A., Yoshida, P., Urrusti, J., Frenk, S. and Velasco, S. (1972). Human fetal growth retardation. II. Energy metabolism in leukocytes. *Pediatrics*, **50**, 559

80. Cathro, D. M., Forsyth, C. C. and Cameron, J. (1969). Adrenocortical response to stress in newborn infants. *Arch. Dis. Childh.*, **44**, 88

81. Stern, L., Sourkes, T. L. and Raiha, N. (1967). The role of the adrenal medulla in the hypoglycaemia of foetal malnutrition. *Biol. Neonat.*, **11**, 129

82. Dacou-Voutetakis, C., Anagnostakis, D., Nicolopoulos, D. and Matsaniotis, N. (1973). Small-for-dates neonates: evidence of defective gluconeogenesis for amino-acids. *Pediat. Res.*, **7**, 55 (abstract)

83. Rosado, A., Bernal, A., Sosa, A., Morales, M., Urrusti, J., Yoshida, P., Frenk, S., Velasco, L., Yoshida, T. and Metcoff, J. (1972). Human fetal growth retardation. III. Protein, DNA, RNA, adenine nucletotides and activities of the enzymes pyruvic and adenylate kinase in placenta. *Pediatrics*, **50**, 568

84. Tremblay, P. C., Sybulski, S. and Maughan, G. B. (1965). Role of the placenta in fetal malnutrition. *Amer. J. Obstet. Gynecol.*, **91**, 597

85. Sybulski, S. and Tremblay, P. C. (1969). Placental glycogen contents and utilisation *in vitro* in intrauterine malnutrition. *Amer. J. Obstet. Gynecol.*, **103**, 257

86. Nitzan, M. and Groffman, H. (1971). Hepatic gluconeogenesis and lipogenesis in experimental intra-uterine growth retardation in the rat. *Amer. J. Obstet. Gynecol.*, **109**, 623

87. Chanez, C., Tordet-Caridroit, C. and Roux, J. M. (1971). Studies on experimental hypotrophy in the rat. II. Development of some liver enzymes of gluconeogenesis. *Biol. Neonat.*, **18**, 58

88. Gruenwald, P. and Connell, J. N. (1958). Chronic fetal distress due to placental insufficiency. *Obstet. Gynecol.*, **12**, 712

89. Naeye, R. L. and Kelly, J. A. (1966). Judgment of fetal age: the pathologist's evaluation. *Pediat. Clin. N. Amer.*, **13**, 849

90. Naeye, R. L. (1966). Abnormalities in infants of mothers with toxemia of pregnancy. *Amer. J. Obstet. Gynecol.*, **95**, 276

91. Naeye, R. L. (1965). Cardiovascular abnormalities in infants malnourished before birth. *Biol. Neonat.*, **8**, 104

92. McLean, F. and Usher, R. (1970). Measurements of liveborn fetal malnutrition infants compared with similar gestation and with similar birth weight normal controls. *Biol. Neonat.*, **16**, 215

93. Oh, W. and Guy, J. A. (1971). Cellular growth in experimental intrauterine growth retardation. *J. Nutr.*, **101**, 1631

94. Zeman, F. J. (1968). Effects of maternal protein restriction on the kidney of the newborn young of rats. *J. Nutr.*, **94**, 111

95. Zeman, F. J. and Stangrough, F. C. (1969). Effect of maternal protein deficiency on cellular development in the fetal rat. *J. Nutr.*, **99**, 274

96. Roux, J. M., Tordet-Caridroit, C. and Chanez, C. (1970). Studies on experimental hypotrophy in the rat. *Biol. Neonat.*, **15**, 342

97. Shrader, R. E. and Zeman, F. J. (1969). Effect of maternal protein deprivation on morphological and enzymatic development of neonatal rat tissue. *J. Nutr.*, **99**, 401

98. Wigglesworth, J. C. (1964). Experimental growth retardation in the fetal rat. *J. Pathol. Bacteriol.*, **88**, 1

99. Roux, J. M. (1971). Studies on cellular development in the suckling rat with intrauterine growth retardation. *Biol. Neonat.*, **18**, 290

100. Oh, W., D'Amodio, M. D., Yap, L. L. and Hohenauer, L. (1970). Carbohydrate metabolism in experimental intra-uterine growth retardation in rats. *Amer. J. Obstet. Gynecol.*, **108**, 415

101. Myers, R. E., Hill, D. E., Cheek, D. B., Holt, A. B., Scott, R. E. and Mellits, E. D. (1971). Fetal growth retardation produced by experimental placental insufficiency in the Rhesus monkey. I. Body weight, organ size. *Biol. Neonat.*, **18**, 379

102. Younoszai, M. K. (1971). Growth of the small intestine in intra-uterine growth retarded and normal rat pups. *Pediat. Res.*, **5**, 386 (abstract)

103. Younoszai, M. K. and Ranshaw, J. C. Perinatal gastrointestinal growth: effects of maternal dietary protein. (Personal communication)

104. Cogneville, A. and Tordet-Caridroit, C. (1972). Étude de la composition chimique du tissu adipeux brun interscapulaire au cours du développement chez le rat ayant subi un retard de croissance intra-utérine. *C.R. Acad. Sci. Paris*, **275**, 2695

105. Hill, D. E., Myers, R. E., Holt, A. B., Scott, R. E. and Cheek, D. B. (1971). Fetal growth retardation produced by experimental placental insufficiency in the Rhesus monkey. II. Chemical composition of the brain, liver, muscle, and carcass. *Biol. Neonat.*, **19**, 68

106. Creasy, R. K., Barrett, C. T., de Swiet, M., Kahanpää, K. V. and Rudolph, A. M. (1972). Experimental intrauterine growth retardation in the sheep. *Amer. J. Obstet. Gynecol.*, **112**, 566

107. Dickerson, J. W. T., Merat, A. and Widdowson, E. M. (1971). Intra-uterine growth retardation in the pig. III. The chemical structure of the brain. *Biol. Neonat.*, **19**, 354

108. Widdowson, E. M. (1971). Protein status of small-for-date animals. In: *Metabolic Processes in the Foetus and Newborn*, p. 165 (Jonxis, J. H. P., Visser, H. K. A. and Troelstra, J. A., editors) (Leiden: H. E. Stenfert Kroese)

109. Widdowson, E. M. (1971). Intra-uterine growth retardation in the pig. I. Organ size and cellular development at birth and after growth to maturity. *Biol. Neonat.*, **19**, 329

110. Adams, P. H. (1971). Intra-uterine growth retardation in the pig. II. Development of the skeleton. *Biol. Neonat.*, **19**, 341
111. Chase, H. P., Dabiere, C. S., Welch, N. N. and O'Brien, D. (1971). Intrauterine undernutrition and brain development. *Pediatrics*, **47**, 491
112. Cassady, G. and Milstead, R. R. (1971). Antipyrine space studies and cell water estimates in infants of low birth weight. *Pediat. Res.*, **5**, 673
113. Cassady, G. (1970). Bromide space studies in infants of low birth weight. *Pediat. Res.*, **4**, 14
114. Cassady, G. (1970). Body composition in intra-uterine growth retardation. *Pediat. Clin. N. Amer.*, **17**, 79
115. Cassady, G. (1966). Plasma volume studies in low birth weight infants. *Pediatrics*, **38**, 1020
116. Usher, R. A. and Lind, J. (1965). Blood volume of the newborn premature infant. *Acta Paediat. Scand.*, **54**, 419
117. Bielecka-Winnicka, A. (1966). Hydration in tissues of newborns with too-low weight at birth. *Ann. Paediat.*, **207**, 125
118. Brasel, J. A. and Winick, M. (1972). Maternal nutrition and prenatal growth: experimental studies of effects of maternal undernutrition on fetal placental growth. *Arch. Dis. Childh.*, **47**, 479
119. Chase, H. P., Dorsey, J. and McKahn, G. M. (1967). The effect of malnutrition on the synthesis of a myelin lipid. *Pediatrics*, **40**, 551
120. Chase, H. P., Welch, N. N., Dabiere, C. S., Vasan, N. S. and Butterfield, L. J. (1972). Alterations in human brain biochemistry following intrauterine growth retardation. *Pediatrics*, **50**, 403
121. Dobbing, J. (1965). The effect of undernutrition on myelination in the central nervous system. *Biol. Neonat.*, **9**, 132
122. Hohenauer, L. and Oh, W. (1969). Body composition in experimental intrauterine growth retardation in the rat. *J. Nutr.*, **99**, 23
123. Lockard, W., Brans, Y., Sumners, J., Dweck, H. and Cassady, G. (1973). Fingernail nitrogen accretion in the fetus and newborn. *Pediat. Res.*, **7**, 176 (abstract)
124. Lockard, D., Pass, R. and Cassady, G. (1972). Fingernail nitrogen content in neonates. *Pediatrics*, **49**, 618
125. Lugo, G., O'Neill, L. and Cassady, G. (1971). Carcass water, fat and chloride in the fetal growth-retarded rat. *Amer. J. Obstet. Gynecol.*, **110**, 358
126. Younoszai, M. K., Kacie, A., Dilling, L. and Haworth, J. C. (1969). Urinary hydroxyproline/creatinine ratio in normal, term, pre-term and growth retarded infants. *Arch. Dis. Childh.*, **44**, 517
127. Zamenhof, S., Van Marthen, E. and Margolis, F. L. (1968). DNA (cell number) and protein in neonatal brain alteration by maternal dietary restriction. *Science*, **160**, 322
128. Young, M. and Prenton, M. (1969). Maternal and foetal plasma amino acid concentrations during gestation and in retarded foetal growth. *J. Obstet. Gynaecol. Brit. Commonw.*, **76**, 333
129. Winick, M. (1959). Malnutrition and brain development. *J. Pediat.*, **74**, 667
130. Benton, J. W., Maser, H. W., Dodge, P. R. and Carr, S. (1956). Modification of the schedule of myelination in the rat by early nutritional deprivation. *Pediatrics*, **38**, 801
131. Winick, M., Fish, I. and Rosso, P. (1958). Cellular recovery in rat tissues after a brief period of neonatal malnutrition. *J. Nutr.*, **95**, 623

132. Winick, M. and Noble, A. (1956). Cellular response in rats during malnutrition at various ages. *J. Nutr.*, **89,** 300

133. Lindblad, B. F. (1971). The plasma aminogram in small-for-date newborn infants, p. 111. In: *Metabolic Processes in the Foetus and Newborn Infants.* (Leiden: H. E. Stenfert Kroese)

134. Lindblad, B. F. (1970). The venous plasma free amino acid level during the first hours of life. *Acta Paediat. Scand.*, **59,** 13

135. Eisengart, M. A. (1970). Reflex arc latency measurements in newborn infants and children. *Pediatrics*, **46,** 28

136. Ellis, R. W. B. and Lawley, D. N. (1951). Assessment of prematurity by birth weight, crown-rump length and head circumference. *Arch. Dis. Childh.*, **26,** 411

137. Bergstrom, A. L., Gunther, M. B., Olow, I. and Söderling, B. (1955). Prematurity and pseudo-prematurity. Studies of the developmental age in underweight newborns. *Acta Paediat. Scand.*, **44,** 519

138. Brody, S. (1958). The intra-uterine age of the foetus at birth. *Acta Obstet. Gynecol. Scand.*, **37,** 374

139. Brody, S. (1960). Further studies on the reliability of a new method for the determination of the duration of pregnancy. *J. Obstet. Gynaecol. Brit. Emp.*, **67,** 819

140. Parmelee, A. H., Stern, E., Chervin, G. and Minkowski, A. (1964). Gestational age and the size of premature infants. *Biol. Neonat.*, **6,** 309

141. Farr, V., Kerridge, D. F. and Mitchell, R. G. (1966). The value of some external characteristics in the assessment of gestational age at birth. *Develop. Med. Child. Neurol.*, **8,** 657

142. Farr, V., Mitchell, R. G., Neligan, G. A. and Parkin, J. M. (1966). The definition of some external characteristics used in the assessment of gestational age in the newborn infant. *Develop. Med. Child. Neurol.*, **8,** 507

143. Labhardt, A. (1927). Zur Frage der Schwangerschaftsdauer, *Schweiz. Med. Wchnschr.* **57,** 729

144. Labhardt, A. (1944). Die Berechnung des Konzeptionstermines der Kinderslänge in Vaterschaftsprozessen. *Schweiz. Med. Wchnschr.*, **74,** 128

145. Farr, V. (1966). Skinfold thickness as an indicator of maturity of the newborn. *Arch. Dis. Childh.*, **41,** 301

146. Gleiss, J. and Hermanns, M. (1969). Ektodermale Kriterien zur klinischen Reifesbestimmung Neugeborener. *Arch. Kinderheilk.*, **179,** 266

147. Mitchell, R. G. and Farr, V. (1965). The meaning of maturity and the assessment of maturity at birth. In: *Clinics in Developmental Medicine*, Vol. 19, p. 83 (Dawkins, M. and McGregor, W. G., editors) (Lavenham: The Lavenham Press Ltd.)

148. Damoulaki-Sfakianiaki, E., Robertson, A. and Cordero, L. (1972). Skin creases and maturity: Caucasian and negro infants. *Pediatrics*, **50,** 483

149. Finnström, O. (1972). Studies on maturity in newborn infants. VI. Comparison between different methods for maturity estimation. *Acta Paediat. Scand.*, **61,** 33

150. Christie, A. (1949). Prevalence and distribution of ossification centers in newborn infants. *Amer. J. Dis. Child.*, **77,** 355

151. Berridge, F. R. and Eton, B. (1958). The accuracy of radiological estimation of foetal maturity. *J. Obstet. Gynaecol. Brit. Commonw.*, **65,** 625

52. Blom, S. and Finnström, O. (1968). Motor conduction velocities in newborn infants of various gestational ages. *Acta Paediat. Scand.*, **57,** 377

153. Dubowitz, V., Whittaker, G. F., Brown, B. H. and Robinson, A. (1968). Nerve conduction velocity—an index of neurological maturity of the newborn infant. *Develop. Med. Child. Neurol.*, **10**, 741

154. Ellingson, R. J. (1958). Electroencephalograms of normal, full-term newborns immediately after birth with observations on arousal and visual evoked responses. *Electroencephalography and Clin. Neurophysiol.*, **10**, 31

155. Kirschbaum, T. H. (1962). Fetal hemoglobin content of cord blood determined by column chromatography. *Amer. J. Obstet. Gynecol.*, **84**, 1375

156. Desmond, M. M. and Sweet, L. K. (1949). Relation of plasma proteins to birth weight, multiple birth and edema in the newborn. *Pediatrics*, **4**, 484

157. Gitlin, D. and Boesman, M. (1966). Serum alpha-fetoprotein, albumin and gamma-globulin in the human conceptus. *J. Clin. Invest.*, **45**, 1826

158. Saito, M., Gittleman, I. F., Pincus, J. B. and Sobel, A. E. (1956). Plasma protein patterns in premature infants of varying weights on the first day of life. *Pediatrics*, **17**, 657

159. Thom, H., McKay, E. and Gray, D. W. G. (1967). Protein concentrations in the umbilical cord plasma of premature and mature infants. *Clin. Sci.*, **33**, 433

160. Nörgaard-Pedersen, B. (1973). Alpha-1-fetoprotein concentration in cord serum as a parameter for gestational age. *Acta Paediat. Scand.*, **62**, 167

161. Berg, J. (1968). Immunoglobulin levels in infants with low birth weight. *Acta Paediat. Scand.*, **57**, 369

162. Hobbs, R. J. and Davis, A. J. (1967). Serum gamma-G-globulin levels and gestational age in premature babies. *Lancet*, **i**, 757

163. King, J. and Morris, B. M. (1961). Serum enzyme activities in the normal newborn infant. *Arch. Dis. Childh.*, **36**, 604

164. Townes, P. L. and Ferrari, B. T. (1972). Pepsinogen 7 as an indicator of neonatal maturity: preliminary studies. *J. Pediat.*, **80**, 815

165. Eggermont, E. (1966). Enzymic activities in meconium from human foetuses and newborns. *Biol. Neonat.*, **10**, 266

166. Sell, E. J. and Corrigan, J. J. (1973). Platelet counts, fibrinogen concentrations, and factor V and factor VIII levels in healthy infants according to gestational age. *J. Pediat.*, **82**, 1028

167. Whitehead, R. G. (1957). Biochemical tests for assessing subclinical nutrition deficiency. *Clin. Pediat.*, **6**, 516

168. Whitehead, R. G. (1957). Biochemical tests in differential diagnosis of protein and calories deficiencies. *Arch. Dis. Childh.*, **42**, 479

169. Whitehead, R. G. (1954). Rapid determination of some amino acids in subclinical kwashiorkor. *Lancet*, **i**, 250

170. Kivirikko, K. I., Koivusalo, M. and Koivusalo, P. (1963). Free and bound hydroxyproline in the human amniotic fluid in early and full-term pregnancy. *Ann. Chir. Gynaecol. Fenn.*, **52**, 350

171. Shah, S. I., Alderman, M., Queenan, J. K., Brase, J. and Winick, M. (1972). Nondialyzable peptide-bound hydroxyproline in human amniotic fluid: an indicator of fetal growth. *Amer. J. Obstet. Gynecol.*, **114**, 250

172. Wharton, B. A., Foulds, J. W., Frazier, I. D. and Pennock, C. A. (1971). Amniotic fluid total hydroxyproline and intrauterine growth. *J. Obstet. Gynaecol. Brit. Commonw.*, **78**, 791

173. Cassaday, G. (1974). Amniocentesis. *Clin. Perinat.*, **1**, 87

174. Nörgaard-Pedersen, B., Klebe, J. G. and Grunnet, M. (1971). Carbonic anhydrase

activity in cord blood from infants of diabetic and non-diabetic mothers. *Biol. Neonat.*, **19,** 389

175. Shelley, H. J. (1964). Carbohydrate reserves in the newborn infant. *Brit. Med. J.*, **1,** 273

176. Shelley, H. J. and Neligan, G. A. (1966). Neonatal hypoglycaemia. *Brit. Med. Bull.*, **22,** 34

177. Larroche, J. C., Herissard, N. and Benoun, M. (1971). Hepatic hematopoiesis in hypotrophic rats. Comparison to growth-retarded infants. *Biol. Neonat.*, **18,** 279

178. Naeye, R. L. (1970). Structural correlates of fetal undernutrition. In: *Fetal Growth and Development*, p. 241 (Waisman, H. A. and Kerr, G. R., editors) (New York: McGraw-Hill Book Company)

179. Sumners, J., Brans, Y., Dweck, H., Lockard, W. and Cassady, G. (1973). A non-invasive approach to body composition in the newborn: dynamic skinfold measurements. *Pediat. Res.*, **7,** 179 (abstract)

180. Enesco, M. and Leblond, C. P. (1962). Increase in cell number as a factor in the growth of the organs and tissues of the young male rat. *J. Embryol. Exp. Morph.*, **10,** 530

181. Winick, M. (1970). Cellular growth in intra-uterine malnutrition. *Pediat. Clin. N. Amer.*, **17,** 69

182. Winick, M. (1972). Cellular growth during early malnutrition. *Pediatrics*, **47,** 969

183. Bangham, D. R. (1960). The transmission of homologous serum proteins to the fetus and to the amniotic fluid in the Rhesus monkey. *J. Physiol.*, **153,** 265

184. Gitlin, D., Kumata, J., Morales, C., Noriegea, L. and Arevalo, N. (1972). The turnover of amniotic fluid protein in the human conceptus. *Amer. J. Obstet. Gynec.*, **113,** 632

185. Schulman, J. D., Queenan, J. K. and Doores, L. (1972). Chromatographic analysis of concentration of amino acids in amniotic fluid from early, middle and late period of human gestation. *Amer. J. Obstet. Gynecol.*, **114,** 243

The authors gratefully acknowledge the artistic talents of ·Mrs P. Bailey and the typographical skills of Miss P. Shook.

CHAPTER 19

The Relation of Deprivation to Perinatal Pathology and Late Sequels

Peter Gruenwald

Acute, subacute, and chronic deprivation, alone or in combination, produce a wide variety of abnormal states. When a viable infant is born in poor condition or stillborn, acute fetal distress perhaps aggravated by earlier deprivation, is the cause in the majority of instances. Clinical and pathological observations suggest a non-specific, shock-like state. At necropsy, a variety of more or less characteristic lesions are seen; their significance is principally that of indicators of severe, acute perinatal distress. This will be discussed in the first portion of the present chapter, along with related placental pathology.

When an infant survives a stormy neonatal course as a result of acute, non-specific distress, a variety of severe abnormalities may ensue; this is not within the province of the present discussion. However, many neonates who had suffered subacute or chronic fetal distress, are born in good condition because they were not severely affected by the birth process. These may show the effects of early and protracted prenatal deprivation in later months and years. Among them are particularly the small-for-dates infants. These late sequels will be reviewed in the second section of this chapter.

Relationships and comparisons of the effects of pre-term and small-for-dates birth need to be considered, not only because both concern infants of low birth weight who need to be differentiated, but also because immaturity and fetal deprivation are the two most important non-specific causes of perinatal damage and late sequels, as opposed to such specific conditions as malformation or fetal disease (infection, isoimmunisation, etc.).

Perinatal and Placental Pathology

It has been claimed that systematic pathological investigation of all perinatal deaths by necropsy would disclose the cause of death in the great majority of instances, and thus lead to preventive or curative measures. Examination of the placenta should, of course, be part of this; it can, in addition, be carried out in cases of non-fatal morbidity in the neonatal period.

First, specific pathological conditions must be identified, such as the large groups of malformation and fetal disease (including infections, isoimmunisation, etc.). Malformations seen externally or at necropsy, need to be recorded with a view to counselling when the parents contemplate further pregnancies. If death was not preventable because of malformation, this enters into the retrospective evaluation of management of pregnancy, labour, and the neonatal period. Fetal disease due to isoimmunisation, maternal diabetes, or infection must be recognised by gross and microscopic examination. Intra-uterine growth retardation is common in malformed and chronically infected infants. As was mentioned in Chapter 1, this must not be chalked up to deprivation.

The placenta may show microscopic evidence of acute or chronic infection. In haemolytic disease of the newborn due to Rh-isoimmunisation the large, soft placenta occurs only in severe cases usually with hydrops fetalis. Vernix granulomas of the amnion indicate oligohydramnios due to urinary tract malformation in the majority of cases; the remainder had prolonged leakage of amniotic fluid. These placental changes, as well as the significance of leukocytic infiltration or a single artery in the umbilical cord, are reviewed in Chapter 15.

There remain now for consideration the two largest groups of perinatal death and morbidity: (1) immaturity, and (2) stress at birth caused by hypoxia which may aggravate pre-existing deprivation, including also an ever-shrinking group of cases of mechanical birth trauma with which we are not concerned here. *Immaturity* cannot be defined strictly in terms of gestational age since maturation has many facets and is a gradual process. In the extreme form the fetus is unable to survive without the protection and supply by uterus and placenta. Beyond that there is a wide range of gestational age during which an otherwise unencumbered fetus can survive if proper conditions are provided, but is unduly liable to a variety of unfavourable influences. This, sometimes in combination with perinatal distress, may lead to characteristic pathological entities such as intraventricular cerebral haemorrhage, hyperbilirubinaemia unassociated with isoimmunisation, or atelectasis with hyaline membranes and inadequate functional residual capacity of the lungs (the respiratory distress syndrome), all of which rarely affect mature neonates. Inadequate adaptation to extrauterine life without any of these characteristic changes leads to a reasonable and realistic necropsy diagnosis of immaturity. (This opinion is not shared by all perinatal pathologists.) Reliable recognition of immaturity by microscopic examination of the placenta is difficult in an intermediate time zone when gestation approaches term. Maturity of the terminal villi by the usual criteria (see Chapters 12 and 14) varies to some extent among pregnancies, and even within one placenta from area to area.

Acute perinatal distress occurs during the birth process, or immediately preceding ante-partum fetal death. It is caused largely by deprivation as a result of reduction of the maternal supply line by compression of utero-placental vessels during uterine contractions, and perhaps also by maternal exertion. Rarely there are such added complications as compression of the umbilical cord, or maternal haemorrhage due to placenta praevia. Acute abruption of the placenta will be discussed later in this chapter. Fetal haemorrhage from laceration of the placenta or vasa previa is a special case. Small numbers of fetal erythrocytes are frequently demonstrable in maternal blood during pregnancy; larger haemorrhages into the maternal circulation may occur during the birth process, and may cause maternal isoimmunisation affecting subsequent pregnancies. Most of these complications which add to the stress of birth, are recognised by the obstetrical history more readily than by examination of the placenta. In the neonate, however, some changes caused by acute perinatal distress are sufficiently spectacular to be considered by some as 'causes of death' in their own right; this accounts for the high proportion of demonstrable 'causes' reported by some. They include, among others, 'abnormal pulmonary ventilation'[1], aspiration of vernix caseosa or meconium into the lungs, haemorrhage into the adrenals, and intraventricular cerebral haemorrhage. The latter two conditions have been mistaken for effects of mechanical trauma. The significance of atelectasis with hyaline membranes (the respiratory distress syndrome) is not clear: some believe that it is related to a form of fetal distress in addition to the above mentioned association with immaturity. Other manifestations of perinatal distress which bear some resemblance to shock lesions, include degeneration of the liver which may culminate in multifocal necrosis, heart failure as evident by dilatation of the ventricles and fatty change of the myocardium, necrosis in the adrenal cortex, esophagitis with ulceration and bleeding, and degeneration in various parts of the brain. These lesions become prominent when the infant survives for several hours after birth. What makes all this potentially significant to our considerations of the placenta, is the relationship to deprivation. If all the lesions mentioned in this paragraph are classified in the analysis of perinatal mortality as items under the heading 'perinatal distress', then attention is drawn to the characteristic shock-like perinatal syndrome with a possible relationship to deprivation. Much of this is presumably due to conditions imposed by labour and thus will not leave characteristic marks in the placenta, but a fetus with a previously compromised supply line is more likely to be severely affected. In addition to marks left in the placenta by maternal circulatory disturbances (Chapter 12), yellow meconium staining of the entire fetal surface (in contrast to spots with the green colour of fresh meconium) indicates distress of some duration.

It now remains to examine the relationship of pathological findings to chronic or subacute fetal distress. This must also include, in addition to the above mentioned pathological lesions, changes in the proportions of weights and measurements of the total body and certain organs. Reliably determined weights and measurements are a very important part of perinatal necropsies. Chronic fetal distress is caused by deprivation of a severity and duration sufficient to result in a small-for-dates infant. This has been defined by a birth weight below mean minus two standard deviations for the respective gestational age (Chapter 1). At the first glance it may seem surprising that the external body proportions of small-for-dates infants do not differ significantly from those of normally grown pre-term infants of similar weight. This is due to the fact that growth slowed and perhaps stopped entirely at a time when no significant amount of subcutaneous fat tissue had developed and also the muscle mass was not very large, so that wasting as a result of deprivation could not occur. Both length and head circumference of small-for-dates infants are on the average 1 cm greater than those of pre-term infants, which is well within the range of variation, and error of measurement[2]. Since deprivation affects maturation much less than growth, the small-for-dates infant shows a wide discrepancy between its body size and its maturity as determined by examination of the living neonate (see Chapter 18), or at post-mortem examination by histological study of organs such as the brain, lungs and kidneys.

Growth retardation affects parts of the body in a characteristic pattern which has been known for a long time. When average organ weights of pre-term and small-for-dates neonates of similar body weight are compared, the brain of the latter is 24% heavier than that of pre-term infants, whereas the liver and thymus are lighter (that is, even more deficient than body weight) by 12% and 24%, respectively. Other organs are less affected[3] (Figure 19.1). The validity of two different patterns depending, respectively, on nutritional and circulatory deficiency[4], is questionable. The small-for-dates condition due to chronic fetal distress can often be recognised at the necropsy table by body and organ weights, combined with development of cerebral convolution out of proportion to body weight, even more readily than by micro-

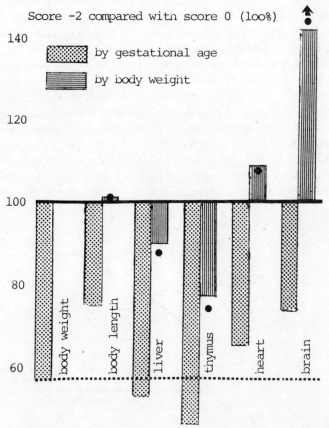

Figure 19.1 Body weight and length and organ weights of small-for-dates infants (score − 2) compared with normally grown (score 0) pre-term infants of similar weight, or gestational age; values of the latter are considered as 100%. The dots give as an example data from the necropsy of one small-for-dates infant.

scopic study (Figure 19.1). The pathologist's ability to make this diagnosis is of practical importance: if an obstetrician terminates a pregnancy resulting in a small infant on grounds of potentially fatal deprivation and growth failure and the infant dies, it should be possible to demonstrate that the infant was not a normally grown pre-term one that should have remained *in utero*.

The placenta in these cases will frequently fail to show any characteristic changes. This is understandable when one remembers that the placenta itself is seldom the primary cause of chronic deprivation. (Chapters 1, 12). Only a small minority of small-for-dates infants have a placenta which is very extensively affected by infarcts, longstanding premature separation, or is excessively small in size. Even some of these changes are caused by maternal circulatory abnormalities and are thus not primarily placental in origin.

In subacute fetal distress growth proceeds normally for a longer period of time. When deprivation becomes severe, days up to a few weeks before birth, and particularly when this happens at or after term, growth has proceeded so far that a deficiency in body length cannot be demonstrated. However, wasting can now occur since considerable amounts of subcutaneous fat tissue and muscle had been formed, and the result is the 'long, thin baby'. The relationship of body weight and length as characterised best by an index relating weight to the third power of length, is abnormal (Figure 19.2), and when the condition is sufficiently severe the appearance may be quite

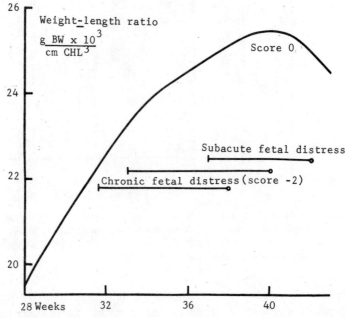

Figure 19.2 Ratio of birth weight to the third power of crown-heel length for neonates with a birth weight within 1 standard deviation from the mean for gestational age (score 0). Data for groups of small-for-dates infants (score − 2), and a representative case of subacute fetal distress are shown by dots in a circle. The horizontal lines connect these with the points on which they would fall if gestational age were commensurate with their actual birth weight. (From Gruenwald, P. (1968). Growth pattern of the normal and the deprived fetus. In: *Aspects of praematurity and dysmaturity* (J. H. P. Jonxis, H. K. A. Visser and J. A. Troelstra, editors), by permission of Stenfert Kroese, Leiden)

spectacular. Characteristic subacute fetal distress occurs most frequently in pregnancies that are prolonged past term. Such infants have been characterised as postmature even though it is well known that the majority of infants born after similarly prolonged gestation do not show severe wasting. It is equally well known that fetal growth begins to decelerate before term, and the abnormally wasted post-term infant represents but one end of a spectrum of variations in the decline of adequacy of the supply line. There are no placental changes characteristic of subacute fetal distress, but there may be visible indications of ageing or a declining maternal supply line (Chapter 12). Empirical standards of fetal growth based on birth weights, include some reduction of fetal growth about term as normal. Yet even fetuses born past term with a body weight within one standard deviation from the empirical mean, show in the growth of their organs a pattern which in its trends is that of deprivation[5] (Figure 11.1). If one wishes to apprehend the entire extent of growth inhibition past term, both in average fetuses and the 'long, thin' babies, one should use extrapolated fetal growth standards as described in Chapter 1.

Body weight deficit in subacute fetal distress is of a magnitude which will not usually place a neonate in the small-for-dates category. So far no objective criteria have been used consistently to define the wasted baby that has suffered subacute distress. The Rohrer index relating weight to length, and skin fold thickness should be used to work out such standards and determine, for instance, whether an infant born with a seemingly respectable weight of a little over 3000 g had in fact lost weight as a result of late deprivation. Figure 19.2 shows the normal changes of the weight–length ratio as well as those in chronic and subacute fetal distress (open and solid circles). When these are transposed to the left to points where they would be if the gestational age were commensurate with the actual weight, those for chronic, but not those for subacute fetal distress approach normal ratios[3].

Acute perinatal distress causing the pathological changes described above, is not characteristically superimposed upon chronic fetal distress. The reason is not known, but it may be suspected that the combination of small body size and advanced maturity is favourable during the birth process. Subacute distress is fairly frequently associated with lesions commonly attributed to acute distress, such as aspiration of vernix caseosa or degeneration in various organs. Then there are those infants who were not known or suspected of chronic or subacute distress, and suffer acutely during the birth process, sometimes leading to intra-partum death. It may be surmised that among them are some whose supply line had been marginally inadequate and was therefore more vulnerable to further reduction during the birth process. The questions of the effect of labour on a previously compromised supply line was discussed above in Chapter 9. No characteristic changes can be expected to occur in the placenta.

There is one group of conditions which may cause any form of fetal distress, and that is *premature separation and abruption of the placenta*. It is obvious that the old retroplacental haematoma lodging in an excavation of the placenta for prolonged periods of time, must be different in its significance for well-being of the fetus from the acute abruption (accidental haemorrhage) which is followed very shortly by natural or artificially induced delivery of the fetus[6]. The former is asymptomatic whereas the latter produces the well known severe clinical signs, but often without any discernible abnormality to be recognised on the delivered placenta. It has been suggested to use the term premature separation only for the pathologically apparent chronic condition, and the term abruptio placentae for the acute condition which may not be pathologically apparent in the placenta[6]. In a study of more than 600 cases with clinical or pathological evidence of either condition, it turned out that each of the two occurred with about equal frequency. Each was associated with the other in somewhat less than half the number of cases, or in somewhat less than one-third the total number of all cases investigated[6]. Premature separation in the strict sense can occur in several bouts and it is assumed that one of these may turn into abruptio, thus combining the pathological findings of previous premature separation with the clinical signs of acute abruptio. Each condition is associated with approximately equal perinatal mortality, premature separation presumably with chronic or subacute fetal distress and abruptio with acute distress. In cases with evidence of both conditions combined, the perinatal mortality is higher[6] (Figure 19.3). It is important to realise that acute abruptio does not leave a recognisable sign on the placenta unless delivery is delayed for a long time.

Multiple pregnancy

Infants and placentas of multiple pregnancies give valuable information on the fetal supply line, as if they were an experiment of nature. A few simple steps need to be taken in order to derive adequate benefit from their studies. The umbilical cords attached to the placentas need to be identified with regard to the twin to which each belongs. The simplest and most reliable method is to tie a piece of cord tape or suture material to the cord of twin A before delivery of twin B. In higher multiple pregnancies other identification should be improvised and explained in writing. Placentas are then identified as A and B as are the twins; if such identification is not made they should be marked in a different manner to avoid false identification, for instance, as X and Y. After delivery of the placentas, the dividing membranes between the sacs are often grossly apparent as being monochorial or dichorial, but this

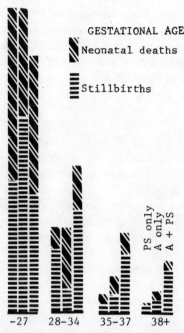

GESTATIONAL AGE

Neonatal deaths

Stillbirths

PS only
A only
A + PS

-27   28-34   35-37   38+

Figure 19.3 Incidence (per cent) of stillbirth and neonatal death in four gestational age groups among cases of premature separation (PS) and abruption (A) of the placenta. The highest columns on the left indicate 100%. From Gruenwald, P., Levin, H. and Yousem, H. (1968). Abruption and premature separation of the placenta: the clinical and the pathological entity. *Amer. J. Obstet. Gynecol.*, **102**, 604, 1968, by permission of C. V. Mosby, St. Louis

should be confirmed by a microscopic section. In monochorial placentas there are always anastomoses of the two circulations and these are usually quite obvious. Unless more detailed studies are planned, injection to demonstrate these anastomoses is not necessary as a rule. Dichorial placentas have, of course, no vascular anastomoses and it is usually quite easy to determine the borderline between the two placentas even if they are fused. In monochorial placentas such a dividing line is absent and no attempt should be made to find one, not only because this would be arbitrary, but also because vascular anastomoses make any separation of the two components an illusion. Even in monochorial twins survival of one twin long after intra-uterine death of the other is quite possible. The weight of the placenta in proportion to that of the fetus is relatively high in twins as compared with singletons[7]. It may seem paradoxical that monochorial twins, even though they are monozygotic, have a greater degree of discordance for birth weight and malformations than do others[7]. Since, however, very small twins and malformed ones have a high mortality, this may no longer be apparent when twin pairs surviving for longer periods of time are considered. The zygosity of twins is obvious in monochorial and in different-sex pairs. In others, which constitute about one-half of the total, somatic characteristics need to be studied in order to establish zygosity.

Examination of the placenta

Suggestions regarding this subject were previously made in more detail[8,9]. It is important that before weighing, the placenta be freed of membranes and cord within 1 cm of their insertion, and also of blood clots. At this point, before fixation, the decision must be made whether clots are significant as evidence of premature separation, or were formed after delivery. Some workers have recommended fixing the entire placenta for weeks and then slicing it in order to recognise the number and age of infarcts. This requires much effort and space which are not available at many institutions; in addition it interferes with preservation of the tissue for histological examination. Each examiner will have to determine what is more important to him, be consistent in the use of his method, and state in his reports what he has been practising.

Pathological examination of placentas without an adequate clinical history of the mother including pregnancy and labour, and of the infant is useless. Since the majority of placentas and pregnancies are normal, a selection usually has to be made except when establishing an unselected series which should be available to check against a questionable abnormal finding. I know of no instance in which this was successfully done by obstetricians, because they are legitimately occupied with other matters when a placenta is about to be discarded. It is therefore desirable to submit to the pathologist all placentas unfixed and refrigerated with a sheet containing the appropriate items of the history. In some hospitals, a form containing obstetrical information to accompany the infant to the nursery is adequate, and a copy can be provided for use with the placenta. Infant and placenta must be weighed on reliable scales which are periodically checked for accuracy within at least 10 grams. The pathologist can very rapidly select certain placentas by preset criteria including certain abnormalities of pregnancy as well as birth weight and infant's condition (Apgar score)[9]. The remaining placentas can be rapidly viewed and those with abnormal features including diffuse meconium staining added to the group to be examined in detail; the rest are discarded. This leaves in the average obstetrical service approximately one-quarter to one-third of all cases to be retained for examination. In addition to weighing there should be a gross description, and pieces from normal and abnormal areas fixed. They should later be trimmed to appropriate thickness in such a manner that the portions cut before fixation and thus distorted, can be discarded. Sections should include both the fetal and the maternal surface, and divided only if too large. Sections of the margin are useless because of the usual degenerative changes, unless a specific abnormality is to be documented.

The necessity of having adequate clinical information also applies to perinatal necropsies, but it is essential that it be kept separate from pathological findings until the final step of evaluation is undertaken[10,11]. This makes it possible to weigh one against the other. If clinical and pathological data are mixed as has frequently been done, then we deprive ourselves of the opportunity of establishing associations and causal relationships between them. As is clear from what was said earlier, much of the pathological information obtained on the infant will fall into the broad category of perinatal distress and much of the data acquired from the placenta will be equally non-specific. This should be faced squarely and not be obliterated by ascribing an independent role of cause of death to some of the non-specific manifestations of distress. In doing this, we arrive at less striking, but more realistic results. This does not negate the value of pathological examination of infant and placenta. As far as the infant is concerned, the pediatrician very frequently has to deal with *perinatal distress, cause undetermined*, and he should learn as much about this as possible. As far as the placenta is concerned, examination will reveal occasional changes indicative of a disturbance in the maternal circulation, and some other features worthwhile from the practical point of view as described in Chapters 12 to 15, but more important, we must learn more about the placenta and this can only be done by examining it carefully. The value of examining fresh placental villi (Chapter 13) has not been established to everybody's satisfaction, largely because it has only been practised by a few investigators.

So-called prematurity, meaning either pre-term birth or growth retardation, has long been known to carry a very high rate of perinatal death, or later sequelae. Consequently, prevention of prematurity became the slogan of those wishing to reduce perinatal loss. We must distinguish fetal deprivation (acute, subacute, or chronic) and its consequences from pre-term birth which may well be considered to be the underlying cause of death in most cases of the respiratory distress syndrome, intraventricular cerebral haemorrhage, and bilirubin encephalopathy. While there can be no doubt in the high *rate* of perinatal death after pre-term birth, few investigators have considered the impact on the total population. Since term birth is so vastly more frequent than pre-term birth, the *numbers* of deaths at various weeks of pregnancy give an entirely different picture. By gestational age, the number

346

of perinatal deaths reaches a peak at term, and by birth weight there is a plateau with a decline only beyond 3000 grams (Figure 19.4). These data from the British Perinatal Mortality Survey of 1958 have been confirmed

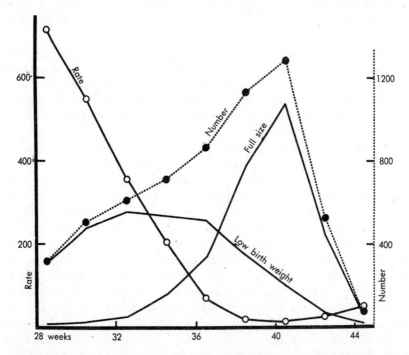

Figure 19.4 Rate per 1000 births and number of perinatal deaths in the British Perinatal Mortality Survey, (a) by 2-week gestational age groups and (b) by 500 g weight groups. Courtesy National Birthday Trust Fund. (From Gruenwald, P. (1970). Perinatal death of full-sized and full-term infants. *Amer. J. Obstet. Gynecol.*, **107,** 1022 by permission of C. V. Mosby, St. Louis)

with material from several other sources[12]. Rates versus numbers of deaths at different ages and weights carry varied implications regarding the role of the fetal supply line and other obstetrical factors, and should therefore be considered seriously when priorities for research, treatment, or prevention are set.

The value of perinatal pathology lies in the assumption that the same conditions which are associated with death, occur to a lesser extent or in different combinations in survivors. Thus, any circumstance of death that can be identified at necropsy, may well cause abnormalities in survivors. That

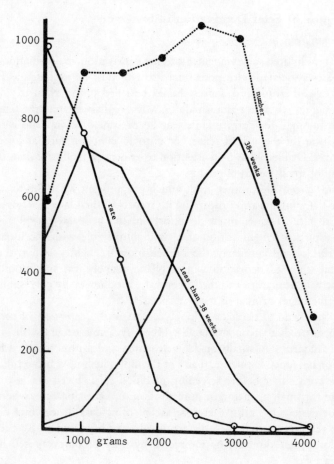

Figure 19.4 (b)

this can be so, is seen in a somewhat crude and non-specific manner in the similarity of trends of perinatal mortality on the one hand, and mental disturbances in survivors on the other, as shown later in this chapter (Figure 19.7).

Perinatal and placental pathology support each other, but can lead to meaningful results only when both their significance and their limitations are understood in the context of the clinical setting. In addition, the placenta must be studied intensively in its own right, as well as for traces left in it by maternal pathological conditions.

Late Sequels of Fetal Deprivation in Survivors

Limiting considerations

In evaluating children surviving intra-uterine deprivation, malformations and fetal diseases associated with poor fetal growth must be excluded as far as possible. Chromosome imbalances should be ruled out, particularly when there are suggestive minor abnormalities. Microcephaly beyond the range of head size in small-for-dates infants can be presumed to indicate cerebral malformation (in the widest sense), or chronic infection such as by cytomegalovirus. Drillien[13] has paid attention to associated malformations in her follow-up of small-for-dates infants.

Drillien[13] also made another point which is significant when pre-term and small-for-dates infants are compared with respect to their later development, namely, that the former often do poorly in the neonatal period and go through a phase of malnutrition at a time comparable with the usual late intra-uterine period. Similarly, the animals most frequently used in the experimental study of deprivation in early life, namely, rat and mouse, are born relatively immature and their neonatal period normally corresponds to intra-uterine stages of man in many respects[14].

Finally, the role of neonatal hypoglycaemia in the causation of cerebral disturbances needs to be considered[15]. Hypoglycaemia occurs with greatly increased frequency in small-for-dates neonates, and is now screened for in better neonatal units. However, many of the individuals now being followed up, were born either before screening of blood sugar levels was a routine procedure for small neonates, or in institutions or other localities where this still is not done. One must therefore accept most data on cerebral defects with the reservation that these defects may have been caused by prenatal deprivation either directly, or indirectly by way of unrecognised hypoglycaemia.

Animal experiments

Large numbers of studies using many different methods have dealt with fetal or neonatal deprivation and its immediate effect on growth. Only a few investigations have been extended to the much more laborious task of detecting late abnormalities of such animals, rehabilitated after the initial experimental period. A few examples will suffice. Rats deprived *in utero* by underfeeding the mother, or during the suckling period by giving one mother too many young to suckle, are permanently well below normal standards in body weight[4,16]. With regard to cerebral function, Barnes *et al.*[17] concluded from behavioural tests that 'nutritional deprivation in early life can cause a long-lasting, possibly permanent retardation in the development of learning behaviour'. Similarly, Simonson et al.[18] found that 'fetal deprivation can cause lasting behavioural damage'. A peculiar metabolic abnormality has been described[19] in the offspring of rats malnourished during pregnancy and lactation: there is poor utilisation of food, so that the early deprived and now normally fed rats require larger amounts for the same weight gain, or gain less at the same restricted level of intake than do normal controls. The same is said to occur in the offspring of women who were inadequately nourished during pregnancy. The existence of this defect which is said to be permanent, needs to be confirmed.

The most spectacular degree of growth retardation occurs in pigs deprived during the first year[16]; this is reversible to a striking extent but not completely, by rehabilitation. One may suspect that the remaining deficit in size is related to deprivation shortly after birth.

Winick et al.[20] have shown that cell division in certain tissues including the nervous system, stops at a specific stage of development, in most mammalian species shortly after birth. This biological clock is not slowed by deprivation, and shuts off cell multiplication even when normal numbers of cells have not formed as a result of this deprivation. At least some of the failure of individuals severely deprived in early life, to catch up when supplies are plentiful later on, can be explained on this basis. Dobbing[21] has championed the additional point that the laying down of various components of the central nervous system has its own time table, and cannot be fully made up at later times. He quite properly holds that the term *retardation* is improper for those defects which are not equal to early stages of normal development, and will not proceed to the normal end point after a longer time. (For the same reason I have been referring to deficit rather than retardation in all considerations of the sequels of deprivation in early life.) The delay of growth of the central nervous system during undernutrition does not affect its chemical constituents to the same relative extent, and rehabilitation also failed to restore near-normal proportions[21]. These experimental observations may be the physical basis of functional aberrations found in animals (see above) and in man to be mentioned below. To what extent degenerative changes augment these developmental aberrations, is not known. It is clear from what has been said about critical periods, that deficient weight at a given age is not a suitable measure of possible deficits since it may have originated at times and intensities differing in relation to one or another process of maturation.

Late human deficits: body size

In one of the earliest studies which differentiated small-for-dates from preterm infants, Drillien[22] found that the former were shorter and lighter at 4 years. Hepner[23] showed the same in representative growth curves, also up to

4 years. Fitzhardinge and Steven[24] extended their study to 8 years. At 4 years, 35% of the small-for-dates infants (gestational age 38 weeks or more, weight deficit at least 30% by Streeter's tables) were below the third centile, and only 8% above the fiftieth in weight. Cruise[25] found infants of less than 2500 g in birth weight and 37 weeks or more in gestational age to be smaller than pre-term infants at 2 and 3 years. Bazso *et al.*[26] showed year-by-year graphs comparing weight and length of small-for-dates and pre-term infants followed for 14 years: the former were consistently smaller than the latter. Babson[27] plotted the growth of pre-term and small-for-dates infants during the first post-term year on a graph representing normal pre- and postnatal growth derived from various sources (Figure 19.5), and also found small-for-dates infants (birth weight less than 2000 g, gestational age 38 weeks or more) well below all others throughout. In another study, Babson *et al.*[28] compared

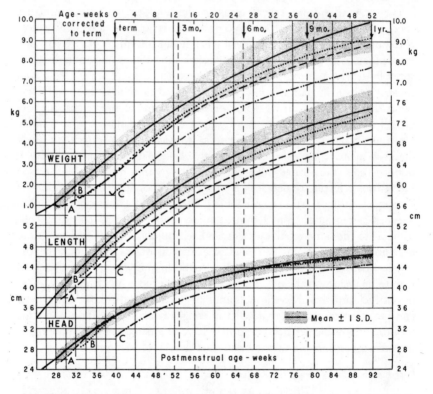

Figure 19.5 Mean growth in weight, length and head circumference of 12 small-for-dates infants during the first year of life. (From Babson, S. G. (1970). Growth of low-birth-weight infants. *J. Pediat.*, **77,** 11 by permission of the author and C. V. Mosby, St. Louis)

twins of whom the smaller one weighed less than 2000 g, and at least 25% less than the larger one. At a median age of $8\frac{1}{2}$ years there was a highly significant difference in height, head circumference, and weight. Thus, the persisting size deficit of prenatally undergrown children is found consistently in humans as well as in experimental animals.

Fetal deprivation and mental deficit

Many laborious studies performed years ago on infants of low birth weight have little value since they do not distinguish pre-term from small-for-dates infants. When the need for this distinction became obvious, there were at first some retrospective studies. Alberman[29] examined the records of 324 cases of cerebral palsy excluding those in whom there was a likelihood of a specific cause, and found that in certain forms such as spastic diplegia and athetosis, there was a dissociation of birth weight and length of gestation suggesting an excess of small-for-dates infants. Barker[30] investigated 607 infants of low intelligence (IQ less than 75) born in Birmingham from 1950 to 1954, also after exclusion of specific causes, and concluded that in this group 'over half the children whose birth weights were $5\frac{1}{2}$ lb or less were born after 37 weeks of gestation', and that the association with slow intra-uterine growth was particularly strong below an IQ of 50.

Next in the study of this problem came the investigation of twins in whom one can serve as the other's control. In the work of Babson *et al.*[28] mentioned above in the context of postnatal growth, significant differences in various psychological parameters were noted at a median age of $8\frac{1}{2}$ years when the smaller twin had weighed less than 2000 g, and was at least 25% lighter than the larger one at birth. Churchill[31] investigated 50 sets of twins at 5 to 15 years, and confirmed a lower IQ in the smaller partner, but only in identical and not in fraternal pairs. Several factors may account for this. In the case of monochorionic pairs, vascular anastomoses in the placenta may favour one over the other as occurs in the 'twin transfusion syndrome' or, since discordance for malformations is relatively frequent and the smaller twin more likely to be affected, there may be an unrecognised brain anomaly.

Finally, prospective studies or those in which accurate records from birth on were available, began to appear; only a few examples will be given. Bazso *et al.*[26], whose growth studies have been mentioned, state that nearly 40% of infants with intra-uterine growth retardation had an IQ below 90, and 20·3% between 70 and 85 when examined at 8 years. (The average birth weight of the growth-retarded group was 2243 g, the gestational age 277·5 days.) In an investigation of fits in children of very low birth weight, McDonald[32] found an association with poor fetal growth. In a series of 52 eight- to eleven-year old children with low birth weight and a gestational age of 37 weeks or more, Horn *et al.*[33] found 24·5% with an IQ of 80 to 89; the proportion was higher with birth weights below 2000 g. Drillien[13] found in 10- to 12-year olds an association of poor fetal growth with lowered IQ only in lower social classes; the original report should be consulted for details. Fitzhardinge and Steven[34] followed up 96 singletons with a gestational age of 38 weeks or more, and a birth weight 30% or more below normal: 50% of the boys and 36% of the girls did poorly in school, without a good correlation with their IQ. Probably the largest study of this kind ever undertaken, and the only one representative of an entire country's population, is that of Davie *et al.*[35] in which nearly 17 000 children born during the

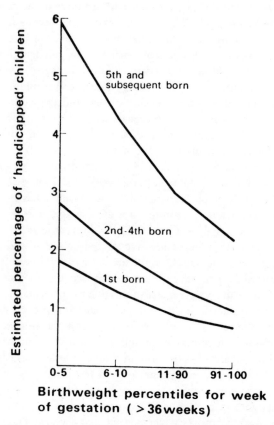

Figure 19.6 Birth weight for gestation, birth order and recognised handicap (children excluded from schooling because of severe subnormality; those already in special schools for the handicapped; and those ascertained by Local Authorities as in need of special schooling). (From Davie, R., Butler, N. and Goldstein, H. (1972). *From Birth to Seven*. London: Longman. With permission of authors and publisher)

control week of the British Perinatal Mortality Survey of 1958 were examined when 7 years old. Only a small sampling of the wide ranging results can be given here. Figure 19.6 gives the proportion of handicapped children as defined in the legend, by birth order and birth weight in relation to gestational age; it is consistently and considerably higher in children with lower birth-weight centiles.

The effect of *subacute fetal distress* with wasting and a minor weight deficit on future well-being is not well known, particularly since this state cannot be sharply defined for statistical analysis (Chapter 11). The effect on body

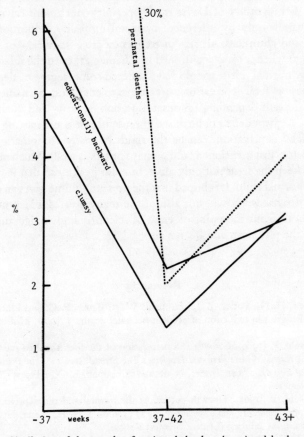

Figure 19.7 Similarity of the trends of perinatal death, educational backwardness and clumsiness. The much higher figure for perinatal deaths is presumably due to the inclusion of early third trimester births which almost all die, and contribute little to the late sequels. (After data of Davie, Butler and Goldstein[35], with permission from the author and publisher)

proportions may have been reached in different ways, some probably quite harmless to the fetus and others with potential significance. Thus, the hunger winter in Holland in 1944–45 produced no subnormal mental performance detectable at military induction examination of 19-year old males[36]. Engleson et al.[37] followed up 'dysmature infants' (by Clifford's definition based on skin changes, with a mean weight about 200 g below normal) at the age of 4 to 5 years, and found that 'more than occasional deviations from the normal were observed'. The authors further state that pooling the results of all tests produced statistically highly significant results, with stage 1 infants often intermediate between stage 0 and the more severely affected stages 2 and 3. The large British study of Davie et al.[35] permits conclusions on moderate, late deprivation only by inference: perinatal mortality, educational backwardness, and clumsiness all rise in frequency after 42 weeks of gestation (Figure 19.7) when, as was mentioned in Chapter 11, even the infants with a statistically 'normal' birth weight have suffered some degree of deprivation.

In conclusion, fetal deprivation can cause transient illness, permanent defect, or perinatal death depending on onset, duration, severity and quality of the deficiency. A given deficit in birth weight, useful as it is as a starting point for studying fetal deprivation, can be the result of many combinations of the kinds of factors just mentioned (and perhaps others as well). Much needs to be learned to keep the fetus not only alive, but also healthy so that it will grow up to be a normal child. It is hoped that the present volume gives an overview not only of what is known, but also of the many aspects which need to be explored both from the point of view of scientific knowledge and for the benefit of the physician and his patients.

References

1. Bundesen, H. N., Potter, E. L., Fishbein, W. I., Bauer, F. C. and Plotzke, G. V. (1952). Progress in reduction of needless neonatal deaths. J. Amer. Med. Assoc., **148,** 907

2. Gruenwald, P. (1969). Growth and maturation of the foetus and its relationship to perinatal mortality. In: Perinatal Problems: The Second Report of The British Perinatal Mortality Survey, p. 141 (Butler, N. R. and Alberman, E. D., editors) (Edinburgh: Livingstone)

3. Gruenwald, P. (1968). Growth pattern of the normal and the deprived fetus. In: Aspects of praematurity and dysmaturity, p. 37 (Jonxis, J. H. P., Visser, H. K. A. and Troelstra, J. A., editors) (Leiden: Stenfert Kroese)

4. Chow, B. F. and Lee, C. J. (1964). Effect of dietary restriction of pregnant rats on body weight gain of the offspring. J. Nutr., **82,** 10

5. Gruenwald, P. (1964). The fetus in prolonged pregnancy. Amer. J. Obstet. Gynecol., **89,** 503

6. Gruenwald, P., Levin, H. and Yousem, H. (1968). Abruption and premature

separation of the placenta: the clinical and the pathologic entity. *Amer. J. Obstet. Gynecol.*, **102**, 604

7. Gruenwald, P. (1970). Environmental influences on twins apparent at birth. *Biol. Neonat.*, **15**, 79

8. Benirschke, K. (1961). Examination of the placenta. *Obstet. Gynecol.*, **18**, 309

9. Gruenwald, P. (1964). Examination of the placenta by the pathologist. *Arch. Path.*, **77**, 41

10. Bound, J. P., Butler, N. R. and Spector, W. G. (1956). Classification and causes of perinatal mortality. *Brit. Med. J.*, **2**, 1191 and 1260

11. Gruenwald, P. (1955). Evaluation of perinatal deaths. *Obstet. Gynecol.*, **6**, 471

12. Gruenwald, P. (1970). Perinatal death of full-sized and full-term infants. *Amer. J. Obstet. Gynecol.*, **107**, 1022

13. Drillien, C. M. (1970). The small-for-date infant: etiology and prognosis. *Ped. Clin. N. Amer.*, **17**, 9

14. Davison, A. N. and Dobbing, J. (1966). Myelination as a vulnerable period in brain development. *Brit. Med. Bull.*, **22**, 40

15. Cornblath, M. and Reisner, S. H. (1965). Blood glucose in the neonate and its clinical significance. *New Engl. J. Med.*, **273**, 378

16. McCance, R. A. and Widdowson, E. M. (1962). Nutrition and growth. *Proc. Roy. Soc. B.*, **156**, 326

17. Barnes, R. H., Cunnold, S. R., Zimmermann, R. R., Simmons, H., McLeod, R. and Krook, L. (1966). Influence of nutritional deprivations in early life on learning behavior of rats as measured by performance in a water maze. *J. Nutr.*, **89**, 399

18. Simonson, M., Stephan, J. K., Hanson, H. M. and Chow, B. F. (1971). Open field studies in offspring of underfed mother rats. *J. Nutr.*, **101**, 331

19. Chow, B. F., Blackwell, R. Q., Blackwell, B. N., Hou, T. Y., Anilane, J. K. and Sherwin, R. W. (1968). Maternal nutrition and metabolism of the offspring: studies in rats and man. *Amer. J. Pub. Hlth.*, **58**, 668

20. Winick, M., Brasel, J. A. and Velasco, E. G. (1973). Effects of prenatal nutrition upon pregnancy risk. *Clin. Obstet. Gynecol.*, **16**, 184

21. Dobbing, J. (1970). Undernutrition and the developing brain. *Amer. J. Dis. Child.*, **120**, 411

22. Drillien, C. M. (1961). A longitudinal study of the growth and development of prematurely and maturely born children. VI. Physical development in age period 2 to 4 years. *Arch. Dis. Childh.*, **36**, 1

23. Hepner, R. (1963). In Gruenwald, P., Dawkins, M. and Hepner, R. Panel discussion: Chronic deprivation of the fetus. *Sinai Hosp. J. (Baltimore)*, **11**, 51

24. Fittzhardinge, P. M. and Steven, E. M. (1972). The small-for-date infant. I. Late growth patterns. *Pediat.*, **49**, 671

25. Cruise, M. O. (1973). A longitudinal study of the growth of low birth weight infants. I. Velocity and distance growth, birth to 3 years. *Pediat.*, **51**, 620

26. Bazso, J., Karamazsin, L. and Gelei, K. (1964). Observations on the physical and mental development in newborn infants of intra-uterine growth retardation. *Internat. Cong. Copenhagen Scient. Study Mental Retard.*, p. 411

27. Babson, S. G. (1970). Growth of low-birth-weight infants. *J. Pediat.*, **77**, 11

28. Babson, S. G., Kangas, J., Young, N. and Bramhall, J. L. (1964). Growth and development of twins of dissimilar size at birth. *Pediat.*, **33**, 327

29. Alberman, E. (1963). Birth weight and length of gestation in cerebral palsy. *Develop. Med. Child. Neur.*, **5**, 388

30. Barker, D. J. P. (1966). Low intelligence: its relation to length of gestation and rate of foetal growth. *Brit. J. Prevent. Soc. Med.*, **20,** 58
31. Churchill, J. A. (1965). The relationship between intelligence and birth weight in twins. *Neurol.*, **15,** 341
32. McDonald, A. D. (1964). Fits in children of very low birth weight. *Develop. Med. Child Neurol.*, **6,** 144
33. Horn, R., Grävinghoff, C. and Wolf, H. (1969). Ergebnisse psychologischer Nachuntersuchungen von ehemals frühgeborenen und ehemals hypotrophen Neugeborenen. *Monstsschr. Kinderheilk.*, **117,** 442
34. Fitzhardinge, P. M. and Steven, E. M. (1972). The small-for-date infant. II. Neurological and intellectual sequelae. *Pediat.*, **50,** 50
35. Davie, R., Butler, N. and Goldstein, H. (1972). *From birth to seven. A report of the National Child Development Study,* (London: Longman)
36. Stein, Z., Susser, M., Saenger, G. and Marolla, F. (1972). Nutrition and mental performance. *Science*, **178,** 708
37. Engleson, G., Rooth, G. and Törnblom, M. (1963). A follow-up study of dysmature infants. *Arch. Dis. Childh.*, **38,** 62

Index